The Green Handbook

earth + health

BOOK I. FOOD

Joanna Kappele
human ecologist, environmentalist, nature and planet advocate

For my dad who often said, Prepare to Rise.

Prepare to Rise + The Adore Foundation,
a 501c3 organization in Chicago.

Library of Congress Control Number:2019908470

Pollinators Edition 2019
ISBN: 978-1-7330884-1-1
The information you've been looking for.

Gratitude and acknowledgements to all the researchers, scientists, journalists, nonprofit organizations, environmentally-minded attorneys, universities, newspapers, leaders and dedicated people throughout the world who've been documenting and working to solve public health and environmental issues. This book is a compilation of information, much of which is based on work conducted by these extraordinary people and organizations. Without their work this book wouldn't have been possible. Many thanks to all my friends and family and loving animals who encouraged me and believed this book could be done.

In memory of my parents, Tom and Betty
and my brother, Chris.

Table of Contents

Introduction

What's in your food?

Do you ever wonder how food might contribute to your health, or to disease? We just want food that tastes good, that's safe, and if it's good for us that's a big plus! But, none of us want food or water that makes us sick! Yet what do we really know about either? What's in our Food? What's in our water? What's the difference between organic, conventional, GMO? Have no fear, this book is here to help unravel the mysteries of these issues for you—what's really going on with food, how it affects you, and why you need to care. You'll learn how to choose food to protect your and your family's health. Bonus--you'll also be helping the planet!

As nature has it, our health and the planet's health are inextricably entwined, and both are in danger. Food is different today than it used to be; it's far more complex now and goes by strange names and labels. Many food items are riddled with pollution like chemicals, fertilizer, pesticides, preservatives, secret ingredients, and disease-causing substances. We've come a long way from the stock yards of a century ago, yet today we have a dangerous rising of antibiotic resistant bacteria due chiefly to conditions at confined animal farms (factory farms). That's not all—in food you can often find pesticide residues, nitrosamines, and synthetic hormones. Water as well is a catch basin for all the agricultural chemicals that don't help us in the least. All these pollutants easily sneak into our bodies through the foods and beverages we eat. They not only can harm us, they harm the planet's resources as well. This book presents the top issues affecting our food and health right now, and gives you solutions and ideas to help change the situation. In a world like we have today, it's helpful to be aware so we can make informed decisions when it matters. And with environmental issues in particular, it truly does.

Food that remains close to its natural state tends to remain healthier for us than food that is refined and processed. Food grown with sustainable methods is also healthier for the earth, whereas industrial agricultural urges extreme use of chemicals that harm people, damage ecosystems, cause severe pollution issues, and play a major role in furthering climate change.

We have to face it, America of 70 years ago is very different than today. The 1950s was a turning point for our country, where we parted ways with the old, with nature, with sensibilities. Chemicals designed for ammunition and killing suddenly became the cornerstones of agriculture. When World War II ended the bomb making facilities left idle began churning their materials into synthetic fertilizer—a product that has continued to cause planetary distress since the very first application. Synthetic fertilizers and pesticides have caused a furor that's been spreading and slowly killing the planet in its wake. Trickling their way down ever so slowly killing soil, crippling and poisoning waterways--is it merely coincidence that our oceans have been warming since the advent of toxic agricultural runoff? We've gone from using weapons of war against each other to using weapons of war against our planet. Our farm fields are doused with poison, the soil is crying for help, our waterways are polluted with toxins—is it any wonder diseases are soaring and humanity's gone astray?

Behind closed doors, a lot of trickery has occurred within the food and chemical sector. From herbicides to fungicides, GRAS additives to endocrine disruptors, the list of health harming toxins infiltrating the food supply keeps getting longer. In conjunction with this dismantling, pollution resulting from modern farming and manufacturing has gotten out of hand. With the loss of safe water and clean food, education has fallen, poverty has risen, violence has risen, crime has risen, disease has risen-- is this all connected? Then by the end of the 20th century we were blindsided with the dawning of a new breed of food never before seen, GMOs. Think of it, before the 1990s we all ate nonGMO food. Now to identify which is real and which is genetically modified, we need labels.

We've been misled into accepting these toxins as normal and told to ignore their relationship with human and animal disease. Unless we act now to change our circumstances and limit toxins in our food and water, the future for humanity may be irreversibly different than today.

What's the Difference? Isn't all food the same?

The differences start with the way food is grown.

Organic: avoids substances known to harm people and animals.

- No synthetic fertilizer is used.
- Organic food is grown with least pesticides, only natural pesticides used if needed
- Animals are not given antibiotics, drugs, synthetic hormones, or GMOs.
- Pollinator-friendly methods, no neonicotinoids, natural fertilizers that nourish soil
- Biodynamics was the origin of organic farming, remains synonymous with organic

Integrated Pest Management: (IPM) uses least toxic pest-removal methods

Conventional: Foods produced using substances + methods that cause harm

- Wide array of toxic pesticides used that harm people, animals, birds and bees
- Neonicotinoids and other pollinator-harming substances used frequently
- Synthetic fertilizer used abundantly, causing disease, air and water pollution
- Monocropping methods cause erosion, habitat destruction, and toxic runoff

GMO (bioengineered): These foods are close to conventional, in addition:

- Biotech seeds & GMO foods are modified with DNA from other plants and animals.
- They're designed to withstand greater amounts of herbicides than other plants
- The seeds can be coated in pesticides or implanted with toxins that never wash off
- GMO crops may require more fungicides than other traditional plants

Through creative collaboration we can reverse the damage inflicted upon us from modern methods of agriculture. Read on to find out how best to keep your family and yourself safe from the unwantedness. Prepare and learn about these issues now so you can bring the solutions home. We have an amazing opportunity before us that if we harness properly will manifest the changes that are needed. Get ready, prepare and have hope. Step by step we'll get our health and our planet in order. For the sake of coming generations, we must act now. Prepare to rise.

ONE

FOOD + FARMING What's in Your Food?

If the People let the government decide what foods they eat and what medicines they take, their bodies will soon be in as sorry a state as the souls who live under tyranny.
President Thomas Jefferson

1. PESTICIDES

> **Pesticides and Disease**
>
> Where do pesticides fit into the picture of environmental disease? Man, however much he may like to pretend the contrary, is part of nature. Can he escape a pollution that is now so thoroughly distributed throughout the world? We know that even single exposures to these chemicals, if the amount is large enough, can precipitate acute poisoning. But this is not the major problem. For the population as a whole, we must be more concerned with the delayed effects of absorbing small amounts of the pesticides that invisibly contaminate our world.
>
> **Rachel Carson** *Silent Spring* 1962

Pesticides are poisonous substances targeted to expel life. They act without discretion, with capacity to harm all. Nonetheless they're used widely and abundantly in the food growing process. As a result, many foods we eat can contain traces of them. Conventional and GMO methods tend to use more pesticides than any other farming style. Pesticides are a broad group of chemicals that include herbicides, insecticides, fungicides, miticides, fumigants—these substances are invisible disease triggers extending far beyond the farm field. They're used extensively in agriculture and beyond-- from sports fields, gardens and lawns to parks and schools, homes and buildings, forests and public spaces. Considering that more than 60% of herbicides are documented endocrine disruptors,[1] do we really need these toxic chemicals, or are we better off without them?

PESTICIDE: "A pesticide is any substance used to kill, repel, or control certain forms of plant or animal life that are considered to be pests. Pesticides include herbicides for destroying weeds and other unwanted vegetation, insecticides for controlling a wide variety of insects, fungicides used to prevent the growth of molds and mildew, disinfectants for preventing the spread of bacteria, and compounds used to control mice and rats. Because of the widespread use of agricultural chemicals in food production, people are exposed to low levels of pesticide residues through their diets."[2]

Admittedly we're only starting to understand the extent of harm pesticides inflict upon us, how harm is accelerated when pesticides are combined, and how the secrecy of inert ingredients continues to deceive the world. We do know human and animal health is deeply affected by pesticides, probably moreso than by any other environmental or agricultural contaminant. As documented throughout this book, scientists the world over consider pesticides neurotoxins, endocrine disruptors, reproductive toxins, carcinogens and tumor promoters. Why then are we using these substances on food? By reducing toxin use on growing food, might we reduce the incidence of cancer, of degenerative disease, reverse the uprising of neurological disorders, of reproductive problems, of mental health disorders and even possibly reverse trends toward violence? Because pesticides are applied to food crops, these chemicals easily seep into our bodies through the food and beverages we consume.

PESTICIDES: "Over 1 billion pounds are used in the United States each year, and approximately 5.6 billion pounds worldwide!"[3] They come by different names, but all are disastrous for our health. Keep children and pets away from pesticides.[4]

WHY ARE THESE CHEMICALS STILL USED IN THE US?

- **Chlorpyrifos:** organophosphate insecticide, was to be banned until EPA reversal in March 2017. In August 2018 Court ordered EPA to withdraw all uses, yet President Trump's administration has appealed the ruling.[5] Used on corn, soy, wheat, almonds, apples, fruit trees, broccoli, brussel sprouts, cauliflower, cranberries, cotton, golf courses, ant & roach bait.[6] Health effects: affects brain, behavior & learning disorders[7]
- **Paraquat:** used for weed control, Health effects: linked to Parkinson's Disease.[8] China is world's largest producer of paraquat. Bans in: Sweden, Austria, Denmark, Finland.[9]
- **Neonicotinoids:** Systemic, persists in environment, Health effects: cholinesterase inhibitor, causes paralysis & death to bees and pollinators[10], ban pending in EU.[11]
- **Fungicides:** Health **effects**: brain impairment, neurodegenerative diseases, disrupts mitochondria causing autism-like conditions & Alzheimer's,[12] reduces bee survival[13]
- **Dicamba**: used for weed control, pesticide drift, Health effects: reproductive toxin, may harm lungs and liver.[14] Damages crops, farmers sought ban, EPA reversed course[15]
- **2,4-D:** covers over 78 million acres of agricultural land,[16] found in many 'weed and feed' fertilizers. Health effects: endocrine disruptor, suspected link with hormone, thyroid, and reproductive disorders, sarcoma, lymphoma, decreased fertility.[17]
- **Enlist Duo:** 2,4-D mixed with glyphosate, very toxic to people and wildlife, threatens to worsen spread of superweeds, combining pesticides together elevates risk of harm[18]
- **1,3-D Telone:** fumigant, organochlorine, widespread water contaminant, Health effects: Cancer,[19] Banned in EU, still allowed as fumigant on strawberries in California.[20]
- **Carbaryl**: insecticide, Health effects: cholinesterase inhibitor, muscle weakness, harmful to kidneys and liver, reduced fertility and mortality of offspring observed in rats,[21] toxic to wild birds,[22] banned in Austria, UK, Germany.
- **Atrazine:** Health effects: potent reproductive toxin, endocrine disruptor, hormonal abnormalities, found in nearly all water supplies,[23] used on corn, sugarcane, evergreen tree farms, golf courses, it persists in soil and the environment, causes harm to mammals, birds, amphibians.[24] Banned in France, Sweden, Denmark, Germany, Italy.
- **Glyphosate:** Health effects: leaky gut syndrome, depression, mineral deficiencies, lowers tryptophan, serotonin, melantonin, dopamine production,[25] non-hodgkin's lymphoma and other (see page 32). Banned in over 27 countries and the list of cities in the U.S is growing,[26] thank God.

"Since 1974 in the U.S., 1.6 Billion Kilograms of glyphosate (or 1.77 million tons) has been applied. Genetically Engineered herbicide tolerant crops now account for about 56% of global glyphosate use."[27]

MOST COMMON PESTICIDES USED in U.S. (based on data from EPA, USDA)

Pesticide	Where Used	Damages
Glyphosate	Used on GMO foods: soy, corn, potatoes, canola as well as other crops through disecation before harvest, residues contaminate food[28] and drinking water worldwide	Roundup™ formulation is deadly to human embryonic cells[29], extended exposure triggers psychiatric illness by reducing serotonin and dopamine--hormones related to happiness[30], harms soil health, interferes with mineral absorption[31]
Atrazine	Used on corn, sugar cane, watermelon, lawns, golf courses, weed & feed fertilizer, prevalent water contaminant	Endocrine disruptor, harms aquatic animals, causes reproductive dysfunction via the hypothalamus-pituitary axis, banned in the EU[32]
2,4-D	Used on GMO crops, contaminates drinking water	Possible carcinogen, may cause reproductive damage, may damage liver and kidneys[33]
Enlist Duo	Used on GMO crops, contaminates drinking water, 2,4-D mixed with glyphosate	Kidney toxin, Possible Carcinogen, reproductive toxin, may cause Parkinson's, hypothyroidism[34]
Paraquat	Used on corn, potatoes, banana, soy, tea, peanuts, citrus, coffee, citrus, sugarcane [35]	Causes Parkinson's disease[36]
Neonicotinoids Clothianidin…	Systemic Pesticide used on fruit crops, corn, potatoes, apples, grapes, rice, spinach, cauliflower, pet flea collars	Does not wash off foods[37], neurotoxin, endocrine disruptor, causes hormonal imbalance, harms bees & pollinators
Fungicides Trifloxystrobin, chlorothalonil…	Used on wheat, corn, soy, grapes, peanuts, nuts, potatoes, tomatoes, coffee, tea shrubs, strawberries	Studies with brain cells showed harm to neurons, similarities with autism and neurodegenerative disease[38], toxic to kidneys, weakens honey bee immunity[39]
Chlorpyrifos organophosphate	Used on peaches, broccoli, cilantro, peppers, strawberries, soy, almonds, apples, corn[40]	Neurotoxin, harms children, causes learning disorders, ADHD, lower birth weight[41]
Glufosinate	Little known herbicide used on GMO crops, market expected to reach 2.34Billion by 2022,[42] very similar to glyphosate	"Inhibits glutamine synthetase in both plants and animals,"[43]causes brain damage, birth defects, cell suicide,[44] used to grow libertylink GMO crops

Cholinesterase Inhibitors: "a chemical that binds to the enzyme, cholinesterase, and prevents it from breaking down the neurotransmitter, acetylcholine. With toxic doses, the result is that excessive levels of the acetylcholine build up in the synapses and neuromuscular junctions and glands."[45] Organophosphorous and Carbamate Pesticides are cholinesterase inhibitors.

Endocrine Disruptors (EDC): "Endocrine disruptors are chemicals that may interfere with the body's endocrine system and produce adverse developmental, reproductive, neurological, and immune effects in both humans and wildlife."[46]

President's Cancer Panel: Reduce Cancer Risk by Reducing Pesticide Exposure

The President's Cancer Panel in 2010 determined that we can reduce our cancer risk by reducing exposure to pesticides. "Individuals can take important steps in their own lives to reduce their exposure to environmental elements that increase risk for cancer and other diseases. Exposure to pesticides can be decreased by choosing, to the extent possible, food grown without pesticides or chemical fertilizers and washing conventionally grown produce to remove residues."[47]

RoundUp, Glyphosate Cancer Controversy

In 2003 Monsanto's leading toxicologist Donna Farmer wrote to the CEO stating,

"The terms glyphosate and Roundup cannot be used interchangeably nor can you use 'Roundup' for all glyphosate-based herbicides any more. For example, you cannot say that Roundup is not a carcinogen. We have not done the necessary testing on the formulation to make that statement. The testing on the formulations are not anywhere near the level of the active ingredient."[48]

Donna Farmer, Lead Toxicologist 2003 Monsanto Company

Since August 2018 the federal court system has officially determined Monsanto's *Roundup* causes cancer. The company was further found guilty of deceiving the world in that they failed to warn consumers of Roundup's cancer risk.[49]. Thanks to the men and women who are coming forward, our hearts go out to you. The first lawsuit involved DeWayne Johnson, who the jury found developed nonhodgkin's lymphoma from exposure to *Roundup*. As a school groundskeeper, *Roundup* was his go-to product. He, like many thought the stuff was harmless; had he been aware it could harm him he could've made an informed decision and avoided it. In fact, if Monsanto had been honest in the beginning and informed the EPA that actually, Roundup can cause cancer-- it may never have been found on store shelves. Alas as court records show, they did not choose the path of truth. May all who have suffered from this exposure, all brave souls coming forward, and all who've been affected by this and similar products, heal from this assault. If you've lost loved ones to cancer caused by Roundup or any other toxic pesticide, please help raise awareness to prevent further loss and pain. Go to www.baumhedlundlaw.com to find out more.

One of the biggest problems with pesticides like *Roundup* is that the EPA relies on testing results provided by the manufacturer, in this case Monsanto. (Monsanto incidentally was bought out by Bayer in 2018.[50]) Secondly, testing submitted for *Roundup,* like lots of other pesticide tests, only consisted of information regarding the primary ingredient, glyphosate—even though Roundup contains many other ingredients. Roundup, like other pesticides contains numerous secret "inert" ingredients that amplify the toxicity of the product. Even though they increase toxicity, inerts are considered "inactive" by the EPA and FDA, thus inert ingredients do not require disclosure. In the underworld of trade secrets and company memos, however, the truth concerning Roundup's health effects, likely caused by the inert ingredients, at last reached the public.

Through the *Roundup* trial internal emails surfaced that reveal serious negligence and criminal activity. The corruption extends all the way to the EPA. Some documents show fear, others serious concern and bribery, as well as lab results documenting tumors and diseases in animals. We now know that for years Monsanto knew there were serious disease and cancer risks from

Roundup, but they did everything in their power to keep that information from us and to keep their products on store shelves. As a result of this evidence, now declassified, we have to ask whether or not there are still individuals at the EPA working in collusion with chemical companies like Monsanto? What can we do to protect ourselves when the government agencies designed to keep us protected from environmental toxins don't do their job?

One of the most important documents showing collusion between the EPA and Monsanto involved Dr. Marion Copley and Jess Rowland at the EPA. "Marion Copley, D.V.M., a 30-year career EPA scientist and recipient of numerous awards, wrote a letter to Mr. (Jess) Rowland in March 2013, two years before the public debate about the carcinogenicity of glyphosate began in earnest. Dr. Copley was a senior toxicologist in the EPA's Health Effects Division, and she worked closely with Mr. Rowland. Diagnosed with terminal cancer, she had to retire for health reasons and passed away in January 2014. Before her death, she voiced her serious concerns to Mr. Rowland about his and EPA's handling of glyphosate. Dr. Copley's dying declaration begins by naming no fewer than fourteen effects of glyphosate known to EPA, all of which are plausible mechanisms of action explaining the increase in lymphoma risk." [51]

In Marion Copley's own words:

"Dear Jess, Since I left the Agency with cancer, I have studied the tumor process extensively and I have some mechanism comments which may be very valuable to CARC based on my decades of pathology experience. I'll pick one chemical to demonstrate my points. Glyphosate was originally designed as a chelating agent and I strongly believe that is the identical process involved in its tumor formation, which is highly supported by the literature.

- Chelators inhibit apoptosis, the process by which our bodies kill tumor cells
- Chelators are endocrine disruptors, involved in tumorigenesis -Glyphosate induces lymphocyte proliferation -Glyphosate induces free radical formation
- Chelators inhibit free radical scavenging enzymes requiring Zn, Mn or Cu for activity
- Chelators bind zinc, necessary for immune system function
- Glyphosate is genotoxic, a key cancer mechanism
- Chelators inhibit DNA repair enzymes requiring metal cofactors
- Chelators bind Ca, Zn, Mg, etc to make foods deficient for these essential nutrients
- Chelators bind calcium necessary for calcineurin-mediated immune response

Chelators often damage the kidneys or pancreas, as glyphosate does, a mechanism to tumor formation -Kidney/pancreas damage can lead to clinical chemistry changes to favor tumor growth -Glyphosate kills bacteria in the gut and the gastrointestinal system is 80% of the immune system -Chelators suppress the immune system making the body susceptible to tumors. Previously, CARC concluded that glyphosate was a "possible human carcinogen." The kidney pathology in the animal studies would lead to tumors with other mechanisms listed above. Any one of these mechanisms alone listed can cause tumors, but glyphosate causes all of them simultaneously. It is essentially certain that glyphosate causes cancer. With all of the evidence listed above, the CARC category should be changed to "probable human carcinogen". Blood cells are most exposed to chelators, if any study shows proliferation of lymphocytes, then that is confirmatory that glyphosate is a carcinogen."[52] Jess disregarded Dr. Copley's warnings and continued doing all he could to shield glyphosate from review by CARC, the Cancer Assessment Review Committee.

Marion Copley was a serious scientist who really tried to get those with power at the EPA to act responsibly. There are many like her, unfortunately there're many people who aren't as concerned. In any event, we can no longer let misbehaving corporations control lackeys in our government, least of all when their decisions affect our health. Monsanto is like the evil emperor and the dark side, we must not forget we are the resistance, the Jedis! Going forward, we must have a strong EPA force, one that conducts its own legitimate safety testing rather than relying solely on information provided by manufacturers. Additionally, when testing pesticides, instead of merely evaluating the primary ingredient, researchers must examine the pesticide formulation in its entirety, including all inert ingredients. Should any formulation endanger the public, people or animals, use must be prohibited, or at very least severely minimized.

Children Need Protection from Pesticides

Children are at a greater risk from pesticides. Children's internal organs are still developing and maturing and their enzymatic, metabolic, and immune systems may provide less natural protection than those of an adult. There are "critical periods" in human development when exposure to a toxin can permanently alter the way an individual's biological system operates. Children may be exposed more to certain pesticides because often they eat different foods than adults. For instance, children typically consume larger quantities of milk, applesauce, and orange juice per pound of body weight than do adults. Children's behaviors, such as playing on the floor or on the lawn where pesticides are commonly applied, or putting objects in their mouths, increase their chances of exposure to pesticides. Adverse effects of pesticide exposure range from mild symptoms of dizziness and nausea to serious, long-term neurological, developmental and reproductive disorders. Americans use more than a billion pounds of pesticides each year to combat pests on farm crops, in homes, places of business, schools, parks, hospitals, and other public places.

www.epa.gov/pesticides/factsheets/kidpesticide.htm

DANGER: SECRET INGREDIENTS

Inert ingredients intensify the effects of chemicals and break down natural barriers of defense. "**Inert** ingredients can increase the ability of pesticide formulations to affect significant toxicologic end points, including developmental neurotoxicity, genotoxicity, and disruption of hormone function. They can also increase exposure by increasing dermal absorption, decreasing the efficacy of protective clothing, and increasing environmental mobility and persistence. Inert ingredients can increase the phytotoxicity of pesticide formulations as well as the toxicity to fish, amphibians, and microorganisms."[53]

Of all pesticide ingredients, inert ingredients may be the most dangerous. Yet in the United States we're prevented from even knowing what inerts are present in a product because inerts are considered trade secrets. Inerts are not tested for safety. From the Presidents Cancer Panel's Report of 2009, "Many of the inert ingredients in pesticides also are toxic, but are not required to be tested for causing chronic diseases such as cancer. For example, xylene is used as the inert ingredient in almost 900 pesticides, and has been associated with increased risk of brain tumors, rectal cancer, leukemia."[54] *Why is it used then*? It may take many more years to uncover all the inert ingredients in pesticide recipes. One by one we must get these substances withdrawn.

In today's world few get away without full disclosure, why do toxic chemical companies get a waiver? Another harmful side effect from Roundup's formulation has been uncovered. "Its inert ingredient, POEA (polyethoxylated tallow amine) is deadly to human embryonic, placental, and umbilical cord cells."[55] How can POEA legally be allowed in a product that is used to grow food? Where's the logic? "Roundup was among the most toxic herbicides and insecticides tested. It is commonly believed that Roundup is among the safest pesticides. However, Roundup was found in this experiment to be 125 times more toxic than glyphosate."[56] Dangerous ingredients are just not acceptable, not on this planet. How is using them legal? The list of allowable inert ingredients needs serious review ASAP.

TOXIC CHEMICAL OVERUSE

Using vast amounts of toxic chemical pesticides to grow food really didn't become mainstream until the mid 1950s. Is it just coincidence that birth defects[57], cancer rates[58] and chronic diseases[59] have been steadily rising since then?[60] "Cancer incidence in the American population has skyrocketed—up 48% from 1950 to 1990 according to National Cancer Institute."[61] There are so many pesticides in use today—the EPA claims pesticide use went down a bit from 948 million to 877 million pounds[62], and another report states over 1 billion pounds are applied annually to crops in the U.S., while worldwide over 5.6 billion pounds of pesticides are used annually.[63] The majority of health studies to date involve synthetic chemical pesticides, but natural pesticides can be as dangerous when overused[64]. As with most substances in this world, moderation is key.

While of course there can be certain instances when pesticides are useful, it's the widespread worldwide overuse prevalent today that's causing catastrophic consequences for all life on this planet. When not just our food but also our drinking water is contaminated, clearly too many chemicals are being used. Such overuse is anti-earth. You may hear that we need these substances, food can't be grown without them. But is that true? There's evidence that yields can be greater and plants can be healthier when soil is healthy. Yet, the chemicals prevent soil health rather than encourage it. Soil is weakened and made less fertile first and foremost by synthetic fertilizer, then pesticides further conflict and restrict soil prosperity. Alas disease sets in and more chemicals are sought, which begets more chemicals still. These chemicals are a dead-end street.

CDC Study: Pesticides in 100% of People Tested

In 2000 the Center for Disease Control began monitoring people for pesticide residues in order to better understand the relationship between chemicals and human health. From data released in 2003 involving testing of 9,282 people in 26 different locations for 34 pesticides and 82 other chemicals they found[65]:

- "One hundred percent of the people tested for pesticides in both their blood and urine have at least three of the 23 pesticides in their bodies. The average person in this sub-group of the study carries 13 of the 23 pesticides measured.
- Ninety-nine percent of all people tested had detectable levels of the breakdown product of the banned pesticide DDT, 93% had detectable levels of chlorpyrifos.

- Among those tested for pesticide residues in both blood and urine, the average person had 13 pesticides in his or her body.
- Two chemicals found in nearly all the test subjects were TCP, a metabolite of the insecticide chlorpyrifos (found in 93% of those tested), and p,p-DDE, a breakdown product of DDT (found in 99% of those tested).
- Based on these data—which present results from testing for only a fraction of the pesticides that individuals are actually exposed to—it is clear that most people in the U.S. carry a significant body burden of pesticides and pesticide metabolites.

Source: Pesticide Action Network presents all this data in their report *Chemical Trespass.*

Fungicides Fungicide use has increased drastically in recent years—estimated to be a $21 billion industry in 2017[66]. Researches have found at least one fungicide in 75% of surface water samples and 58% of ground water tested.[67] Not only do fungicides impact soil microorganisms thereby interfering with nutrient absorption, but researchers have identified fungicides as endocrine disruptors, causing both kidney and liver damage.[68] Carbamate fungicides like organophosphates are cholinesterase inhibitors. Further studies have linked fungicides with weakened immune systems of bees and bats, making them more susceptible to disease and death.[69] Fungicides impact thyroid health and interfere with hormone function. "Thyroid hormones affect metabolism, brain development, breathing, heart and nervous system functions, body temperature, muscle strength, skin dryness, menstrual cycles, weight, and cholesterol levels. The thyroid hormone is essential for normal brain development in fetuses, babies, and young children. Mild hypothyroidism in the mother is known to have harmful effects on her fetus's brain development."[70] Fungicides applied to wood are known as 'wood preservatives.'[71] Most recently, antibiotic-resistant fungus is starting to appear in people.

Neonicotinoids are a newer type of pesticide that presents a troubling dilemma for pollinators, our waterways, and many vital wildlife and insect species. Birds for example eat bugs, but if the bugs gobbled up by the birds have been impacted in anyway by pesticides, the birds' lives will be shortened indeed. Audubon reports that neonicotinoid coated seeds are contributing to dire water contamination. 5% of the chemical may be taken up by the plant, while "the rest leaches off the seed, accumulates in soil, and sluices via snowmelt, rain, and groundwater seepage into ponds and wetlands, where insects like midges and caddis flies—a staple for billions of grassland birds—start their lives."

"A 2015 study by the U.S. Geological Survey found neonics in 63 percent of water samples taken from 48 streams. In Canada, researchers detected at least one neonic—there are seven types on the market—in 91 percent of wetlands. Unlike many liquid pesticides, neonics can persist and accumulate in ponds for months, if not years."[72]

The health of birds is only one of many indications we are harming life on earth with these chemicals. According to the newest report, State of the World's Birds, "Pesticides associated with farming continue to have a big impact. There is mounting evidence that neurotoxic insecticides known as neonicotinoids are having a detrimental impact on farmland birds. Neonicotinoids are widely used across North America, Europe and elsewhere to pre-treat crops, enabling them to collect in high concentrations in surface water and on the surface of seeds."[73]

Atrazine is commonly used on soy and corn crops as well as on golf courses and hidden in fertilizers. It's used so extensively that it has been found in over 90% of waterways tested,[74] and it can easily be found in our drinking water. Atrazine and other triazine pesticides can induce mammary gland tumors and are known to affect sexual development.[75] Atrazine's effects:

- Endocrine Disruption: The science on atrazine's effects on the hormone system continues to grow. It alters levels of key hormones in rats and can delay puberty. In male frogs, exposure to atrazine causes a kind of "chemical castration," causing them to develop female sex characteristics. Researchers hypothesize that atrazine signals the conversion of testosterone to estrogen, demasculinizing the frogs.
- Reproductive Effects: epidemiological studies find associations between exposure and reproductive effects including increased risk of miscarriage, reduced male fertility, low birth weight, increased chance of birth defect, higher incidence of abdominal defects
- Cancer: Evidence for the carcinogenic potential of atrazine is growing — exposure has been linked to elevated risk of breast and prostate cancer. The recent President's Cancer Panel Report notes that atrazine has possible carcinogenic properties.[76]

The US Geological Survey has shown drinking water sources often contain unsafe levels of agricultural chemicals. Urban water systems can contain as much or more herbicide than rural areas. "Glyphosate was detected more frequently in urban streams than in agricultural streams, and at concentrations similar to those in streams with high agricultural land use in the watershed. In contrast, atrazine was detected more frequently and at higher concentrations in agricultural streams than in urban streams."[77]

Organochlorines: Banned but not Gone

"It is believed that every living organism on Earth has a DDT body burden, mainly stored in the fat."[78] Organochlorines are persistent bioaccumulative toxins that have largely been phased out in the U.S, however their use is expanding in other parts of the world. These substances include aldrin, dieldrin, DDT, heptachlor and hexachlorobenzene. Organochlorine pesticides were recognized as persistent organic pollutants (POPs) that harm ecosystems, bioaccumulate in our fatty tissue, damage human & animal health as well as the earth's protective ozone layer.

According to the United Nations and the World Bank, "As you move up the food chain, concentrations of POPs tend to increase so that animals at the top of the food chain such as fish, predatory birds, mammals, and humans tend to have the greatest concentrations of these chemicals, and therefore are also at the highest risk from acute and chronic toxic effects. In fatty tissue, the concentrations can become magnified by up to 70,000 times higher than the background levels."Health effects of POP Pesticides include Death, Cancers, Allergies, Hypersensitivity, Developmental changes, Damage to the central and peripheral nervous systems, Disruption of the endocrine, reproductive, and immune systems, may be linked to Diabetes[79], causes increased frequency of diseases in wildlife species including birth defects, behavior abnormalities, and declines in wildlife populations.[80] They also harm marine life and oceans; "The negative effects of pesticides in the marine and coastal environments include changes in reef community structure, such as decreases in live coral cover and increases in algae and sponges and damage to seagrass beds and other aquatic vegetation from herbicides."[81] Though these substances were banned in the Stockholm Convention and the Montreal Protocol, they can still be found in waterways, soil, oceans, and within our bodies. Persistent chemicals do not go away easily.

Organophosphates: These are "junior-strength nerve agents,"[82] similar to sarin nerve gas. Over the years many have died—25 school children in India, and in Spain a 1000 people died and thousands more were permanently impaired after eating vegetables containing too much residue.[83] In small doses organophosphates can harm the brain & nervous system.[84]

Banned yet Exported With all the evidence documenting healthrisks imposed by pesticides how do they get approved for use in the first place? Contrary to European standards that endorse the Precautionary Principle, in America the chemical approval process requires safety testing and data be provided solely by *the manufacturer*[85]. Thankfully most POPs are no longer in use here, but what of the imported produce and meat products we bring in? Who's watching what other countries are using? Of those pesticides that are banned, such as carbofuran, manufacturers can legally make them for export to other countries.[86] Brazil leads the world as pesticide importer with a big appetite for those banned elsewhere. A Brazilian physician told Reuters, "This is a giant laboratory for the worst of industrial-scale agriculture."[87]

RESIDUES IN FOOD

Pesticide residues, or tolerances, are *supposedly* safe levels of pesticides allowed in food and beverages—these levels are set by the EPA. In its evaluation, the EPA looks at pesticides individually, though they claim to consider data regarding other pesticides that may be present when reviewing foods in question. Most crops and foods are inundated with a wide variety of fungicides, herbicides, insecticides, and pesticides. Many, particularly root vegetables, strawberries and stored grains & nuts are also exposed to fumigants. Nearly all the data the EPA uses in its safety evaluation comes from test results provided by the manufacturer. "Pesticide companies, or registrants, must submit a wide variety of scientific studies for review before EPA will set a tolerance."[88]

Do we really know what manifests from combinations of pesticides, does the EPA? If for instance glyphosate suppresses tryptophan[89], and tryptophan deficiency is linked with schizophrenia, what happens when we have significant amounts of glyphosate in our body? Does that increase our risk for developing schizophrenia? What if we also eat a lot of nuts, dried fruit and cereal from grains that were stored in facilities fumigated with sulfuryl fluoride? Sulfuryl fluoride impacts the white matter in our brain; when brain white matter is compromised that's also a trigger for schizophrenia[90]. So, if our grains are heavily doused with Roundup and then also exposed to fumigating, what happens when we eat these foods?

Everywhere you look in the food supply you'll find extraordinary doses and wild combinations of pesticides used on foods. You have to wonder what we're risking? The likelihood of exposure is reduced when choosing organic, biodynamic, IPM or vertical, hydroponic, aquaponics foods—assuming these foods haven't been contaminated by other sources such as drift, wind and rain. These alternative farming methods combined only represent a tiny fraction of food grown in the US, though the number of organic farms is increasing. The US grows so much GMO that we have to import millions in organic crops[91] to fulfill the needs of the increasingly health-conscious US population.

PESTICIDE RESIDUES ON FOODS

Data collected from EPA, USDA, Toxnet Sources find data at whatsinmyfood.org

Grapes	56 Pesticides[92]	Pesticide Effects & Damages
Imidacloprid	Neonicotinoid	Neurotoxin[93], contaminates baby foods, kills bees, used in flea collars, bed bug treatment, kills cats and dogs[94]
Boscalid	Fungicide	Possible carcinogen, effects liver and thyroid[95]
Pyraclostrobin	Fungicide	Harms brain[96] toxic to bees, hives & health of bee larvae, linked with increasing bee death to fungus[97]
Myclobutanil	Fungicide	Harms brain, reproductive toxin, prevents iodine absorption, harms thyroid[98]
Trifloxystrobn	Fungicide	Implicated in declining bee health, magnifies impact of other pesticides, contaminates water[97]
Tebuconazole	Fungicide	Possible carcinogen, harms thyroid,[95] endocrine system
Fenhexamid	Fungicide	May be toxic to honeybee larvae,[99] can promote ovarian cell proliferation, worsens ovarian cancer[100]
Apples	**47 Pesticides[101]**	**Pesticide Effects & Damages**
Diphenylamine	Fungicide	Banned in EU, applied to apples post harvest in U.S., converts to carcinogen nitrosamines,[102] toxic to aquatic animals[103]
Thiabendazole	Fungicide	Carcinogen, reproductive toxin[98]
Pyrimethanil	Fungicide	Carcinogen, bee toxin, hormone disruptor[98]
Phosmet	Organophosphate	Possible Carcinogen, Neurotoxin, Bee toxin [97,98]
Acetamiprid	Neonicotinoid	Bee toxin[97], toxic to birds, earthworms, bioaccumulates[104]
Imidacloprid	Neonicotinoid	Bee toxin, endocrine disruptor, evidence of cancer risk, notable water contaminant particularly in urban areas[105]
Carbendazim	Fungicide	Possilbe carcinogen, bee toxin, hormone disruptor[99]
Thiacloprid	Neonicotinoid	Probable carcinogen, bee toxin[104,105]
Bell Peppers	**53 Pesticides[106]**	**Pesticide Effects & Damages**
Pyraclostrobin	Fungicide	Harms brain[96] , toxic to bees[95,97]
Boscalid	Fungicide	Thyroid toxin[95], possible carcinogen
Imidacloprid	Neonicotinoid	Bee toxin, endocrine disruptor, evidence of cancer risk, Found in baby food, water contaminant [93,94]
Thiamethoxam	Neonicotinoid	Bee toxin[98], kidney, liver damage, reproductive tox[107]
Acetamiprid	Neonicotinoid	Bee toxin[98], bird toxin, earthworms, bioaccumulates [102]
Myclobutanil	Fungicide	Harms brain, reproductive toxin, harms thyroid[98]
Chlorpyrifos	insecticide	Neurotoxin, toxic to children & bees, endocrine[108]
Bifenthrin	pyrethroid	Possible carcinogen, reproductive + endocrine disruptor[104]
Strawberries	**45 Pesticides[109]**	**Pesticide Effects & Damages**
Captan	Fungicide	Probable Carcinogen,[110] may cause birth defects
Pyrimethanil	Fungicide	Probable carcinogen, bee toxin, endocrine disruptor

Carbendazim	Fungicide	Possible carcinogen, hormone toxin, bee toxin
Bifenthrin	Insecticide	Possible carcinogen, reproductive toxin, bee toxin
Malathion	Organophosphate	Neurotoxin, hormone, bee toxin, possible carcinogen[112]
CORN	**15 Pesticides[111]**	**Pesticide Effects & Damages**
Malathion	Organophosphate	Neurotoxin, probable carcinogen,[112] mosquito sprays
Chlorpyrifos	Organophosphate	Neurotoxin, endocrine, reproductive + bee toxin[108]
Permethrin	Insecticide	Probable carcinogen, endocrine disruptor, bee toxin
Pirimiphosmethyl	Insecticide	Neurotoxin, Bee toxin
CELERY	**64 Pesticides[113]**	**Pesticide Effects & Damages**
Acephate	Organophosphate	Hormone disruptor, neurotoxin, possible carcinogen
Linuron	Herbicide	Hormone + reproductive toxin, possible carcinogen
Propiconazole	Fungicide	Thyroid toxin, possible carcinogen, reproductive + bees
Malathion	Organophosphate	Possible carcinogen, neurotoxin, hormone & bee toxin
WHEAT	**16 Pesticides[114]**	**Pesticide Effects & Damages**
Malathion	Organophosphate	Neurotoxin, hormone & bee toxin, possible carcinogen
Chlorpyrifos	Organophosphate	Neurotoxin, endocrine disruptor, bee toxin[108]
Methoxychlor	Organochlorine	Hormone disruptor, can alter fetal testis development[115]
Piperonylbutoxide	Insecticide	Endocrine disruptor, suspected carcinogen, liver toxin
Pirimiphosmethyl	Insecticide	Neurotoxin, bee toxin
Trifluralin	Herbicide	Endocrine disruptor, suspected carcinogen, bee toxin
PEACHES	**62 Pesticides[116]**	**Pesticide Effects & Damages**
O-Phenylphenol	Fungicide	Carcinogen, reproductive toxin, hormone disruptor
Iprodione	Fungicide	Carcinogen, hormone disruptor
Phosmet	Organophosphate	Neurotoxin, possible carcinogen, bee toxin
Azinphos methyl	Organophosphate	Neurotoxin, bee toxin, hormone disruptor
Chlorpyrifos	Organophosphate	Neurotoxin, endocrine disruptor, bee and child toxin[117]
KALE	**55 Pesticides[118]**	**Pesticide Effects & Damages**
DDE	Organochlorine	Carcinogen, hormone disruptor, reproductive toxin
Dieldrin	Organochlorine	Carcinogen, hormone disruptor, bee toxin
CILANTRO	**68 Pesticides[119]**	**Pesticide Effects & Damages**
Chlorpyrifos	Organophosphate	Neurotoxin, hormone disruptor, bee toxin[108]
DDT	Organochlorine	Reproductive toxin, endocrine disruptor, banned in US
DDE	Organochlorine	Carcinogen, endocrine disruptor, reproductive toxin
CANNIBAS	**Pesticides**	**Pesticide Effects & Damages**
Myclobutanil	Fungicide	Harms brain, thyroid[96], heated converts to cyanide[120]
Imidacloprid	Neonicotinoid	Neurotoxin, toxic to bees[121],[105]

Reproductive Toxins

Reproductive hazards are substances or agents that may affect the reproductive health of women or men or the ability of couples to have healthy children. These hazards may cause problems such as infertility, miscarriage, and birth defects. www.osha.gov

Endocrine Disruptors

Chemicals that may interfere with the body's endocrine system and produce adverse developmental, reproductive, neurological, and immune effects in both humans and wildlife.

Carcinogen

a substance that causes or contributes to cancer

Neurotoxins

poisons that target the brain and nervous system

Cancer

A group of diseases characterized by uncontrolled growth of abnormal cells that can result in death if not controlled—Worldwide, over 14 million cases of cancer occur each year, and this figure is expected to reach nearly 22 million by 2030.Cancer is the second leading cause of death globally, accounting for an estimated 8.2 million deaths in 2012. Source: U.S.Dept of Health & Human Services[122]

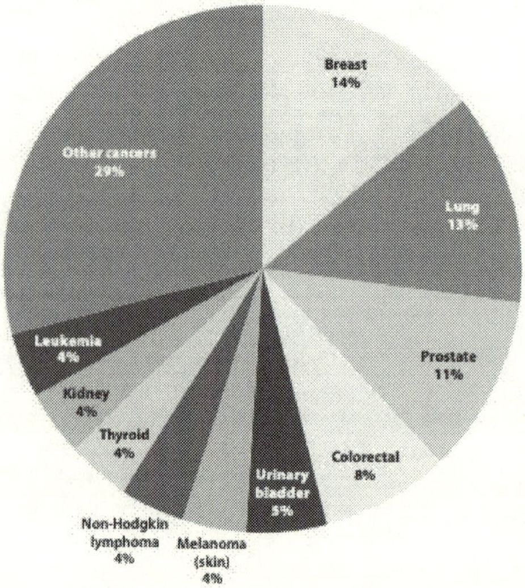

The ten most common cancers in the United States

ORGANOPHOSPHATES

Organophosphates are a group of human-made chemicals that poison insects and mammals. Organophosphates are the most widely used insecticides today. They are used in agriculture, the home, gardens, and veterinary practice. They work by damaging an enzyme in the body called acetylcholinesterase. This enzyme is critical for controlling nerve signals in the body. The damage to this enzyme kills pests and may cause unwanted side effects in exposed humans.

Source: CDC

Neonicotinoids in Baby Foods

Neonics were among the most frequently found pesticide residues in infant and toddler foods. Unlike most other pesticides, neonics cannot be washed off of food prior to consumption. [123]

HEALTH EFFECTS OF PESTICIDES & RESIDUES

Pesticides are toxic to our brains and nervous system[124], they act as endocrine disruptors and are linked with reproductive disorders[125], birth defects[126] and a slew of health maladies. Health effects may include, but are not limited to: reduced IQ, learning disabilities[127], cognitive disorders[128], neurological disorders[129],cancer, lymphoma and leukemia[130], respiratory illness and asthma[131], kidney disease[132], Parkinson's,[133] DNA damage[134], memory loss and Alzheimers[135]; behavioral changes[136]; loss of sense of smell[137], attention deficit disorders[138], autism[139], poisoning and allergies[140], as well as causing and contributing to significant water contamination[141], widespread effects on ecosystems and habitats, drastic declines in wildlife animal populations, pollinators, and climate change.[142]

PESTICIDES CAUSE DISEASE: Pesticides cause disease in children and adults as well as animals. Without herbicides and the prevalence of toxic chemicals throughout the environment, would we be witnessing the surges of disease occurring today?

CHILDREN & CANCER: According to the American Association of Pediatrics, "Epidemiologic evidence demonstrates associations between early life exposure to pesticides and pediatric cancers, decreased cognitive function, and behavioral problems."[143] "For many children, diet may be the most influential source, as illustrated by an intervention study that placed children on an organic diet (produced without pesticide) and observed drastic and immediate decrease in urinary excretion of pesticide metabolites."[144]"Pesticide use in homes may increase the risk of children developing leukemia or lymphoma. Children exposed to insecticides indoors were 47% more likely to have leukemia & 43% more likely to have lymphoma."[145]

ENDOCRINE DISRUPTORS and BREAST CANCER: According to Breast Cancer Prevention Partners, "Atrazine is an endocrine disruptor, and exposure to atrazine has been associated with an increased risk of developing breast cancer."[146] Many herbicides and fungicides are known endocrine disruptors[147], how do all the multiple exposures affect our health?

NEURODEVELOPMENT DISORDERS (NDD): Researchers with Harvard's School of Public Health report, "One out of every six children has a developmental disability, usually involving the nervous system. In recent decades, a gathering amount of evidence has linked industrial chemicals to NDDs. Grandjean and Landrigan conclude that industrial chemicals are responsible for what they call a silent pandemic that has caused impaired brain development in millions of children worldwide. It is silent because the subclinical effects of individual toxic chemicals are not apparent in available health statistics. Testing chemicals for toxicity is a highly efficient public health measure. However, less than half of the thousands of chemicals currently used in commerce have been tested to assess acute toxicity and, although new chemicals undergo more thorough testing, access to the data may be restricted because companies fear exposing proprietary information. Also, current testing rarely includes neurobehavioral functions."[148]

ORGANOPHOSPHATES & CHOLINESTERASE INHIBITORS: In 1981 over 1000 people died in Spain after eating peppers containing high residues of organophosphate pesticides.[149] In 2013 25 children in India died after eating school lunches contaminated with organophosphates[150]. "In 1986, more than 20 people in Sierra Leone, many of them children, died after eating bread made with flour that was transported in a truck that was previously used to carry organophosphates."[151] Cholinesterase inhibiting pesticides include organophosphates, carbamates and neonicotinoids.[152]

CARBAMATES & CANCER: Fungicides and insecticides in the carbamate family have been in use since 1959. "In studies, mice were fed high daily doses of carbaryl for 2 years. Male mice had an increased number of blood vessel tumors at all dose levels. At the highest dose, both male and female mice had an increased number of kidney and liver cancers. Based on these studies, the Environmental Protection Agency (EPA) has classified carbaryl as 'likely to cause cancer."[153] Exposure to Carbaryl has been found to induce skin tumors in mice[154] and increases risk of melanoma in people[155]. Carbaryl is used on food crops as well as golf courses.

GLYPHOSATE, CANCER & DISEASE: 2018 marked a turning point when the verdict came through finding Roundup guilty of causing nonhodgkin's lymphoma and Monsanto guilty of extreme deceptiveness. As court records show, "Monsanto's claim that glyphosate targets an enzyme found only in plants is "false, misleading, and deceptive, as the enzyme that glyphosate targets is found in people and pets—specifically, in beneficial gut bacteria critical to their health and well-being, including their immune system, digestion, allergies, metabolism, and even their brain function."[156] Numerous studies confirm that glyphosate acts as a mineral chelator,[157] perturbs gut bacteria,[158] causes malignant tumors in animals[159], interferes with proper kidney & liver functions in animals, and can damage DNA.[160] Looking back at Dr. Copley's letter (p. 14), she emphasized the mineral chelating properties of glyphosate, in particular Magnesium (Mg), zinc (Zn), calcium (Ca), copper(Cu). How many diseases are linked with deficiencies? If magnesium deficiency plays a role in strokes[161] does that mean glyphosate can cause strokes too?

HAWAII, BIRTH DEFECTS & PESTICIDES: "Exposure to a variety of pesticides have been linked to increased risk of birth defects."[162] Hawaii now contains more GMO testing fields than any other U.S. state. Because of the climate, biotech companies can grow three crops per year from one plot of land instead of only one. That equates to a lot of pesticide spraying and pesticide drift. With this increase the incidence of birth defects and the number of students with learning disabilities have soared. The *Guardian* reported, "the incidence of birth defects in Hawaii is more than 10 times the national rate."[163] "In Hawaii, DuPont-Pioneer sprays pesticides up to 16 times a day, on 2/3 of the days each year, on fields that are often near schools or hospitals. And they do not notify the public of what they spray, or when & where they spray it."[164]

BIRTH DEFECTS IN WILDLIFE: "A suite of reproductive and congenital defects was identified in birds, reptiles, and mammals alike that were attributed to high concentrations of organochlorine pesticides and industrial chemicals. Due to the ubiquitous and persistent nature of many anthropogenic chemicals, these defects, including thyroid dysfunction, hatching success, egg shell thinning, and gross birth deformities, have since been identified in numerous wildlife populations across the world. Certain wildlife such as amphibians are especially vulnerable to chemical perturbation and are suffering alarming population declines. Amphibian field studies have found severe hindlimb and other developmental abnormalities, the greater the agricultural intensity, the greater the number and severity of defects in toad populations." [165]

ANTIBIOTIC-RESISTANT FUNGUS (ARF) and BACTERIA (ARB) ARF is a new, not nearly as prevalent as antibiotic resistant bacteria. Overuse of toxic fungicides on crops is the primary suspect leading to life threatening antibiotic-resistant 'super 'fungus.[166]

CODE RED: CLIMATE CHANGE

Not only do pesticides contribute to the development of many diseases, they also harm the planet, contribute to climate change and deterioration of the earth's ozone layer. During a time when nations are striving to control effects of climate change, shouldn't everything be done to reduce the use of substances that contribute to it? The Montreal Protocol[167] was established to phase out ozone damaging chemicals like fumigants—nonetheless some remain in use. Fumigants are still used to prep soil for crops like strawberries as well as permitted on stored grains, nuts and dried fruit.[168] Here's a look at some of the chemicals used in farming:

SULFURYL FLUORIDE: According to MIT Sulfuryl fluoride contributes *4,800 times more* to global warming than carbon dioxide[169]. Even more troubling, it causes brain lesions and vacuolation[170]—in other words, it causes holes in the brain's white matter. Within the white matter lie the nerve fibers that connect nerve cells. With loss of the white matter, what horrible diseases develop? Think of the spike in Alzheimers and dementia, could this be because of sulfuryl fluoride use in food storage, landscaping, and residential pest control? If a chemical like this isn't banned, what further harm may come to our health & our planet?

METHYL BROMIDE: Methyl Bromide accumulates in the atmosphere, where it destroys the earth's protective ozone layer. It's linked with increased risk of prostate cancer[171], damages to DNA, lungs and liver, and can cause neurological complications. Through the Montreal Protocol, most nations phased out methyl bromide by 2005. However, the United States approved the continued use of the fumigant under the "Critical Use Exemption" clause. Over 4,000 exemptions were granted; most to strawberry and grape growers. Just in 2015, 376 metric tons were used to grow strawberries.[172] Also used when sealing shipping containers. [173]

CHLOROPICRIN: about 10 mill lbs. used annually, often with sulfuryl fluoride[174]

NITROUS OXIDE: In conjunction with synthetic fertilizer, fumigants appear to alter soil biota and release nitrous oxide,[175] which is perhaps the most potent greenhouse gas of all. Nitrous oxide stays in the atmosphere for over 100 years and remains in the soil for decades. According to the EPA, "Nitrous oxide molecules stay in the atmosphere for an average of 114 years before being removed by a sink or destroyed through chemical reactions. The impact of 1 pound of N2O is almost 300 times that of 1 pound of carbon dioxide."[176] Chances are fumigants worsen toxic runoff and water pollution caused by synthetic fertilizer.

ANTIBIOTICS AS PESTICIDES: Citrus growers in Florida struggling to combat citrus greening, a disease spread by an invasive insect known as Asian citrus psyllid. Growers resorted to using 2.23 million pounds of oxytetracylcine and streptomycin to combat the disease- this is 36 times more than that used by humans each year![177] How will this impact agricultural runoff? to antibiotic resistance? What wide-scale destruction could result from this? Does anyone know? Studies show these antibiotic/fungicides have a drastic effect on soil as well as animals.[178] Could using natural means like predatory wasps, the phyllid's natural predator be a better idea?

RESISTANT WEEDS Caused by overuse of pesticides. We're starting to see resistant fungus now from overuse of fungicides. Clearly, the overuse of toxic chemicals is making us very vulnerable; pesticides no longer work, antibiotics can be ineffective. We're on a slippery slope.

SUMMARY OF PESTICIDES MOST WORRISOME FEATURES

1. Pesticides cause harm to people and animals and unintended targets. Many are known endocrine disruptors, neurotoxins, reproductive toxins, complicit in triggering many diseases.

2. Pesticides are killing bees, birds, bats and pollinators. This threatens the entire food supply!

3. Pesticides contaminate water supplies, air, and food worldwide.

4. Inert ingredients increase pesticide toxicity and many are dangerous toxins: The term inert has been changed on labels to "other ingredients."[179] Considered trade secrets, they compound dangerous effects. A refrigerant, Chlorodifluoromethane, was phased out because it depletes the ozone layer, is now starring as an inert pesticide ingredient[180].

5.Agricultural Runoff containing pesticides, synthetic fertilizer and fungicides contaminates water sources, exposes us to toxins, and causes toxic algae blooms, deadzones, and red tides.

6. GMO and Conventional Farming Methods Linked to Climate Change: Fumigants damage the ozone layer. Pesticide overuse contributes to bee and pollinator colony collapse as well as irreversible loss and damage to countless species of wildlife,[181] not to mention the spread of resistant weeds. Fertilizer is responsible for the majority of global nitrous oxide emissions[182]—NO2 is one of the most notorious greenhouse gases. Monocropping results in vast amounts of methane emissions, deforestation, water & air pollution. These are major acts of climate sabotage!

7. More and more pesticides are required on GMO crops despite the fact that genetically engineered crops were touted as needing far *less* herbicides. "Pesticide use has increased by 404 million pounds from the time genetically engineered crops were introduced back in 1996."[183]

8. Superweeds develop from overuse of toxic herbicides: With GMO farming and the increased use of glyphosate, weeds are becoming more resistant than ever. In retaliation, herbicide companies are striving to create more toxic substances capable of outdoing the persistent weeds "To combat the issue of glyphosate-resistant weeds, while maintaining the benefits of glyphosate-tolerant crop technology, seed and agrochemical industries have developed multiple herbicide-tolerant crops by stacking tolerance traits for additional herbicide chemistries."[184]

9. Overuse of fungicides: causing the world's newest threat: antibiotic-resistant fungus[185]

10. Hidden Ingredients added to increase toxin absorbability: Adjuvants are chemical additives like surfactants that increase toxicity & absorption of chemicals. "Despite the known toxicity of adjuvants, they are regulated differently from active principles, with their toxic effects being generally ignored. Adjuvants are not subject to an acceptable daily intake, and they are not included in the health risk assessment of dietary exposures to pesticide residues."[186]

11. Stacking, combining pesticides increases toxicity: Toxic pesticides are more troublesome when mixed. When we're exposed to multiple sources who knows what may result?[187] Manufactures are constantly looking for stronger concoctions. Enlist Duo is one such culprit made of glyphosate & 2,4-D, which the EPA 'unlawfully approved.'[188]

12. Pesticide Drift: Pesticide drift refers to the nature of pesticides to volatilize and disperse through the air after application, contaminating unintended targets such as nearby schools.

13. **Pesticides Linked with Birth Defects:** Hawaii has become a hotbed for GMO testing and with it an unusually abundant amount of pesticides. Birth defects have skyrocketed.[189]

14. Pesticides can persist for a very long time in nature affecting us all. [190]

15. Pesticide residues are found in many of our foods and beverages.

SOLUTIONS Pesticides

PROTECT YOURSELF AND YOUR FAMILY

"Individuals can take important steps in their own lives to reduce their exposure to environmental elements that increase risk for cancer and other diseases. Exposure to pesticides can be decreased by choosing, to the extent possible, food grown without pesticides or chemical fertilizers and washing conventionally grown produce to remove residues."[191]

The President's Cancer Panel May 2010

EAT FOR HEALTH

- Protect your family & yourself: limit exposure to pesticides, herbicides, fungicides.
- Rinse your veges & fruits before eating or cooking.
- When possible seek foods with fewer pesticides, conventional & GMO foods tend to contain higher levels of pesticides than other foods.
- Many grains today are treated with glyphosate before harvest. Organic varieties more likely have no glyphosate; best options include brown rice, amaranth, and quinoa.
- Though pesticide use is saturating our entire world, organic ag remains less toxic.
- These foods can help your body detoxify pesticides and chemicals *just make sure they're organic*: Burdock root, dandelion root, steamed broccoli, cilantro, sauerkraut, kimchi, kombucha, yogurt, apples, chlorella, spirulina, deep green vegetables, organic teas.

PROTECT YOUR KIDS & PETS FROM LAWN CHEMICALS

"Family exposure to numerous occupational chemicals can be reduced by removing shoes before entering the home and washing work clothes separately from the other family laundry."[180]

1. Don't use toxic pesticides, fungicides, or toxic fertilizer on your lawn and gardens
2. Remove Shoes or wash off the bottom of your shoes after being outside. Get in the habit or removing your shoes when indoors.
3. Protect your children and pets from lawn chemicals in your neighborhood. Avoid freshly treated lawns and wash your pet's paws off with water when they come indoors.

Lawn chemicals are especially dangerous for children, animals and people of any age, especially if direct contact occurs. Pesticide Watch created a guide, *The Truth about Cats, Dogs, and Lawn Chemicals*[192] in which they explain the risk to people and pets. Toxics Action Center[193] revealed:

- 53% of ChemLawn's pesticide products ingredients are possible carcinogens,
- 41% of their pesticides include ingredients that are banned or restricted in other countries.
- All 32 of their pesticide products include ingredients that pose threats to the environment including: threats to water supplies, aquatic organisms, and non-targeted insects."[18]

SAFE DISPOSAL OF PESTICIDES: Due to the dangerous nature of these chemicals, we cannot discard of them in the regular trash or pour them down the drain. They must be taken to a hazardous waste facility or back to the manufacturer. To find a specific location close to you call your local household hazardous waste center at 1-800-CLEANUP.

SOLUTIONS Pesticides

PROTECT THE POLLINATORS Reducing and avoiding use of pesticides outdoors greatly helps the birds and the bees! Right now pollinators are in crisis, in serious decline! Only through our reducing all the pesticides and use of toxins do these creatures have a chance.

PROTECT WILDLIFE IN REFUGES: Pesticides and toxic chemicals do not belong in a wildlife refuge. Since 2014 GMOs and neonicotinoids were banned in all wildlife refuges. That made sense since neonicotinoids and nasty pesticides used to grow GMOs are implicated in killing pollinators and wildlife. Of all places on earth, wildlife refuges should be designated safe zones for animals!

Why would GMO farming or neonics be allowed in wildlife refuges anyway? It seems strange but apparently farming has been allowed in refuges for decades. The Department of the Interior (DOI) definitely has its priorities a little mixed up. Public lands that the DOI manage have long been rented and leased away to drilling, oil, fracking, mining, and ranchers' interests regardless of the consequences to the wild animals that call these wildlands home. Wouldn't it be preferable, if before any activity is allowed on wild lands that the lessee promises to present neither risk nor harm to the natural inhabitants of the lands?

President Obama stepped in and made the wildlife refuges off limits to GMOs and pollinator-killing neonicotinoids. But no more. President Trump reversed that course, so now farmers can go back to growing GMOs in wildlife refuges! If you don't know what GMO farming entails, here it is: land conversion, monocropping, inappropriate and excess use of toxic herbicides and synthetic fertilizer, degradation of soil, water pollution, harm to pollinators, harm to wildlife, harm to the planet. Send letters to the Secretary of the Interior to get these special places protected once again so that animals can be safe at least somewhere on this planet.

BRING YOUR YARD BACK TO LIFE WITHOUT CHEMICALS: If you have your own yard you can switch to going nontoxic. Your soil and plants may have put their skills into hibernation after years of toxic assault, but like many things in life, land can rebound back to its former glory if given the chance. As relayed by everyone's favorite, *This Old House*, "The underlying philosophy behind organic lawn care is this: Healthy, chemical-free soil begets robust lawns that can virtually take care of themselves. After years of being inundated by chemicals to fend off grubs, eradicate weeds, and green up the turf, the natural capacity of the soil to perform these tasks itself has ceased operation, practitioners say. Cut it off from the chemicals cold turkey, and you'll get things running again—naturally. And once the soil's healthy, you might never have to deal with pesticides, herbicides, even fertilizers again."[194]

Facts About Lawn Chemicals, source: EPA[195]

- When lawn chemicals are applied improperly, they can run off into streams, harming fish and other animals and contaminating our drinking water.
- Even pets are at risk — studies show that the rates of lymphoma in pets of pesticide users are significantly higher than occurrences in the pets of non-chemical users.

2. GMOs

Genetically Modified Organisms, Bioengineered Food

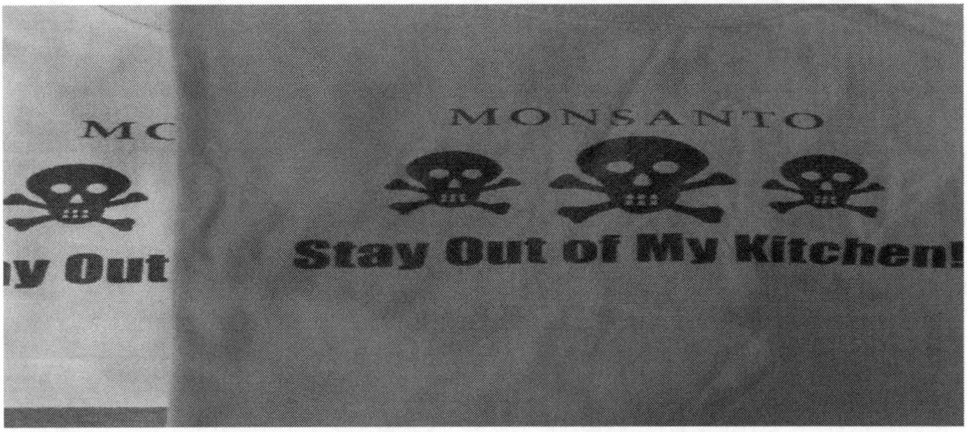

Genetically Modified Organisms, GMOs, are also known as genetically engineered foods (GE), biotech, and the newest name, bioengineered (BE) —these terms all essentially mean the same thing: GMOs. Genetic modification means the food came from a plant whose DNA was modified with DNA from another plant *or* animal. Some GMO plants even have insecticides inserted within their seeds.[196] Because GMO foods have been altered with foreign DNA, these foods lack the integrity inherent in natural foods.

Perhaps what is most dangerous about genetically modified food is not the mixing of the DNA but rather the amount of pesticides used to grow them. The excessive and increasing use of herbicides used to grow GMOs,[197] translates to more foods containing greater pesticide residues. One GMO variety like the Roundup Ready seeds are designed specifically to withstand excessive amounts of *Roundup*, the most used glyphosate-based herbicide. There are many varieties of GMO plants and herbicides to go with them. We're only now beginning to observe the various ways all these GMO seeds and pesticide formulations behave and there's still plenty of unknowns.[198] In a world that already presents an overload of challenges for us all, does any one of us need the additional problems presented when our food contains toxins?

Some argue that genetic engineering has always been going on and that this is nothing new. While it's true farmers and growers have utilized selective breeding and artificial selection techniques to create more desirable foods and crops throughout history, today's biotechnology is quite different.[199] GMOs present a risky combination of herbicides with unnatural and unusual proteins. This can pose a great problem for our bodies, for don't our bodies have an instinctual response to things not recognized?[200] Foods such as GMOs can be interpreted as invaders, causing the immune system to alight and allergic reaction to follow. Beautifully functional and efficient in its design, the human body is incredibly adaptable yet ultimately very sensitive to incoming material it perceives as foreign or strange.

WHAT FOODS ARE GMO?[201]

GMO CORN	GMO SOY
GMO COTTON	GMO CANOLA
GMO SUGAR BEETS	GMO ALFALFA (animal feed)
GMO PAPAYA	GMO ARCTIC APPLE
GMO GOLDEN RICE[202]	GMO ZUCCHINI & YELLOW SQUASH
GMO POTATOES	rBGH MILK, DAIRY[203]
GMO SALMON[204]	GMO SORGHUM

HOW WE ARE EXPOSED TO GMOs

We're exposed to GMOs when we consume any food or beverage product made with GMOs or any derivative of a genetically modified food source such as corn syrup, canola oil, and sugar. GMO foods and ingredients can be found in countless foods: bread, grains, cookies, pasta, pizza, milk, cereal, ice cream, cheese, pie, bakery products, salad dressings, soups, frozen dinners, toaster products, donuts, cakes, pies, ice cream, breakfast bars, candy, sugar, oats, soy, corn, chips, squash, foods containing any type of corn or soy, corn syrup, cornbread, any product containing canola oil, corn oil, cottonseed oil, cornbread, sunflower oil, soybean oil, oats, soy, tofu, tempeh, miso, edamame, soy sauce, deli meat, chicken, pork, turkey, beef, eggs, fast foods, and processed foods. Meat and dairy products derived from animals fed GMO feed, or administered GMO hormones also contain genetically modified ingredients. Salmon is the first animal to be genetically modified, and farmed fish are usually fed GMO feed. Additionally, you may be exposed to glyphosate, if any food you eat is desiccated with glyphosate before harvest.[205] Desiccation is a process used to dry out plants and speed up harvest. Nongmo crops are exposed to this process including wheat, rye, barley, flax, lentils, peas, and many others.[206]

DESICCATION: GLYPHOSATE IN MOST FOODS

In the UK, the Soil Association reported, "Glyphosate can follow the grain into our food. Tests found that almost two thirds of wholemeal bread sampled contained glyphosate."[207] More and more often, farmers are choosing to apply glyphosate to crops not just while growing but also just before harvest. This process, known as desiccation is done to dry out plants and lessen the time it takes to harvest. This results in greater residues in foods and alas, greater exposure to pesticides for us. According to the Soil Association of Scotland, "Glyphosate kills parts of the crop that haven't ripened evenly and dries the crop. This allows Combine harvesters to move more quickly and cover more ground during harvest and may reduce drying cost.

But applying glyphosate so close to harvest makes the likelihood of finding residues in food even higher." Peter Melchett, Policy Director states, "If glyphosate ends up in bread it's impossible for people to avoid it, unless they are eating organic. On the other hand, farmers could easily choose not to use glyphosate as a spray on wheat crops – just before they are harvested. This is why the Soil Association is calling for the immediate ending of the use of glyphosate sprays on wheat destined for use in bread."[208]According to EcoWatch, glyphosate is applied to wheat, lentils, peas, non-GMO soybeans, corn, flax, rye, triticale, buckwheat, millet, canola, sugar beets, potatoes and sunflowers."[209]

RESIDUES IN GMOs: Reports show that GMOs contain higher pesticide residues than non-GMO foods.[210] This is a not a winning scenario for health-conscious people, not to mention the farm animals provided with GMO feed. As revealed by scientists in Norway, "Roundup Ready GM-soy accumulates residues of glyphosate and AMPA, and also differs markedly in nutritional composition compared to soybeans from other agricultural practices. Organic soybean samples also showed a healthier nutritional profile (e.g. higher in protein and lower in saturated fatty acids) than both industrial conventional and GM soybeans."[211]

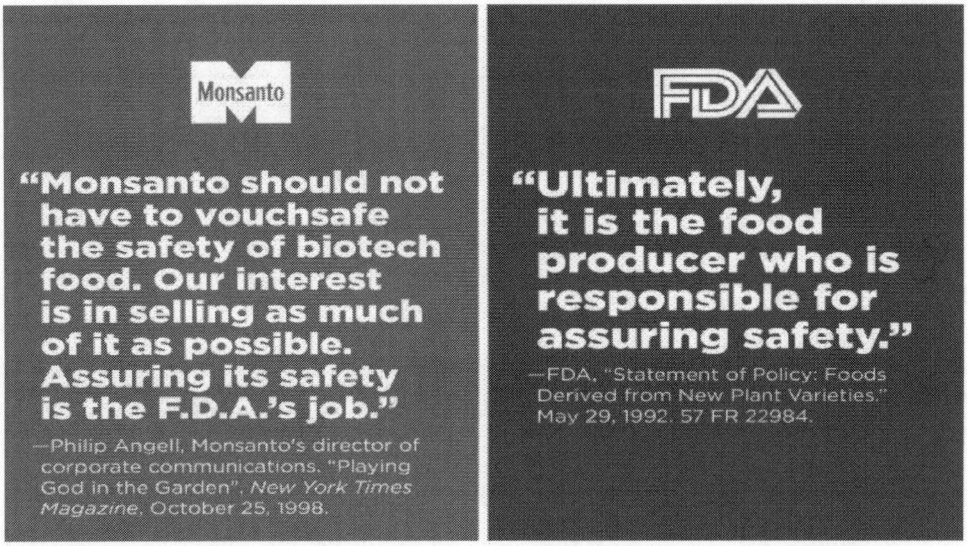

Reprinted courtesy of *Seedy Business*, Report from US Right to Know January 2015[212]

ARE GMOs SAFE? Though genetically modified food may be hailed by their producers as safe, what we've seen from testing tells another story. The US Courts decided last summer that Roundup does cause cancer; they also found that Monsanto covered up that information for years. If the approval process only requires the company to provide its own safety testing, we certainly have reason to worry.

In 1993 the FDA declared GMOs to be generally recognized as safe (GRAS). This decision was based solely on results the manufacturers themselves provided. You might think the FDA and USDA tested GMO foods for safety. That is not the case. As revealed in 2015's US Right to Know Report, *Seedy Business*, "In recent testimony before Congress, the FDA stated that it's "confident that the GE foods in the U.S. marketplace today are as safe as their conventional counterparts."[213] However, FDA does not itself test whether genetically engineered foods are safe. The FDA has repeatedly made this clear."[214]

HEALTH EFFECTS of Glyphosate, and possibly then, GMOs

If there is a risk of health damage from herbicides, it must logically exist whether you're using the pesticides, or you're exposed to them through food or beverages. It's also possible that not only the significant level of herbicide residue, but also the transgenic material found in GMO foods can trigger disease. Recently, it was confirmed[215] that *Roundup* causes cancer. Many studies have provided additional evidence that the pesticides used to grow GMO foods cause major diseases. If the pesticides used to grow these foods are in fact so harmful then GMO foods containing residues of those pesticides can also be harmful.

Deadly to Human Embryonic Cells: "Roundup's inert ingredients amplified the toxic effect on human cells—even at concentrations much more diluted than those used on farms and lawns. One specific inert ingredient, polyethoxylated tallow amine, or POEA, was more deadly to human embryonic, placental and umbilical cord cells than the herbicide itself – a finding the researchers call "astonishing."[216]

Infertility, accelerated aging, liver, kidney, spleen problems, high cholesterol, insulin: From the American Academy of Environmental Medicine: "Several animal studies indicate serious health risks associated with GM food consumption including infertility, immune dysregulation, accelerated aging, dysregulation of genes associated with cholesterol synthesis, insulin regulation, cell signaling, and protein formation, and changes in the liver, kidney, spleen and gastrointestinal system."[217]

Tumors: The *Long Term Study of Rats fed Roundup tolerant Maize (Corn).* "By the beginning of the 24th month, 50% to 80% of female animals had developed tumors in all treatment groups, with up to three tumors per animal, whereas only 30% of controls were affected. The same trend was observed in the groups receiving R (Roundup) in their drinking water."[218]

Rheumatoid Arthritis: From the Agricultural Health Study, "Women who developed Rheumatoid Arthritis were more likely to report ever using the fungicides maneb mancozeb, the herbicide glyphosate, as well as solvents and chemical fertilizers.[219]

Kidney Disease, kidney failure A study of chronic kidney disease amongst farmers in Sri Lanka since the mid 1990s looked at glyphosate found in their drinking water as the primary culprit, "it seems to have acquired the ability to destroy the renal tissues of thousands of farmers when it forms complexes with a localized geo environmental factor (hardness) and nephrotoxic metals."[220]

Liver Disease: decreases levels of CYP enzymes, essential for detoxifyng compounds."[221]

Inhibits Amino Acids, Enzymes, Chelates and Binds Minerals: From the European Food Safety Authority EFSA study: "Glyphosate is known to inhibit 5-enolpyruvylshikimate-3-phosphate synthase (EPSPS), an enzyme of the shikimic acid pathway that leads to the biosynthesis of aromatic acids phenylalanine, tryptophan, and tyrosine and a range of other substances... binds essential minerals effectively, its application could lead to an undersupply of minerals that are essential co-factors in many biological processes in treated plants and potentially also in organisms feeding on such plants. This in turn could impact plant resistance to disease and affect human and animal health. Although the chelating properties are well known, this potential additional environmental risk was never adequately considered in the regulatory risk assessment."[222]

GLYPHOSATE ALERT

Glyphosate is everywhere—including in our bodies. Digging into the secret world of Roundup reveals the darkest of realities. Nearly all food tested contains traces of it.[223] It's found in most food and beverages we consume from bread to beer to water.

What Glyphosate Does:

- Alters the gut microbiome, causes anxiety, depression, and despair behavior[224]
- Glypohosate is an endocrine disruptor[225]
- Glyphosate-based herbicides reduce thyroid function and hormone production[226]
- Glyphosate inhibits apoptosis, the body's ability to fight tumors and microscopic cancers
- Glyphosate impairs the liver's ability to detoxify xenobiotics, and
- Glyphosate suppresses production of serotonin, melatonin, dopamine, and tryptophan[227]

Considering how many foods contain traces of glyphosate, we're likely ingesting quite a bit daily. This comes along with residues of all the other pesticides also used in dramatic amounts—all equally capable of causing detrimental effects to our health. These substances impact our behavior, our mood, our ability to fight disease, and can cause depression[228]. Is it any wonder then that Americans are taking more anti-depressants and anti-anxiety medications? Since 1999, antidepressant use in America has risen 64%.[229] Sleeping pill use is also higher than than ever. The CDC reports that 50 to 70 million Americans suffer from sleep deprivation.[230]

It's effect upon the thyroid gland certainly needs more attention. How does it affect the hormone system? "Thyroid cancer rates are rising faster than any other cancer in the United States, a new study found: Between 1975 and 2013, the number of thyroid cancer cases diagnosed yearly more than tripled."[231] Perhaps the big picture of how glyphosate fully interferes with our health will one day be evident. The combination of toxins has to worsen the impact. We face so many opponents in our quest for health these days; hopefully we will get smarter and stop allowing so many of these substances to be used.

MONSANTO KNEW *ROUNDUP* CAUSED CANCER

Throughout the country we're seeing surges of diseases that run surprisingly parallel with the increased use of poisonous substances, especially of glyphosate-based herbicides. Is it merely coincidence? Is it due to the massive amounts of herbicides needed to grow GMO crops? Are these chemicals more dangerous than others? As reports and hidden emails indicate genuine test results for Roundup and glyphosate were suppressed. "The Monsanto Papers tell an alarming story of ghostwriting, scientific manipulation, collusion with the Environmental Protection Agency (EPA), and previously undisclosed information about how the human body absorbs glyphosate. These documents, which Monsanto did not want you to see, provide a deeper understanding of the serious public health consequences surrounding Monsanto's conduct in marketing Roundup."[232] Some of the secret documents uncovered:

- "Just wanted to let you that what we have long been concerned about has happened. Glyphosate is on for an IARC review in March of 2015."
- "the release of the paper has already had profound impacts…The vivid color photographs of rats with grotesque tumors will not easily be erased from the public psyche... I sincerely hope that the journal will take immediate action by retracting the paper."[233] (see pgs 13-14.)

GLYPHOSATE CREATES NEW HARMFUL ORGANISM!

Dr. Don Huber and fellow scientists from Purdue University discovered something very scary occurring with *Roundup*. In 2011 he wrote an urgent letter to the USDA. Dr. Huber provided me with an updated version of the letter to include here; you can see the original at CBS News.[234]

"Dear Secretary Vilsack, A team of senior plant and animal scientists have recently brought to my attention the discovery of an electron microscopic entity that appears to significantly impact the health of plants, animals, and probably human beings. Based on a review of the data, it is widespread, very serious, and is in much higher concentrations in Roundup Ready (RR) soybeans and corn—suggesting a link with the RR gene or more likely with the presence of Roundup. This entity appears NEW to science! A diverse set of researchers working on this problem have contributed various pieces of the puzzle, which together presents the following.

This is highly sensitive information that could result in a collapse of US soy and corn export markets and significant disruption of domestic food and feed supplies. On the other hand, this new organism may already be responsible for significant harm (see below). My colleagues and I are therefore moving our investigation forward with speed and discretion and seek assistance from the USDA and other entities to identify the pathogen's source, prevalence, implications, and remedies. We are informing the USDA of our findings at this early stage, specifically due to your pending decision regarding approval of RR alfalfa. Naturally, if either the RR gene or Roundup itself is a promoter or co-factor of this pathogen, then such approval could be a calamity.

For the past 40 years, I have been a scientist in the professional and military agencies that evaluate and prepare for natural and manmade biological threats, including germ warfare and disease outbreaks. Based on this experience, I believe the threat we are facing from this pathogen is unique and of a high-risk status. In layman's terms, it should be treated as an emergency.

Unique Physical Properties: This previously unknown entity is only visible under an electron microscope (36,000X) with an approximate size range equal to a medium size virus. It is able to reproduce but doesn't contain DNA or RNA, and in this regard appears similar to a prion. If so, it would be the first such micro-entity ever identified in both plants and animals. There is strong evidence that this apparently infectious agent promotes diseases in plants & mammals.

Linked with Outbreaks of Plant Diseas: The entity is prolific in plants infected with two pervasive diseases that are driving down yields and farmer income—sudden death syndrome (SDS) in soy, and Goss' wilt in corn. it's also found in the fungal causative agent of SDS.

Implicated in Animal Reproductive Failure: Laboratory tests have confirmed the presence of this entity in a wide variety of livestock that have experienced spontaneous abortions and infertility. Preliminary results have also been able to reproduce abortions in a clinical setting.

Recommendations: It is urgent to examine whether the side effects of glyphosate use may have facilitated the growth of this entity or allowed it to cause greater harm to weakened plant and animal hosts. It is well documented that glyphosate promotes soil pathogens and is already implicated with the increase of more than 40 plant diseases; it dismantles plant defenses by chelating vital nutrients; and it reduces the bioavailability of nutrients in feed, which in turn can cause animal disorders. We are now seeing an unprecedented trend of increasing plant and animal diseases and disorders. This *(entity)* may be instrumental to understanding and solving this problem. It deserves immediate attention with significant resources to avoid a general collapse of our critical agricultural infrastructure." The USDA did not reply.

HOW ARE GENETICALLY MODIFIED FOODS MADE?

In addition to concerns with the herbicides used in GMO farming, the process of modifying plants itself is an assault on nature. This is not your traditional plant breeding.

Almost every GM (genetically modified) crop ever created has included a useful little piece of DNA copied from the 'Cauliflower Mosaic Virus' (CaMV). This chunk of DNA is referred to as 'CaMV 35S', and as its name suggests, it is part of the DNA found in a virus which commonly infects cauliflower and related vegetables. In infected plants, its normal function is to switch on the genes needed for the virus to replicate itself. In GM plants its function is to switch on the engineered DNA attached to it, which otherwise would likely remain dormant: effectively it overpowers the host cell's own self-regulatory mechanisms to permanently turn on the inserted genes, which then generate huge amounts of the transgenic proteins.

The value of the CaMV 35S 'promoter' to genetic engineers lies in its promiscuity: it acts on all types of DNA in the genome of all types of plants. Any suggestion that problems could arise from putting millions of copies of an aggressive viral promoter into every mouthful of our food have been reasoned out of existence by the biotech industry and regulators. Their argument goes something like: humanity has been eating such DNA in its natural form forever, besides which it won't survive processing, cooking and digestion, and, even if it did survive, it is plant-specific and so can't turn on the genes in mammals including humans, or gut bacteria, and, even if it did survive and get into such cells, it will only activate the gene to which it is attached.

The Institute for Science in Society and other scientists have been warning of the inherent risk in using CaMV 35S in GM food for a decade. The scientific questions, which GM proponents have reasoned they don't need to ask include, can intact, functional CaMV 35S end up inside our cells and our intestinal flora, and if it gets there can it cause harm? Large chunks of DNA can and do survive digestion and enter animal cells (including human) and can end up in many vital organs; they can also enter microbial cells in the digestive tract. The CaMV 35S promoter can drive genes in any cell it ends up in, not only in plants but also microbes and animals. Engineered genes attached to a universal promoter can be taken up by all manner of living cells and can be functional."[235] **Reprinted courtesy of the Institute of Science in Society**

Today there are more methods used to insert DNA. The institute of Responsible Technology relates: "Other techniques include coating DNA onto tiny metal pellets and firing with a special gun into cells; injecting new DNA into fertilized eggs with a very fine needle. Using electric shocks to create holes in the membrane covering sperm, forcing new DNA into the sperm."[236]

BT TOXINS: Some GMO crops are developed to contain their own insecticide, BT Toxin. While we're supposed to believe there is no danger associated with this, can we trust that these companies fully vetted these foods and they're safe? As explained in *Growing Doubt: A Scientist's Experience of GMOs*, "Bt plants get their name because they incorporate a transgene that makes a protein-based toxin (usually called the Cry toxin) from the bacterium *Bacillus thuringiensis*. Many Bt crops are "stacked," meaning they contain a multiplicity of Cry toxins. Their makers believe each of these Bt toxins is insect-specific and safe. However, there are multiple reasons to doubt both safety and specificity. Bt insecticides share structural similarities with ricin. Ricin is a famously dangerous plant toxin."[237]

BEWARE BT CORN and GMO SOY

GMO soy and BT corn are everywhere. "The fact that genetically modified soy may be present in as much as 70 percent of all food products found in U.S. supermarkets means that a vast majority of Americans may be putting a lot of GM soy into their systems daily."[238] In 2018 94% of the soy and 82% of corn grown in America were GMO crops.[239] There are 20 varieties of GMO soy and 33 different varieties of GMO corn[240] currently approved by the USDA.[241] The biotech industry claims these foods are no different than traditional corn and soy, yet the EPA and FDA admit that they themselves don't test the foods for safety, but merely review data submitted by the manufacturers.[242] Considering the coverups[243] within the biotech corporations, can we really trust any test results they provide? Many independent studies suggest a different tale than what we've been told. Anyone suffering with allergies or digestive issues, take note.

BT CORN

- The BT insecticide is implanted within the seed and the toxin extends to every part of the plant while growing. It remains in all foods developed from the plant.[244]
- Contrary to industry claims when ingested BT passes through the human gut without harm, BT has been found in the blood of pregnant women and their fetuses,[245] thereby demonstrating it does cross through the intestinal wall.
- BT makes holes in insect gut cells and likely does the same in animal and human cells, causing "bowel hypersensitivity,"[246] which is linked with "leaky gut," colitis, gluten sensitivity, acid reflux, reduced enzyme activity and digestive disturbances.
- Rats fed for 90 days on Monsanto's MON863 maize had toxicity in the liver and kidneys.[247] BT pollen kills monarch butterflies[248]

GMO SOY

- Contains residues of glyphosate and its main metabolite, AMPA, a neurotoxin causing glutamate excitotoxicity, oxidative stress, and depression[249]
- GMO soy is nutritionally inferior to organic grown soy[250]
- Soy mimics estrogen and lowers testosterone; eaten raw, soy has an anti-nutrient effect, contains protease inhibitors that inhibit the body's ability to digest protein, and contains phytates which prevent absorption of essential minerals; soy without fermentation also contains goitrogens, which have an ill effect on the thyroid gland.[251]
- Childhood food allergies are a rapidly growing public health problem. Their prevalence in the USA increased by 50% between 1997 and 2011. In the USA, eight foods are responsible for 90% of childhood food allergies: peanuts, tree nuts, cow's milk, chicken eggs, wheat, soy, fish and shellfish.[252]
- Most of the meat & dairy in the US comes from factory-farmed animals that are only fed GMO corn & soy. If you any eat these foods, you are eating lots of GMO corn & soy.
- Rounding out the threats from GMO corn and soy, glyphosate is known to disturb normal gut flora-- the good microorganisms in our digestive tract—and cause anxiety.[253] How does this extra strain on our stomach affect our health? Is it any wonder IBD, colitis and crohn's disease[254] and heartburn[255] are all escalating in occurrence? If we get off all factory farmed meat and dairy and GMO grains and foods, do we become disease free?

CODE RED: CLIMATE CRISIS

Let's look at GMO's contribution to Climate Change.

- GMO Farming requires incredible amounts of pesticides to cope with the persistent super weeds its herbicides have created. This creates an endless loop of toxic exposure.
- Land change for monocropping has devoured countless acres—often land that was once forest, prairie or meadow causing massive shifts in habitats and loss of stored carbon
- Synthetic fertilizer and monocropping cause grave harm to soil life, waterways, people, to countless species and to the planet as we know it.
- Monocropping requires farmers to apply more synthetic fertilizer per acre in attempt to replenish the depleted soil[256]. The nitrous oxide emissions and toxic runoff from fertilizer radicalize climate change, cause toxic algae blooms and are a factor in red tides.
- The deathly use of all these toxic substances terrorizes waterways, air quality, and all creatures including pollinators and beneficial insects, wild animals, pets and people.
- Killing Animals in Waterways: oceans, streams, lakes. rivers, and groundwater are drastically affected by agricultural runoff that not only contaminates drinking water, but also causes dead zones, toxic algae, red tides[257], & warming oceans. When the algae die bacteria take over releasing carbon dioxide & contributing to ocean acidification.
- GMOs and factory farm animals are interlinked, these animals are force fed GMOs rather than the food they'd eat naturally.

GMO & ITS PLANET HARMING FACTORS:

- Overuse of pesticides causes weed resistance
- Toxic herbicides are prone to drift (see page 24, *Hawaii, birth defects & pesticide drift*)
- Toxic pesticides are killing pollinators, beneficial insects, and threatening wildlife.
- Synthetic Fertilizer use has exploded and is a major nitrous oxide (N2O) emitter. N2O is considered "the most potent greenhouse gas"[258], 300x worse for climate than CO2.
- Monocropping & deforestation cause habitat loss, erosion, and loss of carbon storage.
- When soil is sickened, erosion & runoff are promoted, and soil emits carbon dioxide
- Farming chemicals toxify runoff causing lethal toxic algae, algae blooms, dead zones, red tide & ocean acidification
- GMO Soy is likely causing factory farm animals to produce more methane

This anti-earth, anti-life farming practice is not slowing down. Instead our government is subsidizing these farmers and their deadly use of toxins. Our own government encourages other nations to follow our lead, to abandon their traditional ways of growing food for this one. When farmers sign up to try GMO seeds, they enter a binding contract; they're not allowed to replant seeds, the seeds have to be bought every year. The seeds only grow with the herbicides designed to grow with the seeds. Because of the widespread weed resistance that's developed, farmers must keep buying more herbicides to combat them. Though GMO farming was supposed to use less herbicides than all other types of farming, that is far from true. Without sight of common sense, these farming styles and our governments' encouragement of them is misleading us all far away from any climate recovery.

CAN GMOs END HUNGER? Not Likely.

"Despite 20 years of research and 13 years of commercialization, genetic engineering has failed to significantly increase U.S. crop yields."[259]Many scientists argue that GMOS were never intended to yield more, but rather continue providing yields when other crops fail such as in drought conditions. Can GMO crops withstand brutal weather changes as predicted better than traditional or organic plants? And if they could, what nutritional value do those plants offer?

With all the tragic effects brought upon the planet from GMO farming, how can we imagine our food supply dependent on this model? It's only been in use since the 1990s and already we have colossal damage to waterways, soil, air, animals and atmosphere. It's just not sustainable. In poor nations farmers don't have the means to afford GMO farming, let alone get their product to market. Sometimes what is needed most in poverty-stricken nations is not moving away from traditional farming methods, but rather helping improve access so food can get to people.

Above all, the simplest reason to avoid GMOs is often overlooked by GMO enthusiasts. Feeding people, whether 10 or 10 billion requires a continued supply of food—a supply that essentially depends on pollinators. As long as GMO farming continues at warp speed, and with it the increased use of glyphosate and other chemicals, pollinators are at serious risk of going extinct. Without pollinators, game's over. There won't be enough food to harvest. What becomes of us then?

"If we are going to make headway in combating hunger due to overpopulation and climate change, we will need to increase crop yields. Traditional breeding outperforms genetic engineering hands down." Union of Concerned Scientists[260]

SUSTAINABILITY

Sustainability involves nourishing the earth, planting with nature in mind, water conservation, natural pesticide methods, and native planting in sync with each particular climate.

- To feed people there must be food.
- Animals need food.
- To have enough food for all we need bees and pollinators and good farmers*
- Pesticides kill bees and pollinators

***MONSANTO CONTRACTS:** In India many good farmers have lost their lives after signing Monsanto contracts. The contracts have very strict conditions that cripple farmers' hope, "These farmers are losing their lands & their livelihoods, due to the debt they incur trying to afford Monsanto's products. Many of the farmers drink the chemical insecticides in order to commit suicide. Between the years of 1995 and 2013, more than 300,000 farmer suicides occurred, many of which were linked to Monsanto."[261]

Bats, Bees & Birds

Many feel the declining animal and insect populations are attributed to climate change. Though which came first, the warming or the chemicals? Surely the excessive use of pesticides plays a role. Chemicals may reduce insect pests, but they also result in reduced pollinator numbers. This results in a domino effect upon all life. In forests for instance, Carbaryl has been deployed to combat beetles, and fungicides to control tree disease, but these chemicals also harm pollinators and can kill birds—birds are the beetles' natural predator and our most effective weapon. We've entered a global period where we need less chemicals and more common sense.

GMO MILK ALERT

What is GMO Milk? You've probably heard about rBGH or rBST, but what are they? Recombinant Bovine Growth Hormone (rBGH) and Recombinant Bovine Somatotropin (rBST) are genetically modified hormones injected into cows. These cows are also raised at factory farms where they eat only GMO corn and soy. This is how milk becomes GMO milk.

RBGH was designed to increase milk production.[262] Normally cows produce about 70 pounds or 8 gallons of milk daily; rBGH increases that amount 10%. As a result, cows suffer from increased udder and mastitis infections.[263] Cows are treated with antibiotics to fight the infections—an endless cycle that results in milk containing synthetic growth hormones as well as antibiotic residue. Monsanto was the primary manufacturer, and they fought hard to keep GMO milk unlabeled[264]. As a result, any milk product today stating it's rBGH-free must include this disclaimer: *"no significant difference has been shown between milk derived from [rBST]-treated and non-{rBST}treated cows."*[265] While rBGH has been allowed in the U.S. since 1993, it's banned in the entire European Union, Canada, New Zealand, Japan, Israel and other countries.

Some Cafes no longer serve rBGH milk; however, unless they can tell you what organic dairy supplies their milk, the milk they use is still from factory farm cows. (See page 50,51).

HEALTH CONCERNS of GMO MILK

Dr. Samuel Epstein, the late Professor Emeritus at University of Illinois Chicago School of Environmental and Occupational Health, boldly documented the dangers of GMO Milk in his breakthrough must-read book, *What's in Your Milk?*[266] Here are some excerpts:

1. Milk from rBGH cows has much higher levels of the Insulin-like Growth Factor
   - Excess levels of IGF-1 pose serious risks of breast and prostate cancer.
   - Elevated IGF-1 levels inhibit the body's normal ability to protect itself from microscopic cancers by the natural process of programmed destruction, known as "apoptosis." This inhibition of natural cell destruction plus the growth enhancing properties of IGF-1 make it a potent cause of cancer.
   - rBGH milk is likely to spread antibiotic resistant infections in the general population
2. Infants exposed to rBGH milk would consume over 100x the safety margin of IGF-1.
3. High levels of IGF-1 are known to promote both growth & invasiveness of early cancers, and decreases response to chemotherapy!
4. Hazards of rBGH milk: allergic reactions, antibiotic resistance, cancer risk, increase in the long-chain saturated fatty acids resulting in more cardiovascular disease, elevated thyroid hormones, immunological effects from absorption in the digestive tract.
5. The toxic effects of rBGh is evidenced at cattle autopsy: increased organ weights, widespread multifocal adhesions, chronic inflammation of internal organs including heart and lungs, nearly half the cows became infertile, with increased mastitis and anemia.

SOLUTIONS

Protect your health and your family, avoid this milk.
We must get this milk out of school lunch programs.

USDA
(202) 720-2791
1400 Independence Ave. S.W
Washington, DC 20250

SOLUTIONS GMOS

PROTECT YOURSELF AND YOUR FAMILY

GMOs and Bioengineered foods contain pesticide residues and unnatural proteins. To reduce your risk of Cancer, the National Institutes of Health recommends, "Avoid Contact with pesticides." Source: *Cancer and the Environment, What You Need to Know.*[267]

- Limit how many foods and beverages made from GMOs you eat.
- Source rBGH-free dairy products, and milk and meat from animals not fed GMOs
- Free your kitchen, yourself and your family from GMO foods.
- Beware: many grains and other crops are sprayed with glyphosate before harvest
- Support your immune system with nontoxic foods that are rich in nutrients.
- Eat organic green vegetables, chlorella, and yogurt to help rebalance your gut flora
- Supplement with good quality minerals, vitamins and omega oils
- We must help kids: let's get factory farmed milk out of public schools
- Choose Organic Alfalfa for your animals
- Provide full disclosure to Farmers. Synthetic fertilizer and pesticide companies need to provide warnings to farmers and landscapers so they're aware of the harmful nature of these substances. Don't we all deserve the chance to make informed decisions?

GMO Labeling:[268] Some foods derived from GMO plants will still not be labeled, for instance high fructose corn syrup and GMO soybean oil. See page 107 for more info.

GMOs Banned[269]**:** Bulgaria, Croatia, Switzerland, Georgia, Germany, Austria, Greece, Hungary, Italy, Luxembourg, Norway, Poland, Romania, Russia, Scotland, Serbia, Slovenia, New Zealand, Wales

Glyphosate Bans: Argentina, Australia, Belgium, Bermuda, Brazil, Canada, Colombia, Czech Republic, Denmark, El Salvador, England, El Salvador, France (by 2020), Germany, Greece, Italy, India, Luxemburg, Malta, Netherlands, New Zealand, Portugal, Russia, Scotland, Spain, Sri Lanka, Sweden, Switzerland

Countries with partial bans or working toward banning: Albania, Australia, England, Estonia, Finland, France, Ireland, Japan, Latvia, Mexico, Portugal, Spain, Sweden

Glufosinate: Everyone by now may be familiar with glyphosate, but have heard of Glufosinate?[270] It can be used where glyphosate is banned. Research suggests glufosinate does not breakdown in GMO foods and rather regains its pesticidal powers in the 'digestive tract of warm-blooded animals.[271] Due to that and it's threat of reproductive harm, glufosinate is banned in France and under review by the European Parliament.[272]

Meanwhile, in the U.S. GMO crops continue to be planted & ingredients continue infiltrating our foods. In light of the recent revelations regarding Roundup's carcinogen status, if you care to protect your health you may wish to avoid this substance and others like it.

3. POLLINATORS

BEES, BIRDS, BATS in Danger

The food supply depends on Bees and Pollinators—they are essential for producing most of the foods we love to eat. These little creatures are the food makers, pollinating the plants and bringing us all the delicious foods we love. Pollinators include: Bees, Bats, Butterflies, Birds, Beetles, Moths, Pollen Wasps, and even some varieties of flies. These wondrous animals do their work generously and by instinct; work that no man can do. In return for their selfless service, we receive unlimited fruits and vegetables and bounties of food for harvest. Yet today, the survival of the bees and pollinators is uncertain.

The soaring use of pesticides on the very foods they pollinate has made pollinators the casualties of the front line. Unlike any other time in history, bees, birds and bats are dying in record numbers. This is directly related to modern chemicals used in farming. Bees are succumbing to colony collapse disorder, bats are dying off from white nose fungus, and monarch butterfly numbers are dwindling due to loss of the milkweed plant they so vitally depend on during migration. Bats are one of nature's best pest control critters, gobbling up mosquitoes and crop damaging insects. For their pest control skills alone, unless bats are saved North America could experience agricultural losses up to 53 billion/year.[273] As far as bees go, the loss would be insurmountable. "Seventy out of the top 100 human food crops, which supply about 90 percent of the world's nutrition are pollinated by bees."[274]

We truly are in the midst of a crisis. Disease, habitat loss, parasites, fungicides, wind turbines, and exposure to pesticides are all threatening pollinators. Of them all, however pesticides may be the ultimate trigger raising the risk and likelihood of disease. The numbers speak for themselves: US beekeepers lost 40% of their hives last year[275], and nearly 7 million bats have been lost since 2006.[276] Pesticides are lethal to non-targeted species, especially when exposure includes not just one but multiple pesticides. Greenpeace reports that bee pollen can contain as many as 150 different chemical residues.[277] The most dangerous pesticides for bees appear to be neonicotinoids; when combined with fungicides, neonicotinoids kill bees even more swiftly. Equally troubling is that the bees bring the toxins back to their hives where it has multiple effect—One is that more bees get effected; secondly the hive's community instinct to clean out dead and sick bees fades allowing conditions like brood to fester; and lastly in these conditions the director of the hive, the queen bee, is more likely to leave or die leaving a hive without the ability to reproduce.[278] Birds are affected as well. "Forty percent of the world's bird populations are in decline. Agriculture has the biggest impact of all human activities on birds, threatening 74 percent of the 1,469 species at risk of extinction."[279]

WITHOUT BEES WE'LL LOSE: Apples, Avocadoes, Almonds, Alfalfa, Blueberries, Cherries, Apricots, Raspberries, Strawberries, Grapes, Coffee, Coconut, Chocolate, Watermelon, Lemons, Limes, Oranges, Peanuts, Lentils, Legumes, Olives, Onions, Broccoli, Grapefruit, Watermelon, Melons, Carrots, Kiwi, Cucumbers, Cranberries, Celery, Cauliflower,

Macadamia Nuts, Peaches, Sunflowers, Tangerines, Pumpkins, Squash, Peas, Cotton, Soybeans, Beets, Tea, Figs, Vanilla and all the foods and drinks made with these wonderful magical foods like chocolate and wine. Without bees, crop yields can be reduced by more than 90%.[280]

WITHOUT BATS WE'LL LOSE: "Over 300 species of fruit depend on bats for pollination including mangoes, bananas, guavas as well agave, the source for tequila."[281]

WITHOUT BIRDS WE'LL LOSE: Wildflowers, biodiversity, balance in ecosystems, birds help pollinate many plants,[282] without birds, insects will become more obnoxious. [283]

NEONICOTINOIDS: Like other pesticides and toxic chemicals neonicotinoids are allowed to be used widely today despite their danger. Two new studies completed in 2017 confirm that neonicotinoids do in fact harm and kill bees. Exposure results in "decreased survival and immune response, especially when co-exposed to a commonly used agrochemical fungicide." Further, exposure "reduces overwintering success and colony reproduction."[284] As described below*, this dangerous class of pesticides are known neurotoxins that interfere with brain function and harm the nervous system.

HEALTH EFFECTS: "Neonicotinoid toxicity affects the thalamus gland and "has been found to play a role in several central nervous system disorders, including Alzheimer's disease, Parkinson's disease, schizophrenia, and depression. In the developing brain, this subtype is involved in neural proliferation, apoptosis, migration, differentiation, synapse formation, and neural circuit formation. Other studies have found adverse reproductive as well as developmental effects in mammals including reduced sperm production and function, reduced pregnancy rates, higher rates of embryo death, stillbirth, and premature birth, and reduced weight of offspring...."[285]

COLONY COLLAPSE ORDER

"Neonicotinoids act on insect nervous systems. They accumulate in individual bees and within entire colonies, including the honey that bees feed to infant larvae. Bees that do not die outright, experience sub-lethal systemic effects, development defects, weakness, and loss of orientation. The die-off leaves fewer bees and weaker bees, who must work harder to produce honey in depleted wild habitats. These conditions create the nightmare formula for bee colony collapse." www.greenpeace.org

GLYPHOSATE

Researchers studying bees report of fatalities related to glyphosate exposure. "Exposing bees to glyphosate alters the bee gut community and increases susceptibility to infection by opportunistic pathogens. Glyphosate exposure of young workers increased mortality of bees."[286] If glyphosate disturbs the natural balance of their gut bacteria so much as to weaken their immune systems, how many more animals are affected and vulnerable to infection after exposure to the world's most common glyphosate product?

In addition to messing with our gut bacteria, glyphosate disturbs soil health and chelates minerals, which undoubtedly trigger yet more troubles. Dr. Don Huber, explained in his letter to the USDA, "glyphosate promotes soil pathogens and is implicated with the increase of more than 40 plant diseases; it dismantles plant defenses by chelating vital nutrients; and it reduces the bioavailability of nutrients in feed, which in turn can cause animal disorders."[287]

FUNGICIDE THREAT

Though long assumed to be harmless to insects, fungicides are now known to be dangerous to bees and other nontargeted species, including people. Big surprise! Fungicides are endocrine disruptors, neurotoxins, and reproductive toxins. Beyond Pesticides reports, "Hazardous fungicides thiram, ziram and ferbam are teratogens, neuro, reproductive and thyroid toxins, mutagens, and skin sensitizers. These fungicides are used on food crops (strawberries, apples, and peaches) and for seed treatment. Prolonged occupational exposure to thiram increased the incidence of hypertension & diseases of the heart, liver, thyroid and gastrointestinal tract. Ziram causes thyroid cancer in rats and lung and lymph gland cancer in mice."[288]Regarding bees, researchers discovered fungicides interfere with their ability to metabolize and detoxify insecticides thus impacting their energy.[289] Furthermore, fungicides are now found throughout bee pollen samples, and are a suspect in weakening bees to die from nosema fungus.[290] Coincidentally, many species of bats are dying from white nose fungus. Is it the exposure to fungicides that's ultimately weakening bees' and bats' immune systems? What might these substances be doing to us? More troubling news, researchers have found that bees actually are attracted to food tainted with fungicides, [291]which may be why more is found in hives. Exposure to one of these chemicals causes enough trouble, yet pollinators and people are exposed to many of them simultaneously when we're eating. How does this mixture of toxins affect our health?

GMO ALFALFA: In 2014, alfalfa became the first perennial plant approved for GMO.

- Alfalfa is one of the most important crops in the world and it's pollinated by bees[292]
- Cross contamination will occur. Once nongmo crops are affected it's impossible to reverse.
- Most US Honey is derived from alfalfa pollen
- The USDA Animal and Plant Health Inspection Service did not analyze the effect of RR alfalfa on animals and plants before approving of this GMO.[293]
- How might this alfalfa harm animals, cows, horses? Certainly, it can't be good for Bees!

BYE BYE BUTTERFLIES?

Yet more bad news for pollinators-- glyphosate threatens the survival of the monarch butterfly. This is largely because these butterflies rely on milkweed, yet milkweed habitat is vanishing. As caterpillars, monarchs rely exclusively on the milkweed. As GMO fields of corn and soy spread throughout the Midwest, the use of glyphosate has caused milkweed to disappear. Similarly the monarch population has experienced a steep decline. Researches identified both monarch and milkweed losses to run congruent with the increase of glyphosate use between the years of 1996 and 2011. "Glyphosate use on soybeans went from 1.4 million kg in 1994 to 41.7 million kg in 2006; on corn from 1.8 million kg in 2000 to 28.5 million kg in 2010."[294]

Butterflies have existed for 200 million years, they're members of the ecosystem of Earth, plants need them. To think that man's use of chemicals within just the last 30 years could be responsible for making them vanish forever is quite disturbing. What else is at risk of extinction from our use of this chemical? As with all plants and species, losing one forever affects the balance of the planet and can be a striking loss for our own health as well.

SOLUTIONS POLLINATORS

Help the Pollinators & Protect Your Health

Clearly the combination of pesticides, fungicides, and herbicides increases stress on bees and pollinators. Without pollinators pollinating, the availability of food will shift, prices will rise, malnutrition, hunger, and incidences of disease could increase. This is a scenario that will not benefit people or the planet and all its precious ecosystems. As much as possible, do not use pesticides, herbicides or fungicides in your garden or on your lawn.

- Avoid neonics & fungicides by purchasing organic, biodynamic grown foods
- Support local food and farmers markets, foods grown with sustainable methods.

In Your Home and Yard:

1. Use Natural Alternatives to Pesticides: food-grade Diatomaceous earth, ladybugs, companion planting methods. Make your own nontoxic pesticide recipes, see next page!
2. To get rid of weeds consider old fashioned weeding.
3. When purchasing flowers and plants source those that are pollinator friendly
4. If you hire a landscaping company, make sure they use bee-friendly methods
5. Plant your own organic garden. Get ideas and information at www.slowfood.com.

Create a Haven for Pollinators in your Backyard:

- Plant a wide variety of plants native to your region that bloom from early spring to fall. Bees especially need dandelions and butterflies depend on milkweed to survive.
- Avoid modern hybrid plants that don't offer pollen, nectar or fragrance
- Eliminate pesticides as much as possible. If you must please use the least toxic that are pollinator friendly. Only apply in the evening when bees & other pollinators aren't active.[295]
- Protect Birds from Pesticide Poisoning: "Approximately 40 pesticides used in the US are known to be highly toxic to birds. The primary culprits are the organophosphates, carbamate, and organochlorine insecticides."[296]

Help Create Pollinator Protection Laws: Write your Reps and Senators asking that they cosponsor the Pollinator Protection Act of 2019. See what cities and States are leading the way to protecting bees at www.beecityusa.org. Moving forward we can help by demanding the EPA, FDA and USDA do their job and instill better prevention and protective measures for all of us—including honest in-depth safety studies on these chemicals before they're put into market. We cannot simply rely solely on the manufacturer's assurance of safety for approval. Tougher standards can ultimately result in a drastic reduction of disease for both humans & animals.

Help Pollinators and Animals in Wildlife Refuges

In August 2018 the Trump Administration repealed the ban on neonicotinoids and GMOs in U.S. Wildlife Refuges! If even in wild places bees and animals can't be safe from our chemical toxins, what kind of country have we created? **How to Help:** Please urge Congress and Fish and Wildlife Services to reinstate the ban on neonicotinoids and GMOs in U.S wildlife refuges

SOLUTIONS DIY PESTICIDES

PROTECT YOURSELF, YOUR FAMILY & YOUR PETS & POLLINATORS

Fungal Spray

If you notice plants developing fungus or mold, get some baking soda.
Mix 2 Tbsp Baking Soda with 1Gallon Water. Pour into spray container and spray plants where and when needed. Repeat for a few days until resolved.

Safe alternative For Weeding:
Spray white vinegar directly on leaves, or dilute borax with water and spray.

Natural Pesticide Spray:

Mix 1/2 cup white vinegar, 3 Tablespoons food grade diatomaceous earth, ½ cup water, 6 drops each essential oils of orange, lemon, lavender, and peppermint. Add to a spray bottle and spray where needed.

Neem Oil, Mild Insect Spray (Flea Eradicator too)

Neem oil spray
Mix 2 Tbsp Neem oil, dash of mild dish soap with 1quart water
Put in spray bottle and use on plants as needed. Store in refrigerator.

Diatomaceous Earth (Food Grade Quality), natural insecticide

Must use Food Grade quality, very important!
Sprinkle this freely in your garden, it will not hurt your pets or plants.
Sprinkle it around doorways to keep ants out. Works most effectively when dry.
Gets fleas out of your house too, combine with lavender oil and consistent vacuuming.

Rodale's Cayenne Pepper Recipe

Be careful, ingredients can cause sensitivity. Avoid contact with eyes, wash hands when done.
Ingredients:
1 garlic bulb, 1 small onion, 1 teaspoon of powdered cayenne pepper
1 quart of water, 1 tablespoon liquid dish soap
Chop, grind, or liquefy garlic and onion. Add cayenne pepper and mix with water. Steep 1 hour, strain through cheesecloth, then add liquid dish soap. Mix well. Spray your plants thoroughly, including the undersides of the leaves. Store the mixture for up to a week in a labeled, covered container in the refrigerator.[297]

PREVENT POISONING OF WILDLIFE. As senseless and inhumane as it sounds some pesticides have been used by herders and poachers in Africa to kill lions and elephants and other animals. The pesticides are cheap and easily available. One type, Carbofuran was banned in America in 2009 yet still exported to other countries. They sprinkle the odorless substance on dead carcasses that the lions feed upon causing them to die painfully soon after."[298] When we've banned a substance, how can we allow it to still be manufactured and sold to other nations?

4. GMO ALFALFA

"A thing is right when it tends to preserve the integrity, stability, and beauty of the biotic community. It is wrong when it tends otherwise."[299] Aldo Leopold

Alfalfa, in Arabic means the father of all foods. It has long been of tremendous importance to the food chain and to pollinators. In 2014 alfalfa became the first perennial approved for GMO. Real alfalfa is now at risk of contamination from Roundup Ready Alfalfa.
From the report, *Alfalfa, Wildlife and the Environment*[300]

- "Alfalfa is one of the earliest crops domesticated by man and has a long rich history.
- There are about 23 million acres of alfalfa in the US. Alfalfa plus other hay is the third crop in value in the US, behind only corn and soybeans.
- It is worth more than $8 billion annually.
- Alfalfa is a source of incredible insect diversity, which includes many valuable 'beneficial' insects. These, in turn help control many types of insect and mites in alfalfa & other crops.
- Providing Significant Wildlife Habitat: Alfalfa is the beginning of a food chain, and contributes valuable habitat for hundreds of species of herbivores and animals of prey. It hosts several endangered species, plus many familiar ones. Those who love nature should appreciate alfalfa's support of many wildlife species.
- Alfalfa affects many industries from dairying to wool and beef production and horseracing. The many end-uses, such as cheese making and pizza marketing are worth billions of dollars more than the value of the crop itself; they begin with alfalfa
- Protecting the Soil: The deeprooted characteristics of alfalfa and vigorous year-round canopy help protect the soil from becoming airborne and causing dusty conditions, or being washed into rivers as sediment
- Nitrogen Benefits: The biological N2 fixation by bacteria growing on alfalfa roots helps save energy – no N fertilizers are needed! In addition, alfalfa leaves behind nitrogen and improves soil structure for the crop that follows so farmers can apply less fertilizer.
- Alfalfa has tremendous genetic resistance to many pests, a result of traditional plant breeding. Consequently, alfalfa does not need a large amount of pesticides each year compared with other crops."

The plant was perfect, what trait did scientists need to alter? Alfalfa pollen is the source of most U.S. honey (see page 43). We know the pesticides harm bees and pollinators, and the GMO monocropping methods destroy habitats and ecosystems. To what extent will growing this new plant harm animals we do not yet know. If we lose bees, will we lose alfalfa? If we lose alfalfa, what effect will that have on horses and cows, on all the animals that depend on this vital plant?

"A land ethic, then, reflects the existence of an ecological conscience, and this in turn reflects a conviction of individual responsibility for the health of the land. Health is the capacity of the land for self-renewal. Conservation is our effort to understand and preserve this capacity."[301]
Aldo Leopold, *Sand County Almanac*

5. FACTORY FARMS

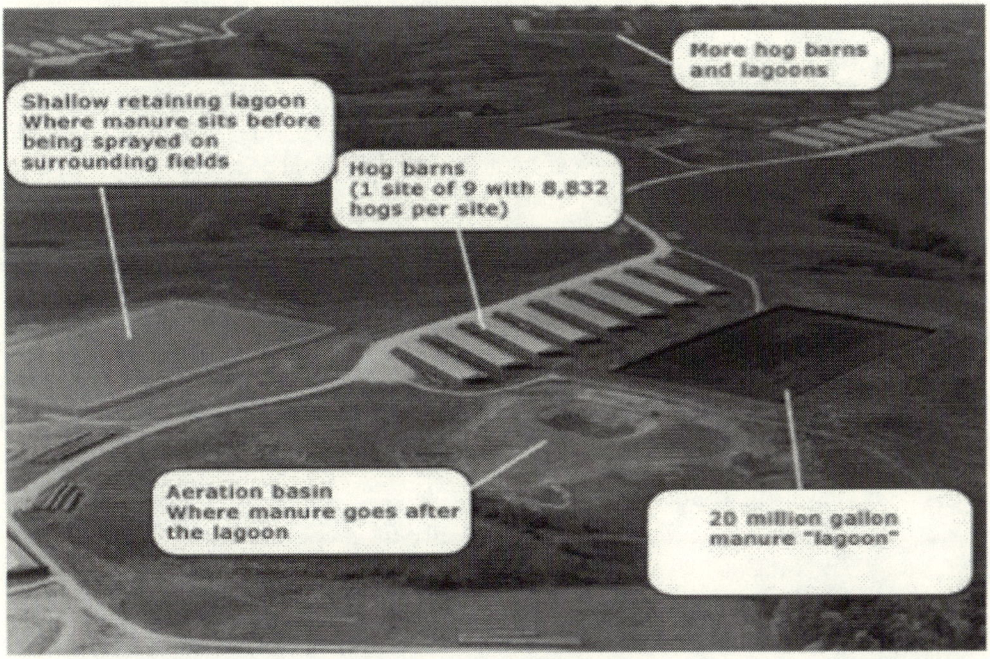
More hog barns
and lagoons
Shallow retaining lagoon
Where manure sits before
being sprayed on
surrounding fields
Hog barns
(1 site of 9 with 8,832
hogs per site)
Aeration basin
Where manure goes after
the lagoon
20 million gallon
manure "lagoon"

Photo courtesy of Grace Factory Farm Project

Thousands of Confined Animal Feeding Operations (CAFOs), otherwise known as factory farms exist in the United States. The majority of farm animals are housed at these farms, which are synonymous with maltreatment of animals and drug culture, as well as unregulated sewage, air and water pollution, antibiotic resistance, and a lingering methane problem. Meat, dairy, and eggs from these farms can impact us in not-so-savory ways when we partake of such foods.

The Center for Food Safety reports, "Animal Agriculture uses over 450 animal drugs, drug combinations, and other feed additives to promote animal growth and to suppress the negative effects that heavily-concentrated confinement has on farm animals. Food animal producers regularly use these drugs for reasons that have nothing to do with medical necessity or animal health—but solely to increase profit."[302] How might these drugs used to promote growth and suppress animal feelings affect human behavior when we consume products derived from these animals? If these drugs cause changes in animals, can they not do the same in us--affecting our mood, suppressing feelings, causing depression, causing weight gain?

FACTORY FARM FACTS

- Over 95% of all farm animals in the US are raised on factory farms.[303]
- In the US there's nearly 10 billion farm animals raised each year in confined animal farms.[304] In 2012, genetically engineered (GE) crops were grown by 17.3 million farmers on over 170 million hectares. Over 70% of harvested GE biomass is fed to foodproducing animals, making them the major consumers of GE crops for the past 15 plus years.[305]

"Factory farms can create health hazards because they are over-crowded and stressful to animals, making it easy for disease to spread. When thousands of beef cattle are packed into feedlots full of manure, bacteria can get on their hides and into slaughterhouses.[306] It only takes one animals to contaminate thousands of pounds of meat inside a slaughterhouse.

These farms have taken the humanity out of animal rearing and created an industry only concerned with quantity of product. Considering all these factors, one might ask how could products from animals raised this way be something we want to eat? Sadly, Europe, Asia and the UK have all adopted the industrial Factory Farm model as a sensible way to raise animals. The Guardian reports, "Nearly every county in England has at least one industrial-scale livestock farm, with close to 800 US-style mega farms operating across the UK."[307]

ANTIBIOTIC RESISTANCE: Most food borne diseases originate at factory farms. Due to crowded confined unsanitary conditions, diseases like E. coli, salmonella and campylobacter are more common in products from factory farms. As the Chicago Tribune reported, "The relatively rapid consolidation of U.S. meat, poultry, egg and dairy production and processing greatly increases the potential for these "problems to spread fast and wide throughout the food system."[308]Graphic Source: CDC.gov[309]

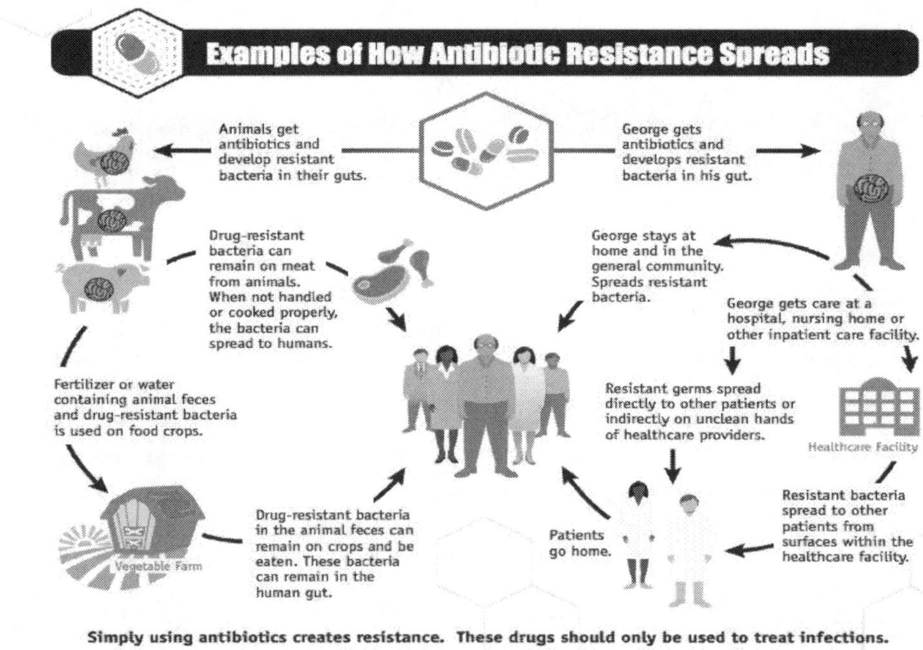

The food-producing animal and poultry industries have undergone a dramatic change that began around 1950.[310] The Centers for Disease Control (CDC) report, *Antibiotic Resistance Threats* cites factory farms as using more antibiotics on animals than are used on people. "Antibiotics are also commonly used in food animals to prevent, control, and treat disease, and to promote the growth of food-producing animals. The use of antibiotics for promoting growth is not necessary, and the practice should be phased out. It is difficult to directly compare the amount of drugs used in food animals with the amount used in humans, but there is evidence that more antibiotics are used in food production."[311] The report further estimates 2 million people a year are infected yearly with food-borne diseases, of which at least 23,000 die annually costing $20 billion in healthcare costs and an additional $35 billion in lost productivity. The people most at risk are those undergoing chemotherapy or complex surgery, those with rheumatoid arthritis or undergoing dialysis, as well as those having organ or bone marrow transplants. Clearly we have a dangerous situation on our hands. The only solution is to seriously reduce the amounts of antibiotics and drugs used on animals.

SEWAGE & POLLUTION

Factory farms produce a staggering amount of sewage waste that's neither treated nor controlled. The waste is contained onsite and outside in stinky, uncovered cess pools. These lagoons emit toxic gases, seep & leak into the ground as well as nearby streams and waterways. The raw manure waste is often applied to farm fields as fertilizer where it can pose additional contamination threats.

If a CAFO is large enough it's supposed to be subject to the Clean Water Act, however this is often neglected. Currently in 2019 there's a battle raging in Iowa. As reported by Food and Water Watch, "Despite over 10,000 factory farms and almost no Clean Water Act regulation, EPA denies petition to withdraw Iowa's pollution program. EPA's petition denial is a whitewashing of Iowa's ongoing failure to regulate factory farms."[312] Despite the ongoing travesty caused by mismanagement, factory farms are even exempt from reporting air contaminants![313]

While we wait for environmental safeguards and regulations to be put in place by an EPA that's short on mindful leadership, these farms under current USDA policy, receive millions of dollars in subsidies.[314] Perhaps that money needs to be earmarked for solving the pollution dilemma. The manure waste poses a great risk to people nearby, even moreso during violent storms. Between the EPA, FDA, USDA and the large corporations who own these harms, they must figure out a better solution for the waste. One idea that could work depends upon them stopping use of antibiotics and hormones as well as investing in better facilities and housing for the animals to prevent illness in the first place. Then instead of pumping the waste to lagoons, or dangerously using raw waste as fertilizer, they could properly compost the animal waste to be resold as legitimate fertilizer—much like the famous "Indore" compost methods of India. This act of return could revitalize our lands, lessen water filtration infrastructure and expense, and actually help make food more nutritious.

ANIMAL WELFARE: Between the crowded conditions and the drug therapy, the suffering endured by these animals is cruel and inhumane. No animal deserves to be so mistreated—locked up in small cages, withheld forever from the outdoors, sunshine and exercise, forced to endure daily administration of antibiotics and growth-enhancing drugs and hormones. Their feed is not from green pasture, but derived from GMO corn and soy, which comes with a whole lot of baggage. Additionally, reports have shown these herbaceous eating animals are often forced to eat the remains of other animals. These animals only experience pain and suffering.

Even when they're transported for slaughter, carriers have up to 28 hours before they have to supply food or water for the animals. Eating meat and eggs from factory farms exposes us to everything the animals were forced to endure. This includes:

- Synthetic growth hormones and steroids
- GMO feed containing GMO corn, GMO soy and pesticide residues
- Drugs, antibiotics, illness and infections and depressing conditions

These animals should be protected under The Animal Welfare Act. The AWA was signed into law in 1966. It is the only Federal law that regulates the treatment of animals in research, exhibition, transport and by dealers. Other laws, policies, and guidelines may include additional species coverage or specifications for animal care and use, but all refer to the Animal Welfare Act as the minimum acceptable standard. The law is enforced by the USDA.[315]

CHICKENS, POULTRY, EGGS and PIGS

Chicken, hens, roosters, turkeys and pigs don't fare well at CAFOs. They're subjected to steroid and antibiotic injections. Chickens painfully get their beaks cut off[316] to prevent injury in their cramped cages, then they're injected with arsenic-laced antibiotics. Being so crowded together, disease is common. The CDC testified in court that overzealous antibiotic injections leads to antibiotic resistance.[317] Even before birth, chicks are injected while still in their shell.[318] Some egg companies claim to treat their chickens well and even claim to be the best, but don't believe it. Unless they're steroid and drug-free and fed real food, you know they're from factory farms.

Pigs and poultry can be subjected to injections of ractopamine, a muscle-enhancing drug that's banned in most of the world. The drug results in muscle gain and reduced appetite. This adds up to a bigger profit for the corporations, for they save on feed and the animals weigh more when they go to slaughter. Cha ching! U.S. meat products containing ractopamine are banned in over 160 countries. Beef and pork contaminated with this drug, a β-agonists can be a risk for people with heart conditions. As the Centre for Food Safety in Hong Kong points out, "Inappropriate usage of β-agonists may leave residues in edible tissues that are of health concern for consumers. For instance, acute poisoning can occur in humans as a result of consumption of meat or offal which contains high levels of clenbuterol. As clenbuterol is heat stable in edible tissues, ordinary home cooking methods such as boiling, roasting, frying and microwaving cannot eliminate its residues. The symptoms of clenbuterol poisoning are rapid heartbeats, dizziness, headache, nervousness, tremor and blood pressure changes. People with heart disease and blood pressure disorder are more likely to be affected."[319] Be careful you source meat that doesn't contain it.

CATTLE, HORMONES & IGF-1: Cows too are mistreated at factory farms. Steroid implants are inserted into cattle intended for beef while dairy cows are subjected to injections of recombinant bovine growth hormone. This rBGH is a genetically engineered hormone that results in mastitis and frequent udder infections for the animals and milk that increases our levels of IGF (insulin like growth factor). It's bad enough that the poor cows are on an endless cycle of antibiotics, which sure enough results in milk with residues, but what does this GMO milk do to us when we consume it? In his book, *What's In Your Milk,* (page 39) Dr. Samuel Epstein revealed, "Levels of insulin-like growth factor-1 (IGF-1) are substantially elevated and more bioactive in the milk of cows hyperstimulated with the biosynthetic bovine growth hormones rBGH.

Converging lines of evidence incriminate IGF-1 in rBGH milk as a potential risk factor for both breast and gastrointestinal cancers."[320]

As more Americans wake up to the danger of rBGH, some big coffee chains are moving away from it, yet their milk is still sourced from farms where cows are confined. rBGH free is good, but not good enough. I'd prefer milk from cows that have access to pasture and real food, not GMO feed. The nutritional quality of milk afterall depends quite possibly and exclusively on how the animals are raised. Cows provided pasture and allowed to graze naturally from fields where natural fertilizers and compost are applied produce milk of superior quality compared to milk from cows imprisoned and fed lifeless GMO food. This type of milk can provide more iron and iodine than milk from cows fed substandard grains, a difference stemming from the food provided to the cows and how that food was grown[321] (see pages 62, 65-66). Omega oils are in better balance in organic milk too! As reported by NBC news, "the reason organic milk is healthier comes down to its ratio of omega-6 to omega-3 fatty acids, which is lower than regular milk. A diet containing too many omega-6 fatty acids and not enough omega-3s has been linked to heart disease, cancer, inflammation & autoimmune diseases."[322]

Before you run out and buy organic milk, you must realize not all organic farms are created equal. The small farms and organic coops that have been producing organic milk and food for ages can be trusted, unless they were bought out by a mega corporation trying to get a piece of the organic bandwagon. There's a whole new breed of colossal mega farms creeping up that claim organic status, yet a lot of these are using monocropping methods and may not be giving their animals very much pasture time. Some of these newer farms are still very much like factory farms confining up to 15,000 cattle at a single farm and providing very little organicness.[323] As in all things, do your research and see if they're really legit or just posers.

FACTORY FARM MEAT and CANCER[324]

The hormones in factory farm meat can cause cancer. According to the late Dr. Samuel Epstein from the University of Illinois at Chicago School of Public Health and creator of the Prevent Cancer Coalition, "Beef produced in the United States is heavily contaminated with natural or synthetic sex hormones, which are associated with an increased risk of reproductive and childhood cancers. Increased levels of sex hormones are linked to the escalating incidence of reproductive cancers in the United States since 1975 - 60 percent for prostate, 59 percent for testis, and 10 percent for breast, warns the Cancer Prevention Coalition.

"The hormones in past and current use include the natural estrogen, progesterone and testosterone, and the synthetic zeranol, trenbolone, and melengesterol. When beef cattle enter feedlots, pellets of these hormones are implanted under the ear skin, a process that is repeated at the midpoint of their 100-day pre-slaughter fattening period. These hormones increase carcass weight, adding over $80 in extra profit per animal. The Cancer Prevention Coalition warned that, "Not surprisingly, but contrary to longstanding claims by the U.S. Food and Drug Administration (FDA) and the U.S. Department of Agriculture (USDA), residues of these hormones in meat are up to 20-fold higher than normal. Still higher residues result from the not uncommon illegal practice of implantation directly into muscle. Furthermore, contrary to misleading assurances, meat is still not monitored for hormone residues." Nevertheless, the FDA and USDA still maintain that hormone residues in meat are within "normal levels," while waiving any requirements for residue testing.

Following a single ear implant in steers of Synovex-S, a combination of estrogen and progesterone, residues of these hormones in meat were found to be up to 20-fold higher than normal. The amount of estradiol in two hamburgers eaten in one day by an 8-year-old boy could increase his total hormone levels by as much as 10%, particularly as young children have very low natural hormone levels. Not surprisingly, the incidence of childhood cancer has increased by 38 percent since 1975. It is well recognized that American women have a greater risk of breast cancer than women in countries that do not permit the sale of hormonal beef."

FARM RAISED FISH: Like the land-based factory farms, farmed fish are contained in cages, and believe it or not, fed GMO feed. They are living so close together that they're more prone to infection and parasites, often loaded up with antibiotics. Farmed fish contain on average 10 times higher levels of PCBs[325] and more persistent organic pollutants (POPs) than wild fish. Due to their GMO diet, they contain less omega oils and higher saturated fat than wild species. GMO salmon is the first animal that's been genetically modified. Approved in Canada in 2017, these fish continually exert a growth hormone that allows them to grow up to twice as fast, as well as weigh twice as much than normal salmon, yet they eat 25% less.[326] If growth hormones make animals heavier, it's not hard to guess what happens to us when we eat them. Again, it's all about quantity, *not* quality with these producers. Sustainable fish farms do exist, choose wisely.

WHERE'S YOUR MEAT FROM & WHO'S INSPECTING IT?

Since country of origin labeling (COOL) was revoked for meat products in 2015, we have no way of knowing where meat originated. This is very troubling, for Ecowatch warns that drug residues in meats could become far worse than we've seen yet. As they report, "in exchange for China agreeing to accept U.S. beef after a long hiatus, the U.S. agreed to import cooked chickens from China. China's food safety record is abysmal, including rat meat sold as lamb and frequent bird flu epidemics." Secondly under the Trump administration, meat inspectors are being phased out in favor of the honor code, USDA's New Poultry Inspection Service."[327]

Right now, inspectors are checking 2 birds PER Second, but the National Chicken Council is trying to make them go even faster![328] Without sufficient time, what good is an inspection? If meat isn't inspected properly, how do we know if the meat is safe? If the meat isn't labeled how do we know where it's from? We already have a dire situation with antibiotic resistance and contaminated meat. These factors ultimately can impact our health. Do we want to take that risk with our family's health?

Information allows us to make informed decisions. As reported by PRI, since the withdrawal of honest meat labeling, "Consumers could no longer differentiate meat that came from animals that were raised in the US from those that were imported. One reason is a loophole that allows beef and pork from outside the country to carry a "Product of the USA" label if it has been processed here."[329] These are truly tragic developments. We must insist on ethics and honesty in meat inspections, and reinstate COOL labeling so we can make informed choices for our health.

CODE RED CLIMATE CRISIS

Animal factory farms push all the climate change buttons and cause significant health problems. Here's some facts from the Food and Agricultural Organization of the United Nations (FAO), the Humane Society, and from the University of Iowa School of Public Health.

Manure and Waste at Factory Farms Emit Significant Air Pollution:

- **Methane** (CH4): 37% of emissions of methane, more than 20 times the GWP (Global Warming Potential) of Carbon Dioxide (CO2)
- **Carbon Dioxide** (CO2) emissions (Source FAO, Livestock's Long Shadow):
    - o Gmo feed requiring vast amounts of synthetic fertilizer. Producing fertilizer for feed crops emits nearly 41 million tons of CO2 around the world each year.[330]
    - o Giant facilities need to vent, cool, heat facilities, operate machinery to grow feed crops amounts to 90 million tons of CO2 globally.
    - o Transporting, processing and slaughtering, packaging animals produces "tens of millions of tonnes" of CO2 annually.
    - o Deforestation and clearing land for pasture, grazing and growing feed crops eliminates carbon sinks and produces 2.4billion tons of CO2 yearly worldwide.
    - o Working the crops and land creates 28 million tons of CO2
    - o Over grazing exhausts the land and provokes erosion. This may apply moreso to ranchers, but it emits close to 100 million tons of CO2 yearly.[331]
- **Hydrogen Sulfide** (H2S): Levels as high as 1,000 ppm have been reported following the perturbation of manure lagoons, and levels greater than 100 ppm are considered immediately hazardous to life and health. Exposure to these elevated levels of H2S can cause rapid loss of consciousness, H2S has been implicated in a number of deaths when encountered in confined environments in agricultural settings.[332]
- **Ammonia** (NH3): animal agricultural operations are responsible for almost three fourths of ammonia air pollution in the United States that can lead to pulmonary disease, scarring of upper and lower airways, lung inflammation, high concentrations can be fatal.[333]
- **Nitrous Oxide (N2O)**: 65% of nitrous oxide emissions worldwide are produced by animal farm operations, this number includes emissions from producing feed crops. N20 is 300 times the GWP of CO2 & it can last in the atmosphere for 150 years.[334] Global farm animal production, including growing feed crops, accounts for 65% of global N2O emissions."[335]

METHANE: While we often hear of methane emissions from cows at factory farms, let's explore a little more. The methane results from the manure lagoons as well as when the cows are digesting food. The majority of GMOs grown in America, particularly GMO corn and soy are provided as feed for the factory farm animals. The farm animals—cows, sheep, goat, buffalo, camels are known as Ruminants. "They have a compartment in their stomach called a rumen where food is broken down through fermentation. This process produces methane gas, which the animals belch out. Enteric fermentation accounts for 18 percent of all anthropogenic methane emissions."[336] Apparently though, the harder food is to digest, the longer it stays in the rumen, and hence more methane is produced. There's evidence that GMO soy is harder to digest[337] than traditional soy. If this is the case, then GMO feed could be contributing to increased methane. "Between 1990 and 2006, methane emissions from pig and dairy cow manure in the United States increased by 34% and 49%, respectively. This increase, according to the U.S. Environmental Protection Agency, is a result of the shift toward confining pigs and cows in larger facilities using liquid manure management systems."[338]

FACTORY FARM HEALTH AND CLIMATE PROBLEMS[339]

MANURE	OVER 300 MILLION TONS,
HYDROGEN SULFIDE	ACID RAIN, SMOG
AMMONIA	RESPIRATORY PROBLEMS,
PARTICULATE POLLUTION	ASTHMA, HEART ATTACKS
VOCs Volatile Organic Pollutants	HEADACHES, NAUSEA, RISK OF CANCER
METHANE	CLIMATE CHANGE
NITROUS OXIDE	CLIMATE CHANGE
CARBON DIOXIDE	CLIMATE CHANGE

HEALTH EFFECTS PEOPLE

- headaches and depression, brain damage[340]
- shortness of breath, wheezing, diarrhea, coughing, sore throats,
- seizures and miscarriages, blue baby syndrome.
- cancer, childhood cancers, reproductive cancers
- high blood pressure, heart problems
- antibiotic resistance, chronic illness
- early puberty, depression

HEALTH EFFECTS ANIMALS

- infections and disease, antibiotic resistance
- depression, anxiety,
- pain, sickness
- vitamin and mineral deficiencies

HEALTH EFFECTS PLANET

- air pollution, acid rain, smog, ammonia pollution, climate change
- toxic runoff, water pollution, nitrate in water,
- antibiotic resistance, harm and cruelty to animals

***METHANE CAPTURE:** Some farms are finally taking action and converting methane for use. Biogas digesters capture methane and convert it to electricity! "Farm digesters are big tanks that contain manure and other waste from barns that house livestock such as cows and pigs."[341] As Farm Journal's MILK magazine reports, in 2018 "Land O'Lakes, Inc. (LOL) and California Bioenergy LLC (CalBio) launched a first of its kind collaboration this summer to finance, build, operate and manage methane digesters on California dairy farms. The project is designed to capture methane from cow manure using on-farm digesters and then compress it into a natural gas pipeline where it can be used by commercial forms of transportation like city buses or heavy trucks in metropolitan areas such as Los Angeles.[342]

SOLUTIONS FACTORY FARMING

PROTECT YOUR HEALTH and YOUR FAMILY

- Avoid artificial hormones and drugs in meat, dairy and eggs, buy organic & biodynamic.
- Ask your favorite restaurants and cafes to source milk & meat from local and organic farms.
- Support local and family farms as much as possible.
- If you're traveling, find good food options at: www.eatwellguide.org
- Eat organic green leafy vegetables and foods rich in chlorophyll, as well as organic yogurt to help your body purge drugs, hormones, and residues found in foods.
- Reducing intake of factory farm foods reduces risk of antibiotic resistant infection

"When animals are given antibiotics for growth promotion or increased feed efficiency, bacteria are exposed to low doses of these drugs over a long period of time. This is inappropriate antibiotic use and can lead to the development of resistant bacteria." CDC[343]

- Reinstate Meat Inspectors: Farms and facilities must be overseen by *ethical* meat inspectors
- Country of Origin Labeling (COOL): Meat must be labeled honestly. Period.
- Support Farm Aid 1-800-FARM-AID
- Massive farms must implement strategies to keep our water and food supply safe.
- Write, call, email your congress people to help get pollution regulations at these farms.

ANIMAL WELFARE ACT of 1966
Isn't it time to get all animals *including* farm animals and any animals trapped or held in captivity included under these provisions?

ANIMAL WELFARE ACT: Let's increase protections for farm animals under the Animal Welfare Act. Why aren't farm animals included? It's unfair that these animals are confined and not allowed to know the minimal comfort provided through adequate sleeping quarters and fresh air. Animals housed in concentrated feeding operations are treated shamefully. The same holds true for wildhorses when captured and corralled, and other wild animals trapped and held in fur farms. Kudos to California--in 2018 they passed a law that improved shelter and arrangements for confined animals.[344]

SMARTER WASTE MANAGEMENT

Can't big farms figure out a less dangerous end game for the waste? If animals were fed and housed wholesomely, and drugs withdrawn, their manure and waste could be composted. Then it could actually serve the soil and be instrumental in revitalizing soil health instead of festering and contributing to climate change and toxic runoff. "Manure and wastewater from AFOs have the potential to contribute pollutants such as nitrogen and phosphorus, organic matter, sediments, pathogens, hormones, and antibiotics to the environment."[345]

"Exposure to antibiotics, growth hormones, and toxic run-off from livestock feed lots can be minimized by eating free-range meat raised without these medications if it is available."
President's Cancer Panel Report 2009[346]

AGRICULTURAL RUNOFF EFFECTS

Agricultural Effects on the Mississippi River

Toxic pollutants can affect human health either because they contaminate drinking water supplies or because they accumulate in the fat or tissue of fish, which are consumed by human populations. Both problems are of concern on the Upper Mississippi River. The primary toxic substances due to fish consumption are currently **PCBs** and **chlordane**. PCBs are the primary reason for fish consumption advisories for the Mississippi River in Minnesota, Wisconsin, and Iowa, while chlordane is the predominant reason for such advisories in Illinois and Missouri. Although **dieldrin** is currently the basis for fish consumption advisories only in Illinois, if other states adopt EPA's risk assessment methods for evaluating fish contaminant data, dieldrin may replace chlordane as a priority for protection of human health. **Mercury** contamination is generally the basis of fish consumption advisories on the Mississippi River only north of the Twin Cities. The second category of toxic pollutants which is of concern to human health includes those substances that pose threats to drinking water. Based upon the fact that they have either shown exceedances of maximum contaminant levels (MCLs) or had a significant impact on water treatment needs, **atrazine** and **nitrate** are considered to be of top priority. Both produce localized and seasonal problems, but are of basin-wide concern. Nitrate is additionally of priority concern because recent research suggests that the Upper Mississippi River is a major source of nitrogen in the Gulf of Mexico.

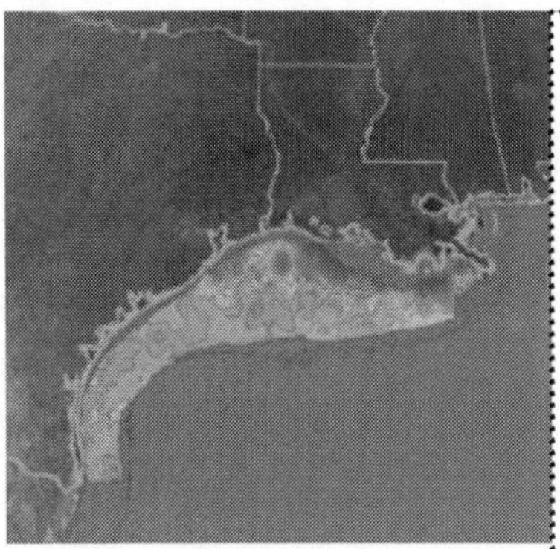

Map Source: NASA
According to the Virginia Institute of Marine Science, there are over 405 Deadzones throughout the world[347]

The Dead Zone

Fertilizer nutrients, notably phosphorous and excess nitrogen cause toxic algae blooms and dead zones. The largest dead zone in the world sits where the Mississippi River meets the Gulf of Mexico. "Scientists have determined this year's Gulf of Mexico "dead zone," an area of low oxygen that can kill fish and marine life, is 8,776 square miles, an area about the size of New Jersey. It is the largest measured since dead zone mapping began there in 1985. This large dead zone size shows that nutrient pollution, primarily from agriculture and developed land runoff in the Mississippi River watershed is continuing to affect the nation's coastal resources and habitats in the Gulf.

6. FERTILIZER

"Fertilizer is the biggest item other than land in an annual budget for farmers."[348] While the pesticide industry may be huge, the fertilizer industry is even bigger. Unlike natural fertilizers of days gone by like manure and wood ash, modern chemical fertilizers sicken soil, contaminate water sources, cause toxic algae blooms, and contribute mightily to climate change and disease. As for our food, synthetic fertilizer seems to weaken soil, which in turn causes plants to be weaker than normal. This can only logically translate to foods with less energy and vitality for us to absorb. More on that in the next chapter devoted to Soil, pages 64-71.

Plants need at minimum, nitrogen, phosphorous and potassium (NPK) to grow, yet to be healthy plants need an array of trace minerals as well. As Julius Hensel decreed in 1892 in his book *Bread from Stones*, "plants need potassium, soda, lime, magnesium, iron, manganese, sulphur, phosphorous and fluorine; and in artificial fertilizers they only receive expensive potassium, phosphoric acid and nitrogen for their nourishment."

The chemical fertilizer industry makes a fortune swindling farmers. Their poisonous concoctions stem from obnoxious chemicals and substances that curse the earth. Their methods of sourcing materials cause widespread water contamination and air pollution. Farming is by no means an easy job, it's grueling and hard labor. Once the farmers are under the control of the chemical companies, it's very hard to break free. The vicious cycle of chemicals that farmers grow to rely upon may be making the farmers' lives even harder. What if we helped the farmers get their land off these substances and get back to nature? Might the farmers' crops have better success? Might the farmers be a little happier, healthier, and richer themselves?

The escalation of synthetic fertilizer use has its roots in war and munition facilities left idle after the World War II. Soon industry and government were collaborating to industrialize agriculture and make use of the bomb-making facilities. Farming was to be reshaped according to their new economic paradigm. "After millennia of ruralities-based agriculture and food production, this all was discarded and governments and their experts emphasized that only an "ecological regime" with industrial foundation will do. They claimed they could relocate agriculture from the ruralities of old to a uniform factory-like environment where industrial fertilizer dominated." Jozef Vissner, *Down to Earth*[349]

Some of the Synthetic Sources:

- Anhydrous ammonia = natural gas + steam + air[350]
- Nitric Acid = ammonia + oxygen gas, or from fossil fuel combustion[351]
- Nitrogen Source: Ammonia, Nitric Oxide, Nitric Acid, Ammonia Nitrate
- Phosphorous: Phosphate + Coal + Sulfur, + Sulfuric Acid, + Nitric Acid
- Phosphate Mining creates tremendous air and water pollution problems, they create huge gypsum mounds that often spill and create sink holes[352].

COMMON SYNTHETIC FERTILIZER ADDITIVES

The connection between the military industrial complex and fertilizer continues. Perchlorate, otherwise known as rocket fuel can be found contaminating some nitrogen fertilizers. Perchlorate is a potent neurotoxin. Already we have problems with perchlorate contaminating drinking water, then the FDA approved perchlorate in food packaging in 2005. How much perchlorate exposure can our bodies handle? Perchlorate targets thyroid function, alters metabolism, and bioaccumulates.[353]Adding to the problem of synthetic fertilizer, Patty Martin, the former mayor of Quincy, Washington discovered that fertilizer throughout the United States is often contaminated with hazardous waste and heavy metals. As reported by the Seattle Times, "they discovered something they found shocking and that they think other American farmers and consumers ought to know: Manufacturing industries are disposing of hazardous wastes by turning them into fertilizer to spread around farms. And they're doing it legally. "It's really unbelievable what's happening, but it's true," Martin said. "They just call dangerous waste a product, and it's no longer a dangerous waste. It's a fertilizer."[354]

The California Public Interest Research Group revealed the dangers of these toxins in their report, *Wastelands, the Threat of Toxic Fertilizer:* "The toxic substances found in the tested fertilizers have been linked to adverse human health impacts. The metals found in these fertilizers are known or suspected carcinogens, reproductive and developmental, liver, and blood toxicants. For example, beryllium is a suspected carcinogen, chromium and arsenic are known to cause cancer and barium can cause kidney and lung damage. Children are most susceptible to the toxic effects of most metals, especially lead, which has been the subject of intense government efforts to reduce lead exposure to children. Products like fertilizer are of great concern as children spend more time on or near the ground and are often exposed to ground level substances through hand-to-mouth behavior."[355]

The late Adrienne Anderson, an environmental health expert and whistleblower also uncovered troubling information. Adrienne was an admired and respected environmental ethics professor at the University of Colorado. In 1998 she was appointed by the Denver mayor to help the Water Reclamation Department. Soon she discovered a major cover up involving a landfill, water contamination, and illegal dumping of munitions and radioactive substances from a Superfund site. She also found out the radioactive sludge was being spread on cropfields like fertilizer.[356] When this situation was brought to the attention of the EPA, the agency decided to make it *legal* to add toxic sludge to fertilizer, radioactive or not! Because of restrictions preventing altering a Superfund clean up that's underway, it took time to remedy the situation.

Yet sewage sludge continues. According to the Center for Food Safety, "Sewage sludge includes anything that is flushed, poured, or dumped into our nation's wastewater system – a vast, toxic stew of wastes collected from countless sources--from homes to chemical industries to hospitals. The sludge being spread on farm fields is a dangerous mix of heavy metals, industrial compounds, viruses, bacteria, drug residues and radioactive material." "The EPA doesn't test for contaminants when they come out the other end of the pipes, where they may be concentrated in sludge. Some scientists are concerned that dangerous levels of contaminants from sludge are passing into crops and groundwater as well as blowing off fields and becoming airborne. Studies have shown that some chemicals in sludge can interact with one another to become more persistent or toxic. Research suggests that the toxins in sludge can pass into milk & meat."[357]

EPA's longstanding policy encourages the beneficial reuse and recycling of industrial wastes. This includes hazardous wastes, when such wastes can be used as safe and effective substitutes for virgin raw materials.[358] Can hazardous waste ever be used safely, especially on our food?
Some fertilizers like the "Weed and Feed" varieties contain atrazine that then leaches into water supplies. Atrazine is an endocrine disruptor,[359] and one of the most common contaminants of

drinking water; an estimated thirty million Americans are exposed to trace amounts of the chemical."[360] Weed and Feeds also kill trees and shrubs.

Nanoparticles are a newer type of agro-additive with relatively little testing. Researchers at Duke University identify nanos as "emerging pollutants." Experiments show nanoparticles in fertilizers and pesticides act as additional stressors to ecosystems and worsen algae blooms. "Big algal blooms were more than three times more frequent and more persistent in tanks where nanoparticles and nutrients were added together than where nutrients were added alone. As much as 80,400 metric tons per year are released into soils, and up to 29,200 metric tons end up in natural bodies of water."[361] That's a lot of nanoparticles.

FERTILIZER'S EFFECT ON THE PLANET Sick soil, water pollution, toxic runoff, toxic algae, algae blooms, dead zones, red tide, ocean acidification, sick and dead animals, air pollution, sink holes, nitrate in drinking water, contaminated ground water, contaminated aquifers, nitrous oxide, methane emissions, ammonia, smog, acid rain, the list goes on and on.

HEALTH EFFECTS: CANCER. Nitrate in water is a causal factor in many cancers including: bladder and ovarian cancers, brain cancer, uterine and rectal cancers, stomach cancer, and nonhodgkin's lymphoma. It also interferes with thyroid gland health.[362], and causes blue baby syndrome. methemoglobinemia.[363] "Populations living in agricultural areas typically have the highest exposures to drinking water contaminated with nitrate, with households using private wells often having exposures several-fold above households using public supplies."[364]

RED TIDE It's not just the toxic runoff from fertilizer that causes horrific water pollution, the phosphate mining facilities in Florida stack their waste, radioactive gypsum, in mounds on site. Approximately 1 billion pounds are currently stored above ground.[365] These produce toxic dust as well as leak and contaminate waterways nearby. They've been known to cause sinkholes and contaminate underground aquifers. While algae blooms are a fresh water issue, red tides are similar dangerous blooms occurring in seawater, most notably the Gulf. Is it because this is where most runoff and deadzones occur? Adding in waste from the phosphate facilities may be the trigger[366]. Scientists are still trying to pinpoint the exact causes.[367]

LOWER YIELDS + LOST SOIL CARBON Soil scientists at the University of Illinois have worked for years with the Morrow Plots, the oldest testing fields in America. They've found that since 1955 when synthetic fertilizers were introduced, both soil carbon and crop production has declined. "We don't question the importance of nitrogen fertilizers for crop production," said Ellsworth. "But, excessive application rates cut profits and are bad for soils and the environment. The loss of soil carbon has many adverse consequences for productivity, one of which is to decrease water storage. There are also adverse implications for air and water quality, since carbon dioxide will be released into the air, while excessive nitrogen contributes to the nitrate pollution problem.'[368]

FERTILIZER'S EFFECT ON FOOD QUALITY Tea is one of the most popular beverages in the world and an example of how fertilizers affect our food. Most tea plants are derived from soils where both synthetic fertilizer and toxic pesticides are applied. These factors impact the tea in your cup. For one, the pesticide residues will get in your tea. Furthermore, new studies reveal that synthetic nitrogen fertilizers may alter the biochemical properties of the tea plant "affecting the quality of specific manufactured tea products."[369]

CODE RED CLIMATE CRISIS

Of all the agricultural chemicals, synthetic fertilizer contributes the most to climate change and it's deathly for people's health. It's also used for sinister purposes such as making bombs, which creates unquantifiable damage to people, places and planet. Further, scientists have discovered that continued use of synthetic fertilizers compromises soil's ability to store carbon, which is essential to mitigate climate change. Excess amounts weaken soil's ability to retain water, increases need for irrigation, worsens agricultural runoff and risks greater erosion. As more synthetics are used on soils, more is needed to make plants grow. It's an endless loop that is devastating for people and planet, yet makes great money sense for the fertilizer industry.

Here are the problems resulting from synthetic fertilizer:

- Nitrous Oxide (NO) Emissions: one pound of nitrogen oxide has a greater effect on climate change than 300 pounds of carbon dioxide.[370] SO2 causes smog & acid rain.
- Sulfur dioxide creates acid rain and has a dire impact on warming the atmosphere, "Large volumes of SO_2 erupted frequently appear to overdrive the oxidizing capacity of the atmosphere resulting in very rapid warming!"[371]
- Methane emissions from fertilizer faciltities are 100x higher than reported[372]
- Fertilizer facilities emit toxic gases: nitrous oxide, ammonia and urea dust, sulfuric acid.
- Ammonia volatilizes from fertilizer on fields & facilities to form particulate matter.[373]
- Fertilizer Runoff and Pollution causes nitrate & phosphorous pollution, causing toxic algae blooms and deadzones, as well as worsens red tides and ocean acidification.
- Fertilizer causes high levels of nitrate in drinking water, causing many types cancer, nitrate transforms to carcinogens upon ingestion and inhibits thyroid function[374]
- Synthetic fertilizer makes soil sick, causes soil acidification, and CO2 emissions[375]
- Phosphate mining creates severe pollution problems: mounds of radioactive gypsum[376] poisoning waterways[377], causing sinkholes and notorious air pollution: radon, sulfur dioxide & fluoride gas (which gets collected & used to fluoridate water), the pollution from these facilities is also a major factor in red tides, killing millions of animals.
- Nitrogen fertilizer facilities have grown significantly in the U.S. due to the expansion of fracking and lower natural gas prices.[378] Fracking processes emit vast quantities of pollutants, greenhouse gases, and their wastewater contaminates waterways and food.
- The Koch Brothers produce fertilizer, now they're moving into the factory farm slaughter business.[379]Already just a few companies control global seeds, pesticides, plastics & pharmaceuticals. Is fertilizer the silent member? Or is the growing cartel of fossil fuel, factory farms, and fertilizer coming next?

NITROUS OXIDE[380]

- Agricultural soil management is the largest source of N_2O emissions in the United States, accounting for about 73.9 percent of total U.S. N_2O emissions in 2017.
- Nitrous oxide is also generated from treatment of domestic wastewater
- "Nitrous oxide is released from bacteria in soil. Modern agricultural practices — tilling and soil cultivation, livestock waste management, and the use of nitrogen-rich fertilizers — contribute significantly to nitrous oxide emissions. A single nitrous oxide molecule has 298 times the global warming potential of a carbon dioxide molecule."[381]

IRRIGATION & WASTEWATER

Hand in hand with fertilizer, farmers irrigate their fields. Irrigation is the process of watering crops. Typically, water from nearby streams, ground water and local sources is used. If water becomes scarce, especially in drought-prone regions, farmers may be forced to source water from anywhere they can get it.

The water drawn for irrigating farms was in the spotlight years ago when it was discovered the Colorado River was contaminated with perchlorate (rocket fuel) from the Lockheed Martin facility[382]. Perchlorate is a potent endocrine disrupter and reproductive toxin. This proved to be a major bioaccumulation problem for foods grown in the southwest.[383] Perchlorate contamination is widespread: it is present in the body of all Americans tested and the majority of foods tested."[384]

Now we have more reasons to be worried! *Food and Water Watch* reports, "Oil companies in California are selling wastewater from their drilling operations to several local irrigation districts, which in turn mix it with the water they sell to growers to irrigate their crops."[385] This means that wastewater, which can include up to 173 different toxic chemicals can end up in irrigation water. Was not the EPA designed to protect us and the earth from toxins of this nature? In this case, we can't blame the EPA, for they were banned from regulating wastewater during the Bush regime (see below).

Contaminants found in fracking and drilling wastewater run the gamut from toxic heavy metals to radioactive waste, endocrine disruptors, neurotoxins, reproductive toxins, major health harming substances. Researchers found many different chemicals in the wastewater, over 100 of which are identified as persistent pollutants. The whole list of substances is hard to obtain because the industry is not required to report chemical use. "More than one-third (38%) were not able to be sufficiently identified for preliminary hazard evaluation, largely due to the withholding of information under proprietary claims!"[386]

Amazingly despite the consequences that may befall such use, laws in the United States do not currently prevent such activities.[387] Untreated wastewater is exempt from regulation, it's even permitted for use on icy roads and as a dust suppressant in many States.[388] To recap, this untreated toxic wastewater can be used to irrigate, to de-ice, and now believe it or not, the EPA is considering letting the oil and gas industry dump it straight into our waterways! The Houston Chronicle reports, "the Trump administration is examining whether to adjust decades-old federal clean water regulations to allow drillers to discharge wastewater directly into rivers and streams from which communities draw their water supplies."[389] We cannot let this happen.

WASTEWATER LOOPHOLE: "The fracking provision, widely known as the Halliburton loophole, after the oilfield services company once run by Bush's vice president, Dick Cheney, is among a host of exemptions to federal pollution rules that Congress and successive administrations have given oil and gas companies over the last 40 years. Oil and gas drilling and production are exempt from laws regulating hazardous waste, chemical-laced runoff from well sites and toxic air pollution from well equipment. In 2005 Congress prohibited the Environmental Protection Agency from safeguarding drinking water that might be harmed by fracking, and even denying the regulator the authority to find out what chemicals companies use."[390]

NATURAL FERTILIZER to the RESCUE!

To be true stewards of the planet we must embrace natural methods of fertilizing and feeding the soil. The point of eating isn't merely for calories and taste, but also for nourishment. Healthy plants from healthy soil logically nourish us better than unhealthy plants from unhealthy soil. Evidence indicates synthetic fertilizer weakens soil, depletes soil of minerals and microorganisms. Such soil is incapable of producing the highest quality plants, if for no other reason than it's lacking in microorganisms essential for the delivery of nutrients and minerals. We can continue feeding soil with synthetic fertilizers that do us absolutely no good, or we can start using real fertilizers that boost soil, plant, animal and human health. Which do you prefer?

Soil quality can vary widely around the world. Soil gets depleted naturally overtime, and without anything added to it, either by nature or by humans, eventually nutrient levels will decrease. This means that the same plants can be produced but can be quite different depending on the mineral profile of the soil they're grown in. This translates to foods of better or lesser quality. As soil expert Dr. Charles Northern exclaimed in the 1930s, "the truth is that these foods vary enormously in value, and some of them aren't worth eating as food. For example, vegetation grown in one part of the country may assay 1,100 parts per billion of iodine, as against 20 in that grown elsewhere. Processed milk has run anywhere from 362 parts per million of iodine and 127 of iron, down to nothing." Clearly vegetable quality depends on soil, and milk quality depends on the quality of the plants the cows are eating. Everything is so deeply intertwined.

So how do we change this and improve food quality? We must start by helping the soil, and to do it properly we must look to nature. Back in the 1880s Dr. Julius Hensel proved that plants need not just 3 minerals, but trace minerals as well. His secret to rebalancing soil was by using rock dust, or mineral manure—basically ground up rocks, granite in particular. Rudolph Steiner, the father of biodynamics developed replenishment methods using antlers and herbal preparations. Another simple way to feed soil is to plant cover crops like legumes, these plants magically convert nitrogen in the soil. Instead of raking up your leaves and throwing them away or using a leaf blower, let the leaves remain on your lawn and garden. Fallen leaves and plants naturally decompose and feed your soil. If you burn wood or plants, don't throw the ashes away but use these as fertilizer too! Lastly, don't forget the compost.

COMPOSTING: Composting is the art of converting food and waste into fertilizer. It's alchemy, turning what once was living sun energy into new life. Almost all your food scraps can be used for fertilizer—everything from fruit and vegetable peels, egg shells, and coffee grounds to natural materials like paper, sawdust, pencil shavings and fallen leaves. Plant matter can go in the compost, some say even bones and fish can go in, just be sure to cover them sufficiently so animals don't dig them up. To make plants really robust and capable of fending off disease and such, manure must be part of the compost, at least so said Albert Howard. This is the classic Indore Method he practiced extensively. He demonstrated conclusively that vegetable-based compost doesn't give plants the same vigor and disease resistance as compost containing both vegetable waste and animal manure. Animals also displayed amazing disease resistance when eating food grown in soils containing both. Today, composting manure is a little bit on the fringe for most of us. But there does seem to be a growing movement. Experts suggest composting manure separately for at least 6 months minimum to allow it to break down sufficiently. Also, the manure generally comes from animals that eat grass and herbs, so dog & cat poop is a no no.

SOLUTIONS FERTILIZER

FOR YOUR HEALTH and the PLANET: Discontinue using synthetic fertilizer. Protect yourself, your family, people and animals by using natural fertilizer that encourages healthy soil: compost, sea minerals, rock dust, wood ash, composted manure, worm casings, vegetable meal, bone meal, kelp, fish emulsion, tea and leaf compost.

- We can grow food and farm utilizing natural, organic and biodynamic techniques
- Avoid Weed and Feed Fertilizers! These contain reproductive toxins, be careful
- Make sure your drinking water is safe and not contaminated, especially if you have a private well. Have it tested regularly for nitrates & lawn chemicals.
- Keep moving toward a more natural farming system—every action counts!
- Compost is great fertilizer and helps saves food from going to waste or to landfill.
- Avoid toxic algae in water, it can kill dogs and animals.

EFFECTS OF SYNTHETIC FERTILIZERS

WATER POLLUTION	TOXIC RUNOFF, TOXIC ALGAE, DEAD ZONES
FERTILIZER POLLUTION	CANCER, DISEASE, BLUE BABY SYNDROME
AMMONIA, SULFURIC ACID	ACID RAIN, SMOG
SICK SOIL	SICK PLANTS, CARBON LOSS, LOWER YIELDS
NITROUS OXIDE	CLIMATE CHANGE
GYPSUM MOUNDS	SINK HOLES, WATER POLLUTION, RED TIDE

These synthetic fertilizers are costing too much sickness to people and planet. Nitrates, Hazardous waste, heavy metals, radioactive sludge, Oil and Fracking wastewater are all unacceptable. We cannot permit such radical pollution to continue. I have no doubt all these industries can afford to filter contaminants out of wastewater before recycling, selling, or injecting it back underground. We need stronger rules, politicians who work in our best interests, as well as an environmental protection force that protects. We can no longer allow dirty wastewater or industrial pollutants of any kind to harm our soil, water sources, or our air.

SOIL ACIDIFICATION: Synthetic fertilizers accelerate and worsen the natural process of soil acidification. Excessively acidic soils lead to a dramatic decline in crop & pasture production, acidic pH alters soil microorganism functioning and reduces mineral availability to plants. "[391]

CLIMATE CHANGE IMPACT: We need a collective approach. If we curb our use of synthetic fertilizer, we'll really minimize the amount of nitrous oxide and other greenhouse gas emissions and air pollutants. If we curb factory farms and fertilizers, we'll see significant results. Reducing use of synthetic fertilizers will help our health, soil, air, and waterways. It'll reduce toxic runoff, dead zones, red tide, sinkholes, which in turn will save people and animals!

GET OFF SYNTHETIC FERTILIZER AND INCREASE YOUR PROFITS:

"In comparing USDA data for Iowa and Illinois, the two states that rank highest in corn production, they found that from 1994 to 2001, annual grain yields in Iowa averaged 1.7 billion bushels with 740 thousand tons of nitrogen, as compared to an average of 1.5 billion bushels produced in Illinois with 847 thousand tons of nitrogen. The difference, Khan said, translates into lower fertilizer efficiency that cost Illinois farmers 68 million dollars per year."[392]

7. SOIL

Soil is the foundation for everything in our lives. It is Earth! Soil health, soil vitality, soil quality is essential to creating nearly all of the food we depend upon for survival. Minerals and micronutrients that plants absorb from soil create healthy plants, which supply us with healthy food in return. For our health it's very important we eat foods of good quality, and that begins with good healthy happy soil.

> "The health of soil, plant, animal and man is one and indivisible."
> Albert Howard

Happy soil is alive with organisms, microbes and bacteria—all working in harmony and synchronicity. Growing healthy plants depends on soil thriving with these beneficial organisms that work their magic and bring us life-sustaining food loaded with minerals and nutrients. Earth friendly methods of farming encourage soil prosperity by continually replenishing soil. Soil in tune with nature stores carbon, grows healthy plants, absorbs water, works with nature to prevent erosion, and resists flooding and drought.

The Food and Agriculture Organization (FAO) of the United Nations states, "Soils are fundamental to life on Earth but human pressures on soil resources are reaching critical limits. Further loss of productive soils will amplify food-price volatility and potentially send millions of people into poverty. This loss is avoidable. Careful soil management can increase the food supply, and provides a valuable lever for climate regulation and a pathway for safeguarding ecosystem services."[393]

SOIL HUMUS, THE SECRET TO HEALTHY SOIL & HEALTHY PLANTS

The organic matter in soil is composed of living microorganisms and mycorrhiza, without which we simply cannot have healthy soil. Synthetic fertilizers, fungicides and pesticides cause unnecessary harm to these microorganisms, and by doing so they threaten the food supply. USDA Soil researcher Rick Haney spoke with Yale Environment 360, "We see that when there is a lot of tillage, no cover crops, a system of high intensity [chemical-dependent] farming, that the soil just doesn't function properly. The biology is not doing much. It's not performing as we need it to. We are essentially destroying the functionality of soil, so that you have to feed it more and more synthetic fertilizers just to keep growing this crop. Our mindset nowadays is that if you don't put down fertilizer, nothing grows. But that's just not true, and it never has been."[394]

Luckily all is not lost, we can rebuild soil. First we have to stop the chemical assault and nurture soil back to health. Rebuilding soil structure requires the help of micro superheros—the soil microorganisms. Without thriving soil organisms, plants won't get fed properly, plants will be weak and prone to disease, soil loses carbon, and all goes downhill. What we seek is healthy humus, the heart of the soil.

"Humus is a product of decomposition of plant and animal residues, through the agency of micro-organisms. Importance of humus in soil processes: The functions of humus in the soil are largely threefold: 1. physical, thereby modifying the soil color, texture, structure, moisture-holding capacity, and aeration; 2. chemical, influencing the solubility of certain soil minerals, forming compounds with certain elements, such as iron, which renders them more readily available for plant growth, and increasing the buffering properties of the soil; 3. biological, by serving as a source of energy for the development of microorganisms, as well as by making the soil a better medium for the growth of higher plants; it also supplies a slow but continuous stream of nutrients for plant life."[395]

Awareness of the importance of soil can be traced back in time circa late 1800s Germany when the relationship between soil health and plant health was emerging. Dr. Liebeg, a chemist developed the theory that plants need nitrogen, phosphorous and potassium (NPK). His theory was accepted widely and helped further the use of artificial fertilizers. At the same time, Dr. Julius Hensel believed in a more natural approach and discouraged chemical manures. Through his experiments with rock dust containing an array of minerals, he proved plants can be healthier and resist both disease and pests without the use of chemicals! Dr. Hensel strongly advocated for soil health and using natural fertilizers. He was perhaps the first to warn of what dangers and diseases could befall mankind from synthetic fertilizer and eating foods grown with chemicals.[396]

Fifty years later Eva Balfour explored Hensel's idea in her book *The Living Soil*. Were modern upticks in illness related to the food people were eating? People in the 1940s didn't have the same robustness, vigor as decades earlier. Could it be related to their food? Was something missing from food that wasn't lacking during their forefathers' time? If so, what was wrong with food?

Before Balfour, however, Rudolph Steiner made a quite a stir in the agricultural world. He was a brilliant scientist who was one of the first, like Hensel to foresee the harm chemical fertilizers would cost the world in lost soil, plant, animal and human health as well as poorer food quality. In 1920s Germany, farmers came pleading to him for help and guidance when their crops and animals withered and suffered from use of synthetic fertilizer. In response, Steiner created the framework for biodynamics, the origin of organic farming. Biodynamics brought the world a more wholistic, planetary and spiritual appreciation for soil, earth, and growing food. Also, of significance the renowned botanist Albert Howard taught agriculture and studied farming in India where he experimented with composting methods. He developed many of the organic farming ideas we have today. These inspiring people were the pioneers that helped develop what we today consider ecological farming methods. They understood that even the tiniest of life forms in the soil are vitally important to our own survival.

Back in America Dr. Charles Northern played a crucial role in helping raise awareness about soil health and how much our own health truly depends on good soil. He was an MD who believed "Sick soils mean sick plants, sick animals, and sick people. Physical, mental and moral fitness depends largely on an ample supply and proper proportion of the minerals in our foods." These minerals can only be found in food if the soil is plentiful with them. Through trial and error, he developed a surefire method using colloidal minerals for crafting perfect soil. He encouraged people to demand quality food, "the growers will quickly respond. They can put back those minerals almost overnight, and by doing so they can actually make money through bigger and better crops. It is simpler to cure sick soils than sick people—which shall we choose?" His findings were shared in the US Senate back in 1936, and they still have a record of it today.[397]

In our modern times it seems much of this earlier wisdom has been lost, for the fertilizer, pesticide, and biotech companies will have you believe that foods can't be grown without their chemical inputs. Looking a little closer, one might find it all very suspect. When speaking of soil quality and fertility, the USDA confirms organic farming practices. "Crops more easily resist disease, survive drought, and tolerate insects when grown in good soil. Organic crop producers build soil quality by adding compost, animal manures, or green manures. As soil organisms break down these inputs, they convert nutrients into forms plants can absorb and create humus that sustains soil quality. Organic producers must not apply sewage sludge or biosolids to soil. Additionally, organic crop producers use cover crops to protect the soil from wind and water erosion. Soil-conserving practices include the use of cover crops, mulches, conservation tillage, contour plowing, and strip cropping."[398] Comparatively, crops grown in soil assaulted repeatedly by synthetic fertilizer produce weaker plants prone to disease thus increasing the need for chemical pesticides. Perhaps farmers are the most wounded by this two-headed monster we've yet to capture.

NUTRITIONAL CONTENT OF PLANTS TODAY

Is there a difference between plants grown with chemicals or without chemicals? The Daily Mail reported, "Nutrients needed to help the body and immune system work properly, balance hormones and produce vital blood cells are dwindling across a wide variety of fruit and vegetables, it emerged. An alarming drop in essential minerals means that the apples and greens of today are nowhere near as good for us as those eaten 50 years ago."[399] If food 50 years ago was already of far lesser quality than 50 years prior to that, that means food nutrient levels have grossly gone downhill over the past 100+ years!

There is research indicating plants grown in composted soil may taste better, have better color and could be more nutritious than plants grown in soil fertilized with chemicals. There is a new study indicating that synthetic fertilizer may lessen the nutrient profile and disrupt the biochemistry of plants.[400] Evidence from the past and present day leans toward naturally grown food being a bit more nutrient packed. Considering the impact of pesticides, fertilizer, and industrial farming methods on soil, perhaps these reports are correct.

In her book Living Soil, Eva Balfour details several instances in 1940's England of people recovering from variance maladies upon ingestion of foods grown not in synthetically-fertilized soil, but composted soil—especially compost made with both vegetable matter and animal manure (the Indore Method). Animals too recovered from ailments when provided compost-derived food, as well as when provided time in the fields without chemicals—but not from food grown or from pastures where chemical fertilizers were used. "Animal instincts may be sound guides to food values, which are actually soil values, because food is nothing more than the conveyancing agent or "agent of transfer" of the soil's qualities into the bodies of man and beast; land in good heart supporting bodily health, vigour and stamina; poor, unbalanced soils producing ill health and debility."[401]

More supportive evidence comes via the British Journal of Nutrition Study from 2014. As reported by National Geographic, the team found that, "Organics contain 18 to 69 percent higher concentrations of antioxidants. The organic eater consumes the antioxidant equivalent of approximately two extra produce portions every day, without altering food intake. Without pesticides to guard against harm, an organically farmed plant will produce more of its own compounds, called antioxidants, to fight damage. And when consumed by humans, these antioxidants also protect our bodies from harm. Notably, when a plant grows organically without pesticides its taste is enhanced as well. Studies considered in the BJN paper show that higher antioxidant levels affect food's organoleptic qualities—taste, aroma, and mouthfeel—

and how the human senses detect a food's unique flavor."[402] This is good news for those who are suffering with disease or those who think today's food has lost its flavor. Look to food grown in healthy soil to make you love food again!

Minerals—are these the essential factors giving foods their flavors and colors? In order to exist in food, minerals and nutrients must first be absorbed by the plant's roots in the soil. Absorption cannot occur unless the organic matter and minerals interact with the beneficial soil microorganisms and fungi. In this process, a unique relationship develops between the fungi and plant roots, where fungi attach to the roots providing nutrient pathways through which absorption can occur. The plant in return provides the fungi with carbohydrates derived from photosynthesis. Like guardsmen, mycorrhizae also offer the host plant increased protection against certain pathogens.[403] Without this essential interaction between plant and soil microorganisms, plants cannot absorb, or therefore contain many minerals and nutrients. This raises questions regarding nutrient quality of plants grown without soil.

PROTECTING SOIL

Soil is like anything else, it needs nourishment and help from time to time. Through natural events soil loses minerals and nutrients, especially at harvest. Unless soil protection methods are enacted and minerals and such are added, soil vitality and nutrient content can get low.

When we help earth we inadvertently help ourselves. Making healthy food relies upon the same tools that make earth healthy, soil healthy. Topsoil is a delicate symphony of humus and organic material gently bound together. Within this hidden habitat are the tiny microorganisms and mycorrhiza that help protect plants and prepare nutrients for absorption. This layer of soil we want to disturb as little as possible. Just before planting when you're preparing the soil it is common to dig and loosen up the dirt. This needs to be done at planting time of course. Doing this too often, though can damage the soil fibers making it less able to hold water or help plants resist disease.

One of the easiest ways to help soil is to encourage earthworms, they're nature's tillers. As Charles Darwin revealed in his book, *The Formation of Vegetable Mould Through the Action of Worms*[404], earthworms play an important role in soil ecology, digesting organic matter, aerating soil and making it more fertile.[405] These substances upset soil health and earthworms: synthetic fertilizer, fungicides, glyphosate, fumigants, pesticides and overtilling.

When soil is compromised, more compounds and chemicals leach during runoff. Water is unable to penetrate the soil so more water, more toxins wash into waterways. As water pollution intensifies, water quality deteriorates, bouts of disease and disorders amongst people and animals increase, toxic algae blooms are more frequent, and dead zones expand. With increased severity of rainfalls more agricultural toxins are leaching into waterways.[406]

Earthworms

Earthworms are a sign your soil is happy and healthy. The more the merrier, there can be as many as 8 million earthworms in one acre! If your soil doesn't have earthworms something's amiss.

Soil is essential for growing healthy plants. Healthy soil protects plants, providing a symbiotic pathway for nutrients between plants and earth. Plants absorb and manifest nutrients through the soil and in return provide the soil life with sugar and nutrients gathered from photosynthesis. It's an exchange between the above ground and the underground. When we ingest plants we partake of this alchemy brew. All the vegetables and fruits, even meat, cheese and dairy contain this special elixir as well--for don't the animals all eat the plants and substances made from the plants, which were grown from the earth?

AVOID BURN DOWN WITH PESTICIDES: Burn down is a no-till strategy that is supposed to be a way to avoid disrupting the soil. Instead of tilling, harsh chemicals are applied to the soil, which then trickle down to 'prep' the soil for planting. This method suggests killer chemicals could help soil. It does not. Typically glyphosate is mixed with 2,4-D for burndown.[407] It's believed that after a certain period of time, usually after a few days up to 3 weeks planting can be done without risk. However, the National Pesticide Information Center reports, "Glyphosate binds tightly to soil. It can persist in soil for up to 6 months depending on the climate and the type of soil it is in."[408] Regardless of how long it takes to exit soil, it leaves a wake of disorder in its path. Any seeds then planted will be at a loss, trying by instinct to absorb substances that have been taken away. Many other herbicides[409] are also used that equally cause damage and harm. Fungicides coupled with use of Glyphosate causes a knockout: colossal damage imbalance, chelated minerals, top soil and fungi in disarray.

HOW CHEMICALS HARM SOIL

One might think chemicals used so extensively may actually benefit people's health. In fact there are no benefits to human health from pesticides or synthetic fertilizer. There's a long list of ailments caused by these substances that linger in our food and water. What they do to soil is most telling, it bears repeating.

"Besides being a broad-spectrum systemic patented herbicide, Glyphosate is also a patented mineral chelator, antibiotic, and desiccant. It disrupts plants' metabolic shikimate pathway, which starves plants of essential nutrients and weakens their immune systems. Moreover, Glyphosate's desiccating effects reduce a plant's ability to uptake water. It essentially gives the plants a condition similar to 'Aids'. As a powerful antibiotic, Glyphosate also kills beneficial bacteria and other microorganisms in the soil. Beneficial organisms fix atmospheric nitrogen for plants' consumption and are necessary for healthy plant growth. Without these beneficial microorganisms in the soil to compete with and suppress harmful plant soil-borne pathogens, the lethal soil-borne pathogens, such as Fusarium* take over, killing the weakened plants."[410]
*Fusarium is a naturally occurring soil fungus and pathogen. When not kept in check by microorganisms, fusarium invades plants' roots, and can kill plants as well as prevent normal growth.[411] There's been a surge in uncurable fungal infections, could that be related to burn down and overuse of soil fungicides and pesticides?

If a garden or field has issues with pests or disease there's likely an imbalance in the soil. Bring the soil to harmony and the natural predators will take care of pest problems, and plants will be more resilient to disease. Chemicals are impartial—harming all life forms. Harm can be imposed on plants, persons, or animals and beneficial insects and pollinators. What the soil needs is proper care, then invaders and pests may not compromise the soil, and plants will thrive again naturally resisting disease and pests. It's like magic, but it's nature, and we opt to end it everytime we use toxic chemicals.

SOIL & CARBON

Healthy soil stores carbon. Synthetic fertilizer, while it may help plants grow does not create healthy soil. In fact, it has the contrary effect of degrading soil. Soil doused repeatedly with synthetic fertilizer, fungicides, fumigants and pesticides breaks down and releases carbon back to the atmosphere. Further, the weakened soil also releases more nutrients i.e. phosphorous, nitrogen into waterways, increasing toxicity of agricultural runoff, water pollution, apoxia (dead zones) and toxic algae blooms. The soil scientists at the University of Illinois confirm that as far as nitrogen fertilizers are concerned: "excessive application rates cut profits and are bad for soils and the environment. The loss of soil carbon has many adverse consequences for productivity, one of which is to decrease water storage. There are also adverse implications for air and water quality, since carbon dioxide will be released into the air, while excessive nitrogen contributes to the nitrate pollution problem."[412] Clearly synthetic fertilizer has surpassed its usefulness.

LOST SOIL CARBON: When Soil is sick it loses its carbon storage ability and in turn, releases carbon to the atmosphere. In order to prevent further release of CO2 from soil we must change our ways and greatly reduce use of synthetic fertilizer, fungicides & herbicides.

SOIL SEQUESTRATION: Healthy soil captures and retains carbon. The microorganisms, soil bacteria and fungi work together nourishing plants, and in the process capture carbon. If we converted all global croplands and pastures to regenerative organic agriculture we could sequester more than 100% of current annual CO2 emissions[413]

SOIL COMPACTION: "The threat of soil compaction is greater today than in the past because of the dramatic increase in the size of farm equipment." Compaction is the reduction of soil volume due to external factors.[414]

DESERTIFICATION: Be it by weather such as drought or by human activities, desertification is what occurs when land once fertile turns to desert.

HELP SOIL: We can help soil retain its vitality by supplying natural nutrients and materials such as leaves and plant waste, compost, rock flour, sea minerals, fish emulsion, kelp, biodynamic methods, biochar. Rotating crops is the proven tradition that keeps soil organisms in balance. Planting peas + legumes over the winter helps enrich and stabilize nitrogen in the soil.

AVOID TILLING TOO MUCH: Soil structure is very delicate and can be damaged easily through tilling. Till only when needed.

SOIL CONSERVATION

Hugh Bennett, the father of soil conservation helped America recover from the Dust Bowl. He raised awareness of better farming techniques to prevent erosion and passed the Soil Conservation Act of 1935. Through his leadership, Congress established the Soil Conservation Service as part of the USDA.

CODE RED CLIMATE CRISIS

"Man sets about his desert-making in various ways. He alters the texture of the soil by using up humus and failing to replace it—by failing to feed the soil with organic matter; livestock are the great converters of otherwise unwanted organic matter to a form in which it can be used by plants. Stockless farming, understocking, burning straw, etc., are all cases of failure to observe the "**Rule of Return**" which is the essence of farming. Only by faithfully returning to the soil in due course everything that has come from it can fertility be made permanent and the earth be made to yield a genuine increase." Lord Northbourne in *Look to the Land,* 1930

To defeat climate change we must protect our allies: healthy soil and healthy forests. The chemical warpath endorsed by the giant industrial farms and biotech has the capacity to destroy both of these. The pollution we're creating from farming is from the chemical inputs and poor land management practices endorsed by conventional and GMO farming standards. Most of our croplands are used to grow GMO feed for animals, while more and more of the food we eat tends to be imported from other countries. Is this a foolish policy? Wouldn't we be wiser to be forging a future where we can be self reliant rather than dependent on other countries to feed us? Currently Russia[415] is determined to be the world's greatest producer of organic food. That's a stand America should consider. Converting to sustainable farming methods not only improves soil health, but it also minimizes carbon and other climate disrupting outputs.

Threats to soil and land include:

- Chemical intensive farming
- Synthetic fertilizer
- Pesticides, fumigants, fungicides
- Unsustainable land management
- Over tillage
- Soil compaction
- Monocropping
- Erosion, Desertification
- Sealing soil, paving over

Climate Change and Soil:

CO2: Carbon dioxide releases from unhealthy soil, when land is cleared or burned
Methane: when soil from forests and peatland is burned and cleared, methane is released
Nitrous Oxide: when soil is saturated with synthetic fertilizer, nitrous oxide is released
Ammonia: when soil is saturated with synthetic fertilizer ammonia is released
Working soil with heavy machinery: soil compaction, releases CO2, fossil fuel emissions,
Monocropping: demands more pesticides, fungicides, fertilizer causing less soil productivity
Runoff: Unhealthy soil can't hold water, more farming chemicals wash away into waterways
Toxic Algae, Water contamination: Results from excessive farm nutrients in waterways
Excessive pesticides: kill off good fungi & cause harmful soil fusarium to dominate soil
Excessive pesticides & fertilizer: Reduces beneficial soil microorganisms and bacteria
Excessive pesticides & fertilizer: sickened soil loses nitrogen-fixating power to help plants
Glyphosate & Roundup: disrupts shikimate pathway, plants lose ability to take up water.

SOLUTIONS SOIL

Without a doubt healthy soil and healthy plants are essential for our health. In today's times when we're forced to contend with so much pollution, soil is more important than ever.
Dear Farmers if you can, please consider taking back your land and your health:

- Avoid using fake fertilizers and toxic chemicals that kill the soil microorganisms
- Some ways to improve and care for Soil; (verify your exact needs with a soil test)
    - Nurture: Add minerals, rock dust, lime, stonemeal, compost
    - Feed it with nature's residues from plants, worm castings, biochar
    - Protect: Cover soil and protect it, don't let it be naked and afraid
    - Treat your yard, your farm as a living organism: www.biodynamics.com[416]
- Let leaves and dead plant material stay & decompose on the soil
- Use natural fertilizers not synthetic chemicals

PREVENT EROSION: Abiding by the natural laws, protecting and nourishing soil, we can keep our soils healthy for generations to come. If we're not careful, the overuse of toxic chemicals combined with overworking soil and clearing land could lead us back to dire times.

WEED MANAGEMENT: Many Weeds are miracle plants in disguise, though many view them as a nuisance. Dousing weeds with herbicides can cause resistance and trouble for your soil and other plants. Contrary to using chemicals, organic farming methods use less harsh methods like mulching to discourage weeds. Many "weeds" like dandelions are super important for bees.

SOIL TEST: Have you experienced problems growing plants? Have you ever wondered why some weeds grow more than others? Instead of fighting weeds with chemicals consider what the soil may need to be healthier to prevent weeds in the first place. In comes the soil test. You can hire someone to test your soil or pick up a test kit, but in many parts of the country you can get your soil tested for free by local experts. Check this site to see if this is offered near you: https://www.gardeningknowhow.com/extension-search.

CLEAN POLLUTED SOIL: PHYTOREMEDIATION

If you have polluted and contaminated soil, you can use plants to pull and remove the toxins. Known as phytoremediation, it takes time and persistence, but can be a lovely way to revitalize your landscape. Sunflowers are some of the best to remove toxins.[417]

EROSION: According to the UN, erosion led to the demise of ancient civilizations.
"When farm productivity declined, usually as a result of soil mismanagement, civilizations also declined - and occasionally vanished entirely. Of the three requisites for a thriving civilization: fertile soil, a dependable water supply and relatively level land with reasonable rainfall which would not cause erosion, it is likely that the third factor was most important, and evidence is mounting that soil degradation has toppled civilizations as surely as military conquest. In countries bordering the Mediterranean, deforestation of slopes and the erosion that followed has created man-made deserts of once productive land. Ancient Romans ate well on produce from North African regions that are desert today."[418] Perhaps the world's most well-known erosion event was the Dust Bowl that plagued America in the 1930's. Through President Franklin D. Roosevelt's and Hugh Bennett's leadership, America thankfully recovered.

8. FUNGUS RESIST*ANCE*

Fungicide use on crops and soil has increased dramatically over the years. This is threatening our food supply and our health. The overuse of fungicides causes imbalance and harm to vital soil life, and it perturbs the planet. Such use has resulted in a new breed of horrors: antibiotic-resistant fungus. Within the past five years the resistant funguses, Candida Auris, have spread slowly around the globe.[419] The CDC recently listed this as an urgent threat!

The azole fungicides may be the root cause for the increasing resistance of the fungus, Aspergillus species. "Similarities between medical and agricultural azoles, and extensive azole use in crop protection, prompted speculation that resistance in patients with aspergillosis originated in the environment. Aspergillus species & Aspergillus fumigatus, are the largest causes of patient deaths from fungi."[420]

These fungal infections are not to be taken lightly. The UK's Independent reports, "Common fungal infections are "becoming incurable"[421] with global mortality exceeding that for malaria or breast cancer because of drug-resistant strains which "terrify" doctors and threaten the food chain."[422] People, animals and crops are all threatened. The most at risk are those with compromised immune systems. CNN reports, "There's not a single vaccine against any fungus at the moment."[423]

Fungicides are used chiefly on:

Soil and crops such as corn, wheat, peanuts, grapes, grains, sugarbeet, potato, strawberries, rice, tomatoes, soybeans, beans,[424]lettuce, apples, almonds [425]

- Golf courses and turf[426], Forest maintenance

Fungicides imperil:

- Bees and Bats, Pollinators, Animals (pollinators make direct contact with plants and fungicides applied to them). Bees are defenseless now against Nosema fungus, bats are dying from white nose syndrome.[427]
- Soil Health
- People!

Despite these dangers, the fungicide market is growing steadily. The triazole class of fungicides leads their competitors. *Market Research Future* reports, "The primary reason for the growth of triazoles is their extensive use for the prevention of soybean rust, which is considered to be a fungal pathogen."[428] Almost all the soybeans grown in the US is GMO soy; is GMO soy more prone to fungus disease? If the soil was healthier would the plants have this disease? Do GMO plants in general need more fungicides than regular crops? Another reason to abandon GMOs!

SOLUTIONS:. If we hope to curtail this unraveling disaster, we must quickly cease using, or at the very least greatly reduce use of toxic fungicides. Scientists state, "significant investment in fungal research, including fungal biology, human and plant pathogenicity, therapeutic agents, diagnostic tools, and vaccines, has the potential to avoid a global catastrophe."[429] Wash hands often with soap and water. Many hand sanitizers actually break down skin defense barriers.

TWO

PLANET + PEOPLE IN DANGER

"We have an obligation and a privilege to preserve
and maintain our planet
and the species we share the planet with."
Ted Turner

CLIMATE CRISIS

Cause and Effect

Monocrops
Land conversion
Overuse of toxic fertilizer
Overuse of herbicides,
Overuse of fungicides
Overuse of pesticides
Resistant weeds
Agicultural runoff
Water pollution
Nitrate pollution
Nitrous oxide (N2O)
Toxic algae blooms
Eutrophication, dead zones
Ocean acidification
Ammonia pollution
Smog
Greenhouse gas emissions
Deforestation
Habitat loss
Loss of wildlife
Pollinator loss
Fungus resistance

Synthetic Fertilizer
NitrousOxide (N2O)
Ammonia (NH3)
Natural Gas
SulfuricAcid (H2SO4)
Acid rain
Smog

Pesticides + Forest Fires

Loss of forests makes air pollution worse

Animal Farming
Methane (CH4)
Water Pollution
Air Pollution
Confinement
Drug Overuse
Antibiotic Resistance
Daily antibiotic
GMO feed = More methane
Manure mismanaged
Zero Grazing
Contaminated water

Wildlife in danger

Tropical Deforestation
10% of Global Climate Change Emissions

What's lost when a forest burns?

GMO soy + cattle
Deforestation
Rainforest lost
fertilizer overkill
Methane
Factory farms

Waste
Food Waste
Packaging Waste
Plastic + Paper
Manure

Pollinators in danger

Palm Oil
Deforestation
Extinction of animals
Native people forced out
67 million acres
forests burned
peatland
Methane
Greenhouse gas emissions

Deforestation
Removal of forests
Land converted to farmland
Expands air pollution
Greenhouse gas emissions
Carbon sink loss
Disposable Paper Products

Conventional Farms
Overuse of fertilizer
Overuse of pesticides
Overuse of fungicides
Overuse of fumigants
Greenhouse.gas emissions
Ozone depleting
Water contamination
Monocropping
Deforestation

Water pollution

Fish + Waterways
Water pollution
Synthetic Fertilizer
Fungicides
Pesticides
Fertilizer Facilities
Endocrine disruptors

Ocean Health: Algae Blooms, Red Tides, Dead Zones, Ocean Acidification, Plastic, Oil Spills, Overfishing

9. CLIMATE CRISIS

If we're serious about helping the planet and turning the tide on climate change we need to honestly examine Big Agriculture. Most of the tragedies we see occurring in the environment, the planetary reactions—are resulting from crimes against nature. A great percentage of these crimes can be traced back to how we grow and produce food today.

Big Ag contributes abundantly more to the climate crisis than traditional and small farms. In the U.S. 42% of greenhouse gas emissions come from Animal Agriculture, globally it accounts for 14.5%.[430] But the damage goes far beyond that. For instance, the chemicals and methods chosen for growing foods are causing soaring numbers of bees and wildlife species to plummet, escalating rates of human disease, plant disease, soil disease, water degradation, and planetary upheaval. Unless we wake up and choose differently, we have little chance to rebound.

Ultimately, we have to stop supporting land use and agricultural methods that promote harm to the planet. Making some modest adjustments can greatly reduce agriculture's contribution to climate change and planetary stress. As an example, nitrogen fertilizers can be scaled back—right now nitrous oxide emission account for roughly 60% of total agricultural emissions.[431]

The companies dominating farming chemicals along with the big conventional and GMO farms—their methods are destructive to the earth, to ecosystems, to pollinators, to animals, to our water and to our air, and to us. Even the farmers themselves are endangered. These methods are destroying the planet and tipping the scales. Their argument that only with their chemical concoctions can we feed a growing population flies right out the window, for surely no one will be eating if the planet is in ruins. The time has arrived--we must adapt to sustainable farming methods.

What's wrong with Big Agriculture?

- Greenhouse Gas Emissions-Agriculture sector emits most nonCO2 emissions globally[432]
- Industrial farming processes—monocropping, factory farming & GMO farming—play a significant role toward furthering planetary distress, habitat loss and climate change.
- Toxic chemicals—fertilizer, fungicides, pesticides, herbicides, insecticides, fumigants—they're outdated and responsible for the collateral damage to the planet and to our health.
- Industrial farming contributes to: sick soil, erosion, deforestation, ozone layer depletion, methane & nitrous oxide emissions, loss of soil carbon toxic agricultural runoff, water pollution, aquatic dead zones, toxic algae, pollinator loss, antibiotic resistance, and more.

Snapshot of Agriculture Emissions Since 1990 interpreted by IATP[433]

CO2	+16.2%	Monocropping, Industrial Farms, GMO
CO2 Urea Fertilizer	+109%	Synthetic Fertilizer
Methane	+14.4%	Factory Farms: waste lagoons + digestion
Manure Emissions	+66%	Factory Farms
Methane Pig Manure	+29%	Factory Farms
Methane Cow Manure	+134%	Factory Farms
Nitrous Oxide	+7.3%	Synthetic fertilizer, manure on fields

From the EPA Report: Inventory of Greenhouse Gas Emission and Sinks 1990-2017[434]

CLIMATE CRISIS + FARMING

"In a time of increasing population growth, climate change and environmental degradation, we need agricultural systems that come with a more balanced portfolio of sustainability benefits. Organic farming is one of the healthiest and strongest sectors in agriculture today and will continue to grow and play a larger part in feeding the world. It produces adequate yields and better unites human health, environment and socioeconomic objectives than conventional farming." *John Reganold, Professor of Soil Science & Agroecology at Washington State University.*[435]

If we're serious about helping the planet & halting climate trends, we need to take a good look at these methods. It all comes down to choices. Some methods make sense, others don't. Let's get real. Industry, government, and those with capabilities have to join in and help resuscitate earth. In helping the planet we truly help improve our own condition. Looking at big agriculture's link with planetary distress, there's tremendous room for improvement:

- **ANIMAL FARMS**: The majority of meat and dairy products come from factory farms--large industrial farms that confine animals to small cages indoors their entire lives. There are approximately 50,000 farms with 1000 confined animals or more, and 400,000 with 999 or less confined animals on site. "The U.S. Environmental Protection Agency defines CAFOs or AFOs (Animal Feeding Operations) as agricultural enterprises where animals are kept and raised in confined situations. Feed is brought to the animals rather than the animals grazing or otherwise seeking feed in pastures, fields, or on rangeland."[436] "Corn and soy that most cows eat makes them especially gassy, so feeding them alfalfa and supplements could reduce how much they belch."[437]
- **CONVENTIONAL FARMS**: This type of farming needs ever more synthetic fertilizer & herbicides, harming the whole planet in the process. Now seeds coated in neonicotinoids are used widely. As more herbicides are applied, life in the soil withers, weeds resist, pollinators die. This is an endless war against nature. Who's winning?
- **GMO FARMS:** Most rely on *Roundup Ready* seeds that have been genetically modified to withstand unconscionable amounts of *Roundup*. Other seeds used for GMO contain the bt toxin that unlike common bt sprays, which can be washed off, GMO Bt infiltrates the plant and remains forever in the food that comes from it.[438] GMO and conventional farming methods involve ungodly amounts of chemicals, pesticides, fungicides, toxic fertilizer, as well as monocropping and other practices that harm ecosystems, destroy habitat, and bring harm and disease to people, animals and pollinators.
- **PALM OIL FARMS**: The lust for palm oil causes massive deforestation and extinction of animals. This is costing the world 500 million tons of $CO2$ yearly,[439] not to mention methane emissions and terror to ecosystems. For the sake of the future of the world, we must realize we need the forests more than the forests need us. Any corporation contributing to or profiting from their loss must be held accountable.
- **LAND COVERSION:** "Heavy tilling, multiple harvests and abundant use of agrochemicals have increased yields at the expense of long-term sustainability. In the past 20 years, agricultural production has increased threefold and the amount of irrigated land has doubled. Over time, however, this diminishes fertility and can lead to abandonment of land and ultimately desertification."[440]

FARMING METHODS

There are two types of farming styles: those that lean toward traditional natural methods, and others that lean heavily toward chemical methods. Farming operations range from small family farms and niche urban growers to giant industrial operations and confined animal farms. The more ecological type of farming uses organic-type methods that strive to avoid toxins while endorsing traditional methods such as crop rotation and symbiotic pest control.

GMO and conventional farming methods, on the other hand involve lots of chemicals, pesticides, dangerous fertilizers, as well as monocropping. These methods harm people, animals, pollinators, and ecosystems. They cause super resistant weeds, toxic water pollution, lower yields, less profits and higher costs for farmers. If it weren't for the subsidies they receive, maybe many of these farmers would switch to sustainable methods and actually be more prosperous.

US Total Farmland	911 million acres[441]
Total Cropland	389 million acres
GMO cropland	182 million acres
Organic Farms	5 million acres
Total pasture	415 million acres
Government owned pasture	155 million acres[442]
Confined Animal farms in US	450,000 farms without pasture[443]

The majority of meat and dairy products in the US come from factory farms—large industrial farms that confine animals indoors their entire life. There are approximately 50,000 farms with 1000 confined animals or more, and 400,000 with 999 or less. "The U.S. Environmental Protection Agency (EPA) defines AFOs as agricultural enterprises where animals are kept and raised in confined situations. AFOs congregate animals, feed, manure, urine, dead animals and production operations on a small land area. Feed is brought to the animals rather than the animals grazing or otherwise seeking feed in pastures, fields, or on rangeland."[444]

GMO farming relies on "*Roundup Ready*" seeds that have been genetically modified to withstand unconscionable amounts of *Roundup*. Other seeds used for GMO contain the bt toxin that, unlike common bt sprays, they can never be washed off.[445] Conventional farmers use seeds coated in neonicotinoids—pesticides largely implicated in colony collapse disorder. Without bees and pollinators, what kind of food supply can we have? On top of this, their monocropping methods require vast amounts of synthetic fertilizer, leading to who knows how many victims of disease. All in all, these methods of farming cause endless harm, perhaps nearly irreversible. As more herbicides and fertilizer are applied, life in the soil withers and weeds resist, plants get weaker and prone to disease, pollutants in water increase. Yet the corporations and manufacturers' solutions, as if they have blinders on, is more and more chemicals. In this scheme there is no end, it's an endless war against life. The Union of Concerned Scientists confirms, "Monsanto's Roundup Ready system, which involves applying glyphosate herbicide to crops genetically engineered to tolerate it, was supposed to decrease herbicide use—and for a while, it did just that. However, this has changed drastically in recent years."[446]

Methods taking us further away from nature

Methods of farming can either benefit the planet or harm the planet. The following methods contribute the lion's share of pollution from agriculture that's affecting the atmosphere and the climate (not to mention our health!) As long as these farming methods are kept in use, attempts to mitigate climate change will be futile.

- **Synthetic Fertilizer** causes cancer,[447] damages soil & destroys its ability to store carbon, and makes plants unhealthy and less vigorous. Nitrate and excess phosphorous contaminate our water sources triggering cancer and disease, toxic algae blooms, dead zones, red tide, and ocean acidification. Fertilizer manufacturing is also a huge problem emitting sulfur dioxide, ammonia, nitrous oxide, fluoride, and methane.
- **Pesticides, Herbicides:** These toxic substances are designed to kill bugs and plants yet they're harming people and animals. They're used abundantly in both GMO and conventional farming. The more we're exposed to them, the more damage can be done. Health effects can be immediate if exposure is significant, or health effects can slowly appear if exposure is minimal yet continuous. Pesticides are killing off bees, bats, and pollinators, this alone could cause our entire food supply to collapse.
- **Fungicides:** Overuse of fungicides is leading to deadly antibiotic-resistant fungus.
- **Fumigants:** Fumigants are pesticides injected into the soil. The most widely used fumigants endanger our health and damage the earth's protective Ozone Layer, thereby increasing climate warming effects. Ozone depleting substances are banned worldwide through the Montreal Protocol. Nonetheless a few remain in use on certain crops.
- **Factory Farms:** "The reality is an increasing number of livestock are "zero graze", spending all or almost all of their time indoors in large warehouse-type facilities."[448]
- **GMO Animal Feed:** Factory farm animals are victims fed only GMO soy and corn.
- **Deforestation, Desertification:** land loss and catastrophic conversion
- **Erosion**— overuse of land, infertile, not replenishing soil, using too many chemicals
- **Monocropping** methods of farming contribute to loss of significant portions of native forest, prairie and grasslands. Monocropping refers to the practice of growing the same crop over and over in a large area of land, year after year. This is devastating for the environment and the atmosphere, for often forests and grassland habitats, home to flora and fauna plus serving as carbon sinks get cleared to make room for these crops.
- **Soil loses ability to store carbon**: With excess exposure to toxic chemicals as well as land transformation—the soil loses its ability to store carbon and store water. This leads to greater greenhouse gas emissions as well as more severe agricultural runoff decimating our health, animals, the waterways and habitats for years to come.
- **Conventional & GMOs**: Whether you believe these foods are safe or not, the methods by which they must be grown are not. These farms combine all the above: synthetic fertilizer, monocropping, deforestation, excessive amounts of pesticides, herbicides, fungicides. "Over 70% of harvested GE biomass is fed to food-producing animals, making them the major consumers of GE crops for the past 15 plus years."[449]

STATUS OF THE WORLD'S SOIL RESOURCES

Report by the UN, **TOP TEN THREATS TO SOIL**[450]:

- Nutrient Balance: insufficient nutrients or excess
- Soil Acidification: pH lowered, leaching or removal of minerals, imbalance
- Soil Biodiversity Loss: decline of soil micro- and macro-organisms
- Soil Compaction: Too much pressure on soil reduces soil porosity
- Soil Contamination: Pollutants, chemicals causing adverse soil health
- Soil Erosion: removal of soil from the land by water, wind, or tillage
- Soil Organic Carbon (SOC): loss of organic carbon stored in the soil
- Soil Salinization: salt accumulation occurring within soil
- Soil Sealing: When soil, earth is permanently sealed over, i.e. with roads, parking lots
- Soil Waterlogging: excess water reduces soil oxygen content, harms plant roots

Methods bringing us back to Nature

ORGANIC and SUSTAINABLE ECO-FRIENDLY FARMING

Growing foods can be done without deadly herbicides and toxic fertilizer. We can grow food and farm without contributing to climate change. We can provide food for an ever-growing population. Farms can convert to organic methods; the USDA has programs to assist farmers making the switch plus there are organic farming mentors available through your State's extension services.

Since most of our farmland is occupied by Big Ag, we're importing most of our organic food. "With demand outpacing domestic supply, the country imported more than $2 billion in organic food last year, and likely significantly more—USDA tracks only 40 imported foods. Organic corn is at the top of that list, with imports jumping more than 200 percent in 2015, according to USDA; the vast majority of that is to feed animals raised for organic meat or dairy operations."[451]

Shouldn't we start planting more organic so we can be self-reliant? Unlike conventional and GMO, organic and biodynamic farmers use sustainable methods, they're ecologically minded and more aligned with nature, striving to prevent harm by avoiding use, minimizing use of toxins. This style endorses use of natural methods that benefit the planet including:

- Soil conditioners and natural fertilizers—ones that produce healthy strong plants
- Such fertilizers include compost and trace minerals, stone meal, biodynamic preps
- Pest and weed control is more strategic with less toxic solutions and outcomes
- Soil is cared for, so beneficial microorganisms flourish rather than get defeated
- Pollinators are cherished, not poisoned
- Farmers rotate crops and plant cover crops to help soil recover in down time.
- Farmers do their best to not contaminate or harm sources of water
- Energy-minded farmers use drip irrigation to use water most efficiently

Simply put, farmers who have a passion for the environment specialize in providing nourishing food without harming the planet in the process. At least they strive to do their best. Many farmers all over the world utilize natural methods such as these. It can be done, and in today's world with its growing population we can use these methods to maximize the land to grow the most without exhausting the land in the process. Of all the sustainable farming styles using soil, organic and biodynamic involve the least harmful pesticides; therefore, foods grown this way will contain less pesticide residue than others. Close to organic farming is IPM—Integrated Pest Management techniques. Also, it's worth noting that sustainable farms are apt to employ more people since many tasks like weeding require people, not chemicals.

- **ORGANIC & BIODYNAMIC FARMING:** "Organic farmers are permitted to use just 20 pesticides, derived from natural ingredients including citronella and clove oil, but only under very restricted circumstances. This means that organic farms are a haven for wildlife and these toxic pesticides can't make their way into the food chain and into us. Organic farming reduces disruption to the natural environment. By rotating crops and selecting crop varieties with a natural resistance to particular pests and diseases, organic farmers are able to reduce or avoid disease problems and the need to control them with chemical inputs."[452] Source: The Soil Association
- **IPM:** Integrated Pest Management: farmers and growers evaluate pest problems that arise and determine the best earth-friendly solution involving the least toxic remedies.
- **URBAN GARDENING:** There is a renaissance of growers bringing life to rooftops, vacant lots and under-used areas of cities across the country. They're usually small plots where neighbors gather & grow their own food. Typically, less chemicals are used.
- **VERTICAL FARMS, HYDRO & AQUAPONICS:** These growers use water rather than soil to grow plants. Farms are usually indoors and protected from the elements. Really don't have to worry about toxic chemicals with these farms.

Earth Friendly Farming or	**Conventional, GMO, CAFO**
Soil Protection and nourishment	Sick soil, Soil depletion, loss of carbon
Nontoxic pest management	Toxic poisonous pest management
Natural fertilizer, compost	Synthetic fertilizer, chemicals
Healthy soil makes plants healthy	Unhealthy soil makes plants weak
Healthier soil holds water, less erosion, runoff	Unhealthy soil, erosion and runoff
Moderate tilling	Burn down tilling killing
Wholesome Animal Rearing	Animals confined & mistreated
Animals eat in the fields, pasture	GMO feed, no outdoors
Sustainable	Nonsustainable
Does not harm habitats, land and water	Harms habitats, land and water
Minimal greenhouse gas emissions	Major contributor to climate change
Doesn't contribute to deforestation	Causes deforestation
Helps soil store carbon	Makes soil release carbon
Decreases greenhouse gases	Increases levels of greenhouse gases
Doesn't harm wildlife	Harms wildlife
Food is full of nutrients	Nutrient quantity compromised
Little or no residues	Lots of pesticide residues

"Overall, organic operations must demonstrate that they are protecting natural resources, conserving biodiversity, and using only approved substances." USDA[453]

CLIMATE CRISIS + FARM SUBSIDIES

The Farm Bill, 2018: "The U.S. Department of Agriculture (USDA) uniquely touches the lives of all Americans daily, through the food they eat."[454] The Farm Bill is decided by Congress. The time has come to embrace sustainable farming and move away from the chemical intensive model. "Better alignment of agricultural and nutritional policies may potentially improve population health."[295] Currently, the overwhelming bulk of U.S. Government farm subsidies go to mega farms and wealthy ag corporations. Very little is directed to the small farms and organic farms because the subsidies are largely pinned for crops grown on the most land: corn, soy, wheat, rice, cotton. These corporations work on an industrial scale using intensive toxic chemicals and planet-harming methods. This is the sector responsible for farming's contribution to climate change. They are the monocroppers, the conventional farmers, the GMO farmers, and the industrial animal factory farmers who use: synthetic fertilizer that's depleting soil and water, toxic unfriendly pesticides that kill pollinators and harm children, GMO seeds & monocropping methods that ruin land, release greenhouse gases and cause massive water pollution problems as well as ocean acidification. Synthetic hormones and misuse of animal drugs cause antibiotic resistance, and now we have fungus resistance to worry about. Is this really the farming model the government should be supporting?

Open the Books' recent study exposes the misdirection of funds to the wealthiest of farmers, most of whom are millionaires. Money also goes to their relatives who may not have anything to do with the farm. As the Balance reports, "Subsidies act like a regressive tax that helps high-income businesses, not poor rural farmers. Most of the money goes toward large agribusinesses. Between 1995 and 2017, the top 10 percent of recipients received 77 percent of the $205.4 billion doled out. The top 1 percent received 26 percent of the payments. That averages out to $1.7 million per company. Fifty people on the Forbes 400 list of the wealthiest Americans received farm subsidies. On the other hand, 62 percent of U.S. farms did not receive any subsidies."[455]

Subsidies were originally created by President Franklin Delano Roosevelt to help farmers struggling during the Dust Bowl and Great Depression.

- The government awarded $13.2 billion in farm subsidies to 957,109 recipients in FY2017.
- 389 recipients received $1 million or more in FY2017 farm subsidies. These top recipients ranged from Pinion Farms in Iowa ($9.9 million) to Pushed & Pullen Farm in Missouri ($1M)
- $626 million in farm subsidies flowed to urban areas with populations of 250,000 or more (FY2015-FY2017). Affluent cities such as Aspen, Colorado ($278,000); Palm Springs, California ($310,420); and Park City, Utah ($1.8 million) reaped large amounts of subsidies.
- Nearly one quarter of all FY2017 farm subsidies ($3 billion) went to just 5,952 recipients who received $250,000 or more each. The top recipients: Pinion Farms in Iowa ($9.9 million); Heard Family Farm in Georgia ($8.9 million); and Hader Farms[456]
- Former USDA Secretary Tom Vilsack received subsidies for his farm in Iowa while in office.
- Should wealthy corporations receive subsidies? "In 2011-2012 Riceland Foods sales were 1.16 billion, their fifth consecutive year of billion-plus revenue. Between 1995 – 2012 they collected $554,343,039 in subsidies."[457]

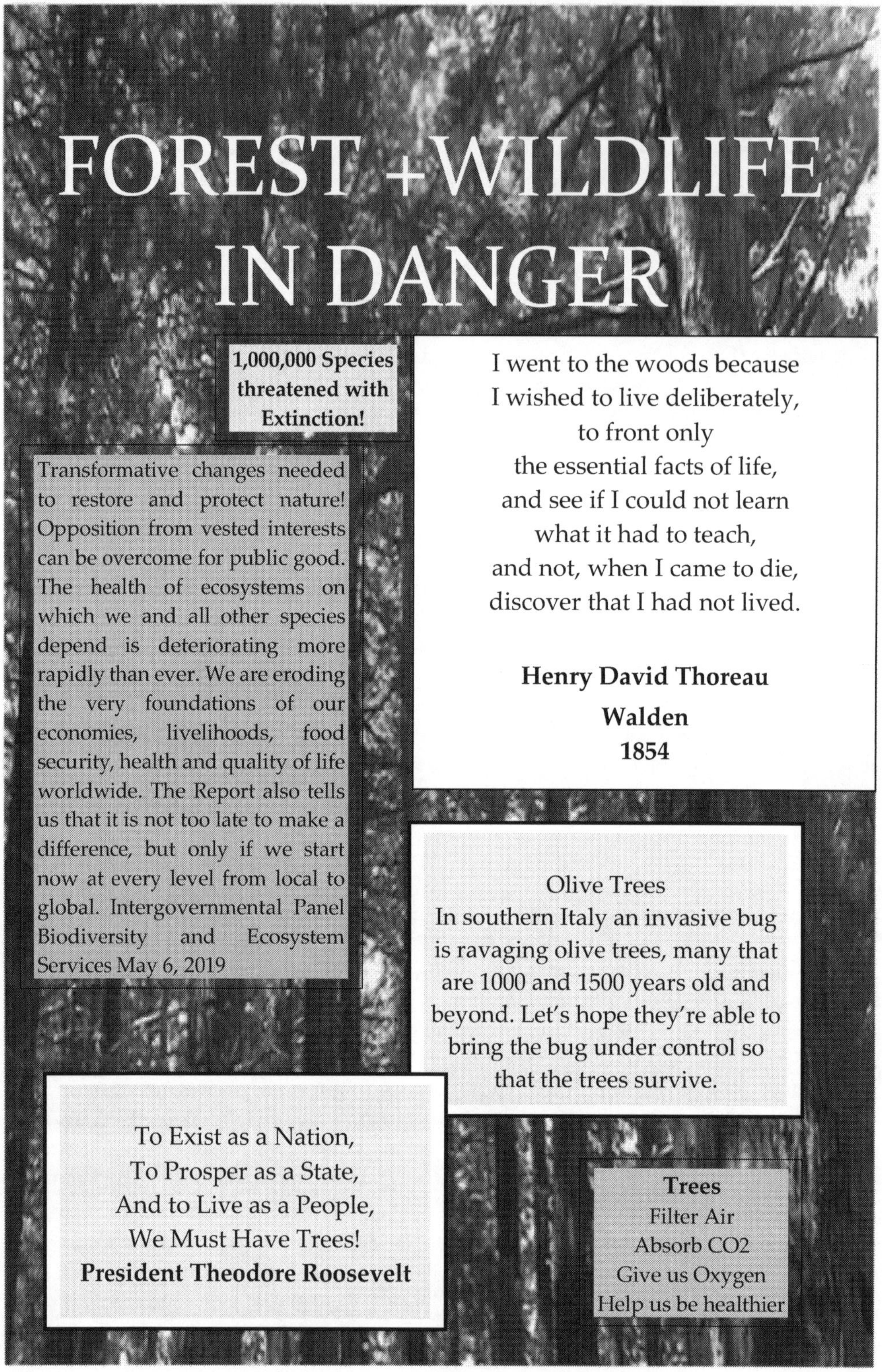

FOREST + WILDLIFE IN DANGER

1,000,000 Species threatened with Extinction!

Transformative changes needed to restore and protect nature! Opposition from vested interests can be overcome for public good. The health of ecosystems on which we and all other species depend is deteriorating more rapidly than ever. We are eroding the very foundations of our economies, livelihoods, food security, health and quality of life worldwide. The Report also tells us that it is not too late to make a difference, but only if we start now at every level from local to global. Intergovernmental Panel Biodiversity and Ecosystem Services May 6, 2019

I went to the woods because
I wished to live deliberately,
to front only
the essential facts of life,
and see if I could not learn
what it had to teach,
and not, when I came to die,
discover that I had not lived.

Henry David Thoreau
Walden
1854

Olive Trees
In southern Italy an invasive bug is ravaging olive trees, many that are 1000 and 1500 years old and beyond. Let's hope they're able to bring the bug under control so that the trees survive.

To Exist as a Nation,
To Prosper as a State,
And to Live as a People,
We Must Have Trees!
President Theodore Roosevelt

Trees
Filter Air
Absorb CO2
Give us Oxygen
Help us be healthier

10. DEFORESTATION

RAINFORESTS + GMOs + CATTLE

While forests are vital for our survival, they continue to be treated as disposable commodities. Forests are home to thousands of species of animals, insects, plant life, and indigenous people. At least since the 1960s tropical rainforests have been targeted for massive clearing and deforestation. Today these trends continue. Annually, deforestation of tropical rainforests costs the world 15% global greenhouse gas emissions. This is more than from all of the cars, trucks and buses worldwide combined![458]

Some of the Forests in Danger[459]:	Cause
▪ Amazon Rainforest, South America	Agriculture, cattle
▪ Atlantic Forest, Brazil, Argentina, Paraguay	Agriculture, cattle
▪ Boreal Forest, Canada	Toilet paper[460]
▪ Borneo and Sumatra Forests, Indonesia	Palm Oil
▪ Cerrado Forest, Brazil	GMO soy, cattle
▪ Choco-Darien, Ecuado, Panama, Columbia	Mining and oil
▪ Tonga's Temperate Rainforest, Alaska	Clearcutting

Rainforests cleared to make room for:

- Grazing cattle
- GMO soy crops

Trees are logged to make:

- Toilet paper, tissues
- Paper
- Fabric (rayon, viscose)
- Cellophane

Effects of Deforestation

- Harm to animals, plants, native people
- Loss of forest habitats, ecosystem imperiled
- Harm to waterways,
- Loss of biodiversity
- Loss of soil carbon

The Soy Moratorium[461]

In 2006 Greenpeace helped show the world that the beef they were eating was raised on soybeans grown on former rainforest land. This led to the Soy moratorium, a pact involving people, industry and government that restricted further deforestation.

SOLUTIONS

- Plant Trees
- Avoid supporting companies whose products conflict with saving forests
- Recycle all things paper: paper and paper bags
- Avoid paper & tissue products from old growth forests or chlorine-bleached
- Soy Moratorium is an example of how we can bring an end to the reckless deforestation caused by Palm Oil.

PALM OIL + EXTINCTION

Trees and forests are essential for human survival. They're here on purpose, they absorb carbon dioxide, and provide us with oxygen. Right now there are forces intent on taking the world's forests down. Over 27 million hectares (almost 68 million acres) of tropical rainforest have already been cleared to make room for palm oil farms.[462] Countless species and native peoples have been forcibly removed in the process and counter on the brink of extinction. Clearing forests is literally a dead end resulting in ghastly releases of greenhouse gas emissions.

PALM OIL'S COST:

- Kills animals, many species are now on the brink of extinction.
- Indigenous and native people inhabitants have been forcibly driven from their lands
- Corporate domination of what that was once precious rainforest ecosystems
- Greenhouse gas emissions: Methane and CO2

ANIMALS FACING EXTINCTION: Sumatran Orangutan, Bornean Orangutan, Sumatran Tiger, Bornean Pygmy Elephant, Sumatran Rhinoceros, Malayan Sun Bear

WHERE IS PALM OIL HIDING?

As a replacement for trans-fat, palm oil is now found in the majority of all supermarket foods! It's found in: biofuels, detergents, soaps, donuts, pastries, biofuels, biscuits, dough, peanut butter, margarine, popcorn, salad dressing, condiments, shampoo, soap, and detergents.

Its secret names include: Palm Oil Kernel, Ealey's genesis, Panmictic Acid, Palmate, Palmitate, Hydrogenated Palm Glycerides Hexadecenoic, Vegetable Oil, Sodium Lauretha Soleplate, Sodium Lauryl Soleplate, Stearate, SDS Sodium, Nards Sodium, Calcium Sterol Lactylate Stearate, Stearate -20 Emulsifier. [463]

Reckless expansion of palm oil has created severe everlasting damage upon our fragile earth. Merciless methods of clearing and burning forests puts animals at risk of extinction and drastically impacts climate change. To make matters worse, most of these forests sit on peatland, which when burned intensifies the amount of methane and carbon dioxide released. This notably reverses the peat's natural role as carbon sink to a role of carbon outputted. When burned the peat releases thousands of years' worth of carbon.

The good news is palm oil farming can be done considerately and sustainably. Support the shift to sustainably grown by becoming aware of the countless products you come across every day that contain palm oil. Where does that palm oil come from? Does that company earth friendly or not? If you care about forests, about protecting animals and the earth, you must stop supporting corporations that contribute to deforestation.

SOLUTIONS

- SEEK SUSTAINABLE PALM OIL OR AVOID IT IN PRODUCTS
- Certified palm oil is grown on land that is not involved with the deforestation
- Every company that uses palm oil, should ONLY use sustainably grown.
- Use healthy oils and fats for cooking: virgin olive oil, unrefined coconut oil, butter, ghee
- We need to create a Palm Oil Moratorium like the Soy Moratorium in 2006 (prior page

FORESTS + FIRE + PESTICIDES

Forests are the allies that we need to combat the effects of our current climate crisis. Without forests our days are numbered. Forests and trees filter pollution, reduce air pollutants, and make it easier for us to live. Instead of days of old when forests maintained themselves naturally, today men insist on managing forests. And how do they do it you ask? Why, with chemicals of course!

'It blows my mind that nobody is talking about this,' said James Steidle, a member of the anti-glyphosate group Stop the Spray B.C."[464]

Researchers from the University of Montana looked at the USDA Forest Service and concluded that in 2010 alone, "1.2 million acres of U.S. federal and tribal wildlands –an area the size of 930,630 football fields was sprayed with 200 tons of herbicides. By far the most commonly used active ingredient was glyphosate –most commonly known to consumers under the brand name Roundup – which is a nonselective herbicide that also kills native grasses and herbs. The U.S. Forest Service, which oversees 193 million acres in the U.S—a quarter of all federal lands declined to share its data on herbicide use. Mike Ielmini, the Forest Service's National Invasive Species Program Manager, told the researchers that he had concerns about his agency's data quality."[465]

The United States is not alone in practicing chemical forestry. In Canada, forests are also targeted. The Canadian Broadcasting Corporation reported in 2018, "It's an annual event — a mass extermination of broadleaf trees mandated by the province. The eradication of trees like aspen + birch on regenerating forest stands is meant to make room for more commercially valuable conifer species like pine and Douglas fir. But experts say it also removes one of the best natural defenses we have against wildfire! When aspen and other broadleaves are allowed to flourish, they form "natural fuel breaks" if their leaves are out, according to Lori Daniels, a professor of forest ecology at the University of B.C. That's why aspen stands are often referred to as "asbestos forests" in wildfire science circles."[466]

Rather than being helpful at all, the use of glyphosate in forests is likely a big factor in the intensity and extent of damage caused by wildfires. As mentioned previously, it's used to intentionally kill young Aspens and Birch trees and other broadleaf species, trees, which serve as a natural fire wall. If that's not bad enough, tree health of those remaining is diminished because the herbicides prevent trees and plants from absorbing and holding water, making them dry as matchsticks. From the Sierra Club: "Glyphosate is a patented desiccant. Its desiccating effects reduce a plant's ability to uptake water. Glyphosate has non-target impacts. Glyphosate use could lead to Sudden Oak Death, Oak Wilt, and a host of Scorch Diseases in which plants can no longer absorb sufficient water and thereby become very flammable. More dry and dead non-target vegetation increases the risk of fire."[467] This is devastating news for not only more risk to habitats results, but wild fires contribute vast amounts of the greenhouse gases and air pollutants: CO2, methane, particulate matter, and nitrous oxide[468]—all crippling climate change instigators. Why are chemicals allowed at all if they can set up forests for failure like this? What people are making these decisions? Back in 2005, whistleblower Doug Parker, who had worked with the USDA Forest Service for over 40 years was fired after reporting misuse of pesticides by Forest Service employees.[469] Why weren't the ones misusing pesticides fired instead?

For anyone who's read *Silent Spring,* this all may sound like deja vu. As is often seen when humans attempt to manage wild places and wild animals, what may have started out with good intentions almost always results in worsened conditions, or people get too much power that they forget the original aim. Read *Sand County Almanac* and *Playing God in Yellowstone* to see what I mean, or read about the USDA's Wildlife Services--a sick branch of government that shouldn't even exist. Regarding the forests, Rachel Carson described an awfully similar situation to what we currently have in the West:

> "This is what happened in some of the western national forests a few years ago, when in 1956 the United States Forest Service sprayed some 885,000 acres of forested lands with DDT. The intention was to control the spruce budworm, but the following summer it was discovered that a problem worse than the budworm damage had been created. In surveying the forests from the air, vast blighted areas could be seen where the magnificent Douglas firs were turning brown and dropping their needles. In the Helena National Forest and on the western slopes of the Big Belt Mountains, then in other areas of Montana and down into Idaho the forests looked as though they had been scorched.
>
> It was evident that this summer of 1957 had brought the most extensive and spectacular infestation of spider mites in history. Almost all of the sprayed area was affected. Nowhere else was the damage evident. Searching for precedents, the foresters could remember other scourges of spider mites, though less dramatic than this one. There had been similar trouble along the Madison River in Yellowstone Park in 1929, in Colorado 20 years later, and then in New Mexico in 1956. Each of these outbreaks had followed forest spraying with insecticides. (The 1929 spraying, occurring before the DDT era, employed lead arsenate). Chemical pest control in the forest is at best a stopgap measure bringing no real solution, at worst killing the fishes in the forest streams, bringing on plagues of insects, and destroying the natural controls and those we may be trying to introduce."[470]

So little has changed. Is the USDA or the chemical industry calling the shots? Is the misuse of herbicides and fungicides also contributing to the spread of tree disease by weakening tree immunity—causing trees to lose their natural resistance to invasive beetles, for instance? Or to white pine blister rust, to aphid infestations, to fungus disease? Is the overuse of these chemicals having an inverse effect by interfering with the beetles' natural predators, in particular killing off birds? Are the massive amounts of herbicides and fungicides used harming soil quality so far as to make the trees not just unable to absorb water, but unable to absorb nutrients as well? This alone no doubt causes sick trees. Without our meddling, would the forests throughout the west be thriving and more fire-resistant today? Nature is after all very capable of surviving on its own, better usually *without* human interference. What on earth are we doing to these majestic places and to the animals that dwell within when we keep using these deadly chemicals?

SOLUTIONS

Help get the pesticides out of our forests before it's too late! www.stopthespraybc.com.

In America urge the USDA Forest Service to cut the use of pesticides in our forest

USDA Forest Service
1400 Independence Ave, SW
Washington, D.C. 20250-1111
Telephone: (800) 832-1355

LAND COVERSION: We're in Critical Times.

Prairies, forests, wetlands, fields, grasslands, public lands, peatlands are all in danger of land grabs and conversion. These irreplaceable ecosystems provide immeasurable benefits to us and to animals: oxygen, water purification, carbon storage, wildlife habitat, peace, and undisturbed oases. Be it for development, cropland, farmland, pasture, palm oil, drilling or fracking—the world cannot afford to lose any more of these irreplaceable open spaces.

Peatlands and Climate change

Peatlands are a type of wetlands which are among the most valuable ecosystems on Earth: they are critical for preserving global biodiversity, provide safe drinking water, minimize flood risk and help address climate change.

Peatlands are the largest natural terrestrial carbon store; the area covered by near natural peatland worldwide (>3 million km^2) sequesters 0.37 gigatonnes of carbon dioxide (CO_2) a year storing more carbon than all other vegetation types in the world combined.

Damaged peatlands are a major source of greenhouse gas emissions, annually releasing almost 6% of global anthropogenic CO_2 emissions. Peatland restoration can therefore bring significant emissions reductions.

Countries are encouraged to include peatland restoration in their commitments to global international agreements, including the Paris Agreement on climate change.

What is the issue?

Peatlands are a type of wetlands that occur in almost every country on Earth, currently covering 3% of the global land surface. The term 'peatland' refers to the peat soil and the wetland habitat growing on its surface.

In these areas, year-round waterlogged conditions slow the process of plant decomposition to such an extent that dead plants accumulate to form peat. Over millennia this material builds up and becomes several metres thick.

Peatland landscapes are varied – from blanket bog landscapes with open, treeless vegetation in the Flow Country of Scotland – a tentative World Heritage site – to swamp forests in Southeast Asia. New areas are still being discovered such as the world's largest tropical peatland discovered beneath the forests of the Congo Basin in 2017.

International Union for Conservation of Nature[471]

www.iucn.org

11. WASTE: PAPER &PLASTIC

PAPER PRODUCTS: Paper products are derived from trees, and too much of it's derived from endangered forests! This is a planetary problem. Trees and forests filter the world's air pollution and they're nature's carbon sinks. When trees and forests are removed to make disposable paper products, humanity and the planet suffer for centuries to come. Right now, the majestic Boreal Forest in northern Canada is being decimated to make toilet paper.[472] This is the world's largest intact forest. What a misuse of resources!

Bleached paper products create yet another problem—dioxin pollution in our waterways. When I worked for Greenpeace in 1989 this was my first campaign —ending chlorine bleaching at the paper mills. Since then paper mills have cleaned up their act somewhat, yet dioxin is a persistent pollutant and remains a big problem. Today you can find advisories against eating fish in many rivers and lakes throughout the country due to dioxin & other persistent pollutants.

PAPER PRODUCTS TO AVOID if from endangered forests or chlorine bleached:

Paper napkins
paper plates
tissue
writing paper
wrapping paper
Paper towels
toilet paper
tissue paper
copy paper

Thank you
Las Vegas MGM
Hotels for banning
plastic straws!!

PLASTIC and FOOD PACKAGING: Plastic is a huge problem, especially when it doesn't get thrown away or recycled. Plastic packaging leads more often than not to litter and pollution in the oceans. Once in the water, plastic gets swallowed by whales, turtles, dolphins, fish, birds and others who mistake it for food. Any animals that eat plastic will suffer starvation and death. Avoid using these:

Straws
plastic cups
plastic lids, caps
plastic water bottles
plastic bags
Styrofoam (polystyrene)
plastic utensils fork, knife, spoon
plastic cups
six pack rings
single use plastic

New York City + Maine
Thank you for banning
Styrofoam in 2019!

SOLUTIONS

- Don't purchase bleached paper products, or those from endangered forests
- Use cloth napkins, handkerchiefs, dish towels, wash cloths
- Use real dishes, metal utensils, reusable cups
- Avoid using single use plastic and Styrofoam
- Be sure to throw garbage away properly, recycle it, or reuse it. Don't be a litterbug.

Let's go big and encourage all companies to reduce their plastic packaging, as well as bleached paper products. Be part of the solution and reduce or ban your own personal use of each. It's going to take practice, we're so used to getting a straw in our drinks, for instance. We have to start somewhere. Next time you're out, just say no straw please, *unless* it's a paper straw from an *un*endangered forest.

FOOD WASTE

So many people throughout the world are hungry, yet we're wasting so much food. We have to find ways to divert food to those who need it. Globally our food waste problem is pretty severe. Key points from the FAO of the United Nations:[473]

- Roughly one third of the food produced in the world for human consumption every year — approximately 1.3 billion tons — gets lost or wasted.
- Food losses and waste amounts to roughly US $680 billion in industrialized countries and US $310 billion in developing countries.
- Fruits and vegetables, plus roots and tubers have the highest wastage rates of food.
- Global quantitative food losses & waste per year are roughly 30% for cereals, 40-50% for root crops, fruits and vegetables, 20% for oil seeds, meat and dairy plus 35% for fish.
- Large quantities of food are wasted due to standards that over-emphasize appearance.

What's lost when food is wasted?

- All the plant, sun, soil energy and resources used to produce the food
- All the water used to grow and produce the food
- All the human energy and labor to produce the food
- All the energy and fuel used to manufacture and transport the food
- All the packaging that has gone into bringing the food to you
- All the nutrients and energy the food had to offer
- The opportunity to nourish and relieve someone's hunger

Where does food go when it's thrown away:

- **Landfills:** Food rotting at landfills emits methane and carbon dioxide. A good solution at landfills: Anaerobic methane digesters that convert methane to usable electricity.
- **Garbage Disposals:** Throwing food down the drain isn't the best solution. It's not good for our water resources, it demands greater water filtration energy, and takes away the food's opportunity to contribute back to hungry people or to the earth
- **Compost:** convert your dated and left-over food scraps. **Benefits of Composting:**.
    - Encourages beneficial soil organisms that break down organic matter
    - Reduces methane emissions and CO2 emissions from landfills
    - Can replace toxic fertilizers, cut nitrous oxide and greenhouse gas emissions,

SOLUTIONS

- Donate extra food to food pantries, homeless shelters, churches, the poor and hungry
- Conserve how much you purchase, increase your awareness of how much you need to prepare meals at home so you only buy what you really need.
- Freeze foods if you can't use them in time, reduce how much gets forgotten & rotten.
- Instead of tossing food scraps in the garbage, start composting them.

SOLUTIONS CLIMATE CRISIS

- We must stop all the nonsense that's put 1,000,000 species on the brink of extinction! There're other ways we can exist, without harming anyone or any species in the process.
- Avoid products containing palm oil derived from sensitive deforested areas
- If we reinvent animal farms, we can make huge strides toward resolving our climate crisis. This will reduce methane, nitrous oxide, ammonia, hydrogen sulfide, as well as water pollution and toxic runoff, acid rain and smog—helping earth heal.
- If we reduce chemicals used in big ag and other farms, we can help habitats, animals, people, pollinators, and ecosystems recover. Let's help farmers make the switch for their health and ours! Fumigants—do we really need them? "More than 200 million pounds of agricultural pesticide-active ingredients are applied to California fields each year, of which more than 40 million pounds are fumigants."[474]
- Move away from GMO corn and soy for farm animals, it increases methane emissions![475]
- Protect & Nurture soil with compost, plant material, cover crops, natural fertilizers
- Help get pesticides and fungicides out of our forests
- Avoid plastic, Styrofoam, and suspicious food packaging
- Avoid bleached paper packaging, products and tissue & those from old-growth forests
- Choose real organic, biodynamic, or IPM foods when and where available
- Eat less meat and when you eat meat, choose humanely-raised products.
- GMO soy & corn grown for animal feed uses excess fertilizer, pesticides and fungicides!
- Factory farm products put us at greater risk for infections that are resistant to antibiotics

Agriculture's contributions to Planetary Harm & Climate Crisis include:

TYPE	Green House Gas (GHG) EMISSIONS,
Big Farming, Industrial Farming	GHG, CO2, Methane, Nitrous Oxide, Loss of Soil Carbon Storage, fungicides, monocropping, synthetic fertilizer, pesticides, fungus resistance, weed resistance
Factory Animal Farming (CAFOs, AFOs)	GHG, Methane, Hydrogen Sulfide, Ammonia, Air and Water pollution, GMO animal feed, nitrous oxide emissions, antibiotic resistance
Palm Oil Farming	GHG, Methane, Deforestation, Lost Carbon Storage
Monocropping	GHG, Deforestation, loss of habitats, lost carbon storage, increased agricultural runoff, fungus resist
Synthetic Fertilizer	GHG, Nitrous Oxide, soil harm, toxic water runoff
Pesticides and Big Ag	GHG, Ozone layer depletion, harms pollinators
Pesticide manufacturing	GHG, toxic air and water pollution
Synthetic fertilizer facilities	GHG, Nitrous oxide, ammonia, SO2, smog
Industrial Ethanol facilities	Carcinogens, Volatile Organic Chemicals
Corn for ethanol in gasoline	GHG, N2O, ethanol in gasoline ups smog,[476]
Food Waste	GHG, Loss of resources, methane, CO2

SOLUTIONS CLIMATE CRISIS

We have the power, every action counts and builds upon another. Maybe through our actions, we'll mobilize great forces of good energy and great people and accomplish tremendous things.

Problem	Action	Results
Pesticides	Ban Fumigants	Helps soil, reduces nitrous oxide
	Restrict Pesticide use	Reduces superweeds, helps bees
	Restrict Fungicide use	Reduces fungal resistance
	Ban Chlorpyrifos	Helps children, protects brains
	Ban neonicotinoids	Helps pollinators and animals
	Reduce use in forests	Helps forests, reduces fire risk
	Ban most toxic pesticides	Reduces toxic runoff, toxic algae
	Limited pesticide use	Improves water, ocean health
	Ban Chlorpyrifos	Helps children, protects brains
GMOs	Reduce, eliminate GMOs	Reduces herbicide use
	Reduce monocropping	Resuscitates land
	Reduce GMO crops	Reduces synthetic fertilizer use
	Reduce synthetic fertilizer	Reduces toxic runoff
	Ban GMO alfalfa	Protects Bees and food supply
	Plant less GMOs	Reduces herbicide + fertilizers
	Ban GMOs in wildlife refuges	Protects animals, pollinators
Industrial Farms	Reduce pesticide use	Helps pollinators, wildlife
	Reduce synthetic fertilizer	Reduces nitrous oxide
	Reduce fungicides	Stops fungicide resistance
	Reduced pesticides, fertilizer	Reduces runoff, acidification
Synthetic Fertilizer	Restrict synthetic fertilizer	Reduces Cancer and N2O
	Reduce use	Soil rebounds, reduces disease
	Reduce use	Improves plant health
	Reduce use	Reduces toxic runoff, red tide
	Reduce use	Curbs toxic algae, dead zones
	Reduce use	Curbs ocean acidification
Factory Farms	Transform, clean up CAFOs	Cleans water, air, helps all life
	Stop daily antibiotic feeding	Curbs antibiotic resistance
	Stop feeding animals soy, corn	Reduces methane, N2O
	Improve conditions for animals	Reduces antibiotic
	Improved manure mngmt	Reduces pollutants, ammonia
		Protects water, reduces runoff
		Improves food safety

SOLUTIONS CLIMATE CRISIS

Soil	Restrict use of synthetic fertilizer	Soil revives, stores carbon
	Stop allowing fumigants	Helps soil microorganisms
	Restrict use of fungicides	Reduces toxic runoff, toxic algae
	Nurture soil, cover, compost	Helps soil, reduces runoff
Forests	Limit, ban pesticides, fungicides	Helps forests recover resilience
Palm Oil	Ban unsustainable palm oil	Helps curb deforestation
Bees +Pollinators	Ban neonicotinoids Restrict, ban GMO alfalfa	Save pollinators and wildlife Saves pollinators and wildlife
Food Waste	Wastes less, compost, donate	Conserves resources, helps soil,
Food Packaging	No more plastic, bleached paper	Prevents pollution
Plastic	Ban Styrofoam worldwide Ban single use plastics	Prevents water pollution Helps oceans recover
Water, Oceans Fish	Don't litter, don't pollute Don't support overfishing	Helps animals + waterways Lets fish populations recover
Litter	Help clean up garbage	Prevents pollution in oceans

The Magic Formula: If we cut the toxins applied to plants, land, soil, as well as those forced unto farm animals, we automatically reduce toxins flowing in runoff, in stormwater, as well as those charging into the atmosphere. Start by reducing synthetic fertilizer and all else gets better. Without question such changes improve our water, air and food which results in reduced exposure to toxins. Do we become healthier? More clear-headed? More at peace? More compassionate and understanding? The planet and animals surely will benefit as will the oceans and forests, and soil microorganisms, kind insects and pollinators. The whole planet could resonate in harmony if we wanted, if we believe. Are we ready to make this happen?

Don't litter, show kids and others that littering is not cool. If you see garbage on the ground on the beach or in parks, anywhere, please help divert it from going in the waterways. Please pick it up and stuff it in the bin so it can get disposed of properly. Then wash your hands.

In other sectors, solutions to curb pollution involve carbon taxes and carbon trading. Considering farming, only modifying the processes can make any true difference. Taxes may incentivize some to cut their emissions, but not necessarily all. What about the other pollutants besides carbon dioxide, are they included in trading or taxes? Only true cutbacks in toxic pollution make a difference. Let's have measurable and effective means starting with no more payouts to Big Ag and the industrial farms using dire amounts of toxic fertilizer and pesticides. Who do these payouts benefit most anyway—the farmers or the chemical companies? These code red times demand a shift in operations ASAP. Government money can be better diverted to people and causes that need it—pollinator protection, climate change prevention, ocean clean up, nourishing school kids, littering education programs, nontoxic food assistance for people in poverty + those less advantaged, protecting animals, back-to-nature programs & urban gardening. I'm sure you have some ideas too, lets pick the best ones and make it happen.

THREE

FOOD PRODUCTION

This country will not be a permanently good place
for any of us to live in unless
we make it a reasonably good place for all of us to live in.
President Theodore Roosevelt

12. ADDITIVES in FOOD

GRAS: *Generally* Recognized as Safe

Food isn't as simple as it used to be. Food is not just grown differently, it's made differently. When we go grocery shopping some of the food going in our cart may come in a can or a box; or at a fast food restaurant it's all wrapped up cozy in a bag for us. Have you ever wondered what's tagging along with these foods? These are processed foods that can contain all sorts of unusual and manmade substances. Anytime we eat processed foods we may be consuming lots of additives made from ingredients that are considered GRAS, "generally recognized as safe." From preservatives to nanoparticles, fats and flavors, what's really in our food?

As the guardian of the food supply, the FDA (Food and Drug Administration) is supposed to be responsible for making sure ingredients in the foods in the U.S. are safe. Yet at this very time there are thousands of additives in foods that have not been tested, some that haven't even been acknowledged, and many that may never be identified on food labels. This breach puts people and animals in harm's way every day.

"A 2016 survey by the Consumer Reports National Research Center found that the term GRAS can be misleading for consumers: 77 percent of respondents believed that 'GRAS' means the FDA has evaluated the ingredient and deemed it to be safe; and 66 percent believed that the agency monitors GRAS ingredients' safety and use. Neither statement is true."

"It's the unknown ingredients—that have never been reported at all, let alone publicly evaluated—that most worry scientists and advocates. Food additives have multiplied exponentially in the past half-century, from a few hundred chemicals to several thousand. They can be found in virtually any processed food—from breakfast cereals and energy drinks to frozen dinners and all manner of snacks."[477]

The GRAS designation is generally a black hole for food ingredients. Originally created in 1958, GRAS was intended for additives that were well known already at that time, and that as minor ingredients didn't necessarily require testing. These were items such as baking soda. Over the years, however the FDA determined that manufacturers and food producers could submit their own safety testing and determine on their own which ingredients qualified for GRAS status. The result is that today we have a significant loss in food transparency with thousands of products in the market place containing ingredients that are unidentified, untested & without labeling.

In 2014 the FDA issued a final rule on GRAS that resulted in little change, however working together we can change this and make our foods safer. It's a no brainer, food manufacturers have to let us know what they're putting in the food! Senator Markey of Massachusetts is on the case, "The health and well-being of the American people depend on a meaningful food safety regulatory policy. The FDA missed an opportunity to strengthen the GRAS process by requiring mandatory reporting of GRAS substances."[478] With our encouragement and persistence though, we can help Congress to push the FDA on this to get the improvements we need. In the meantime, here's a look at what's going in processed foods.

Additives and Preservatives: Mysterious additives and preservatives run the gamut from fungus and antimicrobials to dough conditioners and enzymes derived from pigs' blood. Many of these substances are banned in other countries over health concerns, yet permitted in foods in the U.S. Until the FDA steps up, it's up to us to scout the labels to the best of our ability and avoid the foods/ingredients that harm us. Better yet, make food from scratch with wholesome ingredients. This is a short list of all the many additives out there. If you spot any of these on a label, may be best to avoid them:

- BHA, BHT: a fat preservative, linked to cancerous tumorous growth
- Sodium nitrate: added to processed meats, linked to cancer in humans
- Sodium benzoate: used in carbonated beverages, known carcinogen,
- MSG: causes headaches, linked in to nerve damage, heart problems & seizures
- Disodium guanylate and Disodium inosinate: flavorings, contains MSG
- Propyl gallate: added to fat-containing products, linked to cancer in humans
- Paraben: used to stop mold & yeast, can disrupt hormones, linked to breast cancer
- Polysorbate 60: thickener in baked goods, can cause cancer in laboratory animals
- Camauba wax: used in chewing gum
- Carrageenan: thickening agent, can cause ulcers and cancer
- Chlorine dioxide: used to bleach flour, can cause tumors and hyperactivity in children
- Magnesium sulfate: used in tofu, can cause cancer in laboratory animals
- Potassium bromate: added to flour and breads, linked to cancer in humans
- Brominated vegetable oil (BVO), soft drinks, can cause organ damage & birth defects
- Propyl gallate: found in popcorn, soup mixes, frozen dinners, causes cancer in rats
- Sodium carboxymethyl cellulose: salad dressing thickener, maybe carcinogenic
- *Above & below information source: MPH Programs Advocates for Public Health Education*[479]

Artificial Colors: Studies involving artificial colors and dyes have demonstrated a connection to asthma, behavioral issues, hyperactivity and cancer. Eliminating these things from your diet may result in favorable changes to your health. "Food manufacturers still use plant-based colorings in some countries. For example, in the United Kingdom *Fanta* orange soda is colored with pumpkin and carrot extracts, while the U.S. version uses Red 40 and Yellow 6. McDonald's strawberry sundaes are colored only with strawberries in Britain, but Red 40 is used in the United States."[480] What's the deal with that? Most synthetic dyes are derived from crude oil.[481]

- Red #40: linked to cancer in some studies, can cause hyperactivity
- Blue #1: in candy, bakery goods, soft drinks, can damage chromosomes and lead to cancer
- Blue #2: in candy and pet foods, can cause brain tumors
- Citrus red #1: sprayed on oranges to make, can damage chromosomes and lead to cancer
- Citrus red #2: used to color oranges, can cause cancer if you eat the peel
- Green #3: used in candy and beverages, may cause bladder tumors
- Yellow #6: used in sausage, beverages, baked goods, carcinogen, may cause kidney tumors
- Red #2: may cause asthma and cancer
- Red #3: cherry pie filling, desserts, carcinogen, may cause nerve damage, thyroid cancer
- Caramel coloring: soft drinks, sauces, bread, when made with ammonia can cause cancer
- Brown HT: used in many packaged goods, can cause hyperactivity, asthma, cancer

- Orange B: hot dog and pork casings, high doses bad for liver and bile duct
- Bixin: causes hyperactivity and asthma
- Norbixin: causes hyperactivity and asthma
- Annatto: causes hyperactivity and asthma

Artificial and *Natural* Flavors: If you see "Natural flavors" on an ingredient label it's a red flag. This term is a random designation the FDA allows and companies use to avoid listing "chemicals" on an ingredient label. Flavor companies develop flavors and fragrances from a variety of chemicals to taste or smell like something real and natural. GRAS is such an unregulated area that when you see "natural flavors" on a label it could represent a couple chemicals or hundreds of them. FDA rules as they exist do not require manufacturers to disclose what GRAS ingredients or chemicals may be present. You'll find the term "natural flavors" not just on food and beverage labels but also e-cigarettes, candy, cured meats, etc.

Artificial Sweeteners: In a world that encourages transparency, sugar and artificial sweeteners fail time and time again. Artificial sweeteners can affect your health and may indeed be behind many of the diseases, attention disorders, and weight issues we see today. Avoiding these little monsters can be tricky since they are hidden in many foods and beverages, and they're not always identified on the label. As reported in Time magazine, "Unlike fats, which are broken down into saturated, trans and cholesterol on nutrition labels, sugars are listed in one sweet lump, combining both naturally occurring forms such as sucrose (sugar cane), fructose (from fruit) and dextrose (from corn) as well as the lower calorie substitutes like aspartame, saccharin, sucralose (Splenda), (Truvia), acesulfame potassium (Sunett, Sweet One, Ace K), neotame (Newtame) and Advantame. To find the latter agents, you'll have to hunt in the lengthy list of ingredients on the label."[482]

- **Aspartame** is a neurotoxin[483] causes brain tumors, seizures, and much more[484]
- **Fructose** is a natural fruit sugar, however when it appears without the fruit its sweetness is nonnutritive. Pure fructose is the sweetest of all sugars.[485]
- **High Fructose Corn Syrup, HFCS** is a potent unnatural sugar that overloads the liver and causes heaps of problems for our hearts and arteries.[486] Hidden in soft drinks, protein drinks, condiments, salad dressings, and countless foods, high fructose corn syrup is everywhere. According to Dr. Mark Hyman[487], the average person consumes 20 teaspoons a day! This contributes to nonalcoholic fatty liver disease, diabetes, steatohepatitis, cirrhosis, obesity, bowel cancer & tumors[488]--overall not a good health forecast. HFCS may also contain mercury[489] and influence drug addiction and delay recovery.[490] Free yourself from foods containing this unnatural ingredient.

  When my mom was spending her final days in the hospital, she wasn't able to hold anything down, so the hospital provided her with Ensure. Little did we know that it contained HFCS and probably hastened her death. Today, cancer organizations advise cancer patients to avoid these hyped-up drinks loaded with HFCS: "Ensure and Boost, the two most popular liquid nutritional supplements recommended to cancer patients, may worsen their situation due to certain ingredients they contain."[491] Additional worries accompany the fact that corn syrup production facilities emit significant levels of toxic air pollution linked with learning disabilities, disease and cancer.[492] The fact is no company needs to include this ingredient in their product. It's only used instead of sugar to save a few pennies & increase company profits. What does it cost us in exchange?

- **Neotame:** This newer sugar substitute is derived from aspartame and added to numerous foods and animal feed. Neotame blocks the production of phenylalanine,[493] and it breaks down into formaldehyde after ingestion, yet the FDA approved it! "Neotame is sold under the brand name Newtame and is approximately 7000 to 13,000 times sweeter than table sugar. Advantame is a similar substitute approved for use as a non-nutritive sweetener."[494]
- **Sucralose:** *Splenda* is sucralose, it contains chlorine and is technically a pesticide. It can cause migraines, blurred vision, weight gain, increased blood sugar,[495] and affects the gut microbiome.[496] According to Diabetes Daily, Splenda causes organ damage and shrinks the thymus gland by 40%.[497] In studies with animals, researchers found "Splenda may play a role in certain cancers. Researchers found a higher incidence of Leukemia, and greater incidence of malignant cancers with consumption of Splenda."[498]
- **Saccharin:** Saccharin is used in many diet and sugar-free foods and beverages. It's found in *Sweet and Low*. Studies reveal, "Saccharin is carcinogenic for the urinary bladder in rats and mice, and most likely is carcinogenic in human beings."[499] Because of saccharin's danger, in 1977 labeling was enforced for any product containing it. The Saccharin Labeling Act of 1977 (Sen Ted Kennedy) was signed into law on November 23, 1977 by President Jimmy Carter. USE OF THIS PRODUCT MAY BE HAZARDOUS TO YOUR HEALTH. THIS PRODUCT CONTAINS SACCHARIN WHICH HAS BEEN DETERMINED TO CAUSE CANCER IN LABORATORY ANIMALS.[500] The Saccharin law was repealed in 2000.
- **Truvia** is an artificial sweetener that's marketed as derived from stevia, though it is not. Real stevia is a plant made by nature. Truvia is a combination of chemicals--only one of its ingredients, rebiana,[501] is from stevia. Truvia and similar stevia-based sweeteners only contain rebiana combined with other ingredients. Stick with unrefined, unprocessed Stevia, it's a real plant, nontoxic, and has health benefits.

Nanoparticles have also entered our food supply without testing or labeling, and they're in thousands of products! Yet there's no regulation or actual record of just how many products might contain them! They're added to medicines, cleaning products, sunscreen sprays, lotions, toothpaste, cosmetics, supplements and clothing, as well as food packaging! Virtually there are multiple ways we can be exposed. According to the U.S. Government Accountability Office, "FDA's approach to regulating nanotechnology allows engineered nanomaterials to enter the food supply as GRAS substances without FDA's knowledge."[502] Nanoparticles that we know of: Titanium Dioxide, Iron Oxide, Gold, Silver, Nickel, Silicate, Copper, Platinum Cobalt.

SOLUTIONS

- Avoid processed and suspect foods, read labels
- Go old school, grow your own food and buy from local, small producers when possible.
- Make your own foods from scratch with wholesome, untainted ingredients
- Food-making companies: Please replace HFCS in your products with real & safe sugar

13. FATS & OILS

Traditionally our grandparents and people of generations gone by grew up on animal fats, like butter and lard, and traditional olive oil. Somewhere along the line people were led to believe that they needed to use vegetable oils instead, yet many of these fats and oils can be suspect. Your best bet is to opt for expeller or cold pressed, unrefined, organically grown oils. **Beware of:**

- **Canola oil** (1985 FDA granted GRAS status) is said to be good for the heart though there are concerns that it's really a genetically engineered version of rapeseed oil. Rapeseed oil was banned by the FDA in 1956 because it had high levels of euric acid that caused damage to the heart and high levels of glucosinolates that prevented iodine absorption.[503] If you use it look for organic expeller-pressed or pure press brands that won't include solvents like hexane.
- **Palm oil** is farmed recklessly causing catastrophic damage to the planet, and while for health reasons it should only be consumed moderately, it's found in thousands of products. Do you know how much palm oil you eat everyday? It's disguised as Palm Oil Kernel, Elaeis gunieensis, Palmicitic Acid, Palmate, Palmitate, Hydrogenated Palm Gylcerides Hexadecanoic, Vegetable Oil, Sodium Laureth or Lauryl Sulphate, Steareth, SDS Sodium, NaDS Sodium, Calcium Stearoyl Lactylate Steareth, Steareth -20 Emulsifier."[504] Palm oil is high in saturated fat and increased intake is linked with: higher mortality from heart disease, increased cholesterol levels, and cardiovascular disease.[505] Palm oil use skyrocketed when health effects of partially hydrogenated oils became well known.
- **Partially Hydrogenated Oils** (hardened fats like shortening) went through a popular era but are largely being removed from products due to the trans fat damage they inflict, such as high cholesterol, heart disease, diabetes and stroke.
- **Interesterified Fats** are replacing Trans Fat yet the verdict is still out on their safety. Like partially hydrogenated, they're vegetable oils infused with hydrogen.
- **Trans Fat**: These fats occur naturally in some foods, but the trans-fat of concern is manufactured. It's the worst type of fat you can eat according to the Mayo Clinic[506]. In 2013, trans fats were removed from the GRAS list of substances allowed in food. While many manufacturers have cut back or replaced trans fat, it is still found in some foods.

  BEWARE: Trans Fat, Trans Fatty Acids, otherwise known as partially hydrogenated oil--these can be found in many foods including: doughnuts, fried foods, shortening, margarine, pie crusts, pizza dough, biscuits, cakes. Usually transfat will be identified on labels, *unless* contents are less than .5 grams in which case labeling is *not* required. Eating trans fats can increase risk of heart disease, raise bad cholesterol (LDL), and lower good cholesterol (HDL).[507]

SOLUTIONS

Use healthy fats when cooking at home such as virgin olive oil, unrefined coconut oil, butter (rBGH free) and ghee (rBGH free), lard or tallow (from humanely-raised animals).

14. PROCESSED FOOD

You may hear of processed food a lot, but what does it mean? Processed food in general is food that's strayed from its natural origins—food that has been manipulated in some way by people, at a facility and repackaged to be sold to restaurants or grocery stores.

"According to the United States Department of Agriculture (USDA), processed food is defined as any raw agricultural commodity that has been subject to washing, cleaning, milling, cutting, chopping, heating, pasteurizing, blanching, cooking, canning, freezing, drying, dehydrating, mixing, packaging, or other procedures that alter the food from its natural state. This may include the addition of other ingredients to the food, such as preservatives, flavors, nutrients and other food additives or substances approved for use in food products, such as salt, sugars and fats."[508]

Processed food can be synonymous with junk food, food that has been stripped of its nutrients and native identity. Once stripped of nutrients the food can no longer offer us much other than simple sugar, carbs and potentially, fat.

Some examples:

- Corn gets shaved off the cob and converted with chemicals into corn syrup
- Wheat gets stripped of its bran and germ and transformed into white flour
- Sugar cane gets the life boiled out to become refined white sugar.

These refined foods then get turned into millions of products we see at fast food restaurants, on grocery store shelves, and candy aisles. Instead of building health, when we eat foods like this our bodies absorb calories composed of sugar and empty carbohydrates rather than nutrients. This isn't the best quality fuel for our bodies or minds. If you eat mostly processed foods, you may be setting the stage for disease rather than optimum health. Unfortunately, it seems the government is backing processed food over health. "Government-issued payments *(subsidies)* have skewed agricultural markets toward the overproduction of commodities that are the basic ingredients of processed, energy-dense foods."[509]

Of all processed foods, minimally processed foods are the closest to keeping food in its natural state. As the Academy of Nutrition and Dietetics confirms, "anytime we cook, bake, or prepare food, we're processing food."[510] How we do it and the methods of preparation make all the difference.

Meats can also be found in the processed food category. Meat that is raw, fresh and at the butcher shop is barely processed. Deli meats and packaged meats like hot dogs and bacon, on the other hand are processed extensively. Many meats sealed in plastic have added nitrates—unless the company is using natural aging techniques. Few companies today use the old methods to age meat, though because it takes too much time. While the nitrate commonly found in vegetables is useful for our bodies, in meat nitrates transform into nitrosamines. Therein lies the problem, for nitrosamines are carcinogenic.

NITRATES + NITRITES IN MEAT

Nitrates added to meat form nitrosamines. "Nitrosamines are carcinogenic in more than twenty different animal species, and no species has been found to be resistant."[511]

These substances are typically not present in natural foods and vegetables containing nitrate, but rather form in manufactured foods due to a reaction of additives.

"The typical pink-red color of cured meat is due to the interation of nitrite, formed by the reduction of nitrate, with myoglobin—a muscle protein related to the blood pigment hemoglobin—to form colored derivatives.

Nitrate has a general anti-bacterial action, besides being particularly effective in inhibiting the outgrowth of spores of Clostridium botulinum...Over the years, the meat packing and processing industries have found that certain nitrate/nitrite ratios were ideal for preserving meat and also producing the reddish color which consumers have grown to expect as visual proof of so-called "freshness." As the necessity for preservation has diminished, largely owing to modern refrigeration methods, the "cosmetic" use of nitrite has assumed greater importance to the meat industry.

Nitrosamines have been found in many different meat and fish products, as expected from the content of natural constituent amines and nitrite food additives. The highest concentrations of nitrosamines in food are found in cooked bacon. Nitrosamine carcinogens have also been found in various other foods such as cheese, salami, hotdogs, nitrate cured fish." Nitrosamine formation in food can largely be avoided by banning the use of nitrate as a food additive. Whenever feasible nitrite should be replaced by other effective preservatives, including common table salt." Dr. Samuel Epstein, *The Politics of Cancer*

Health Effects: NDMA (*N*-nitrosodimethylamine) is a potent carcinogen that can induce malignant tumors in the liver, lung, stomach,[512] and lymph system.[513]

Back in the 1977 when nitrosamines were first linked with cancer, the FDA and USDA were on the brink of banning the use of nitrates in meat. They gave the meat industry 3 months to prove nitrates didn't cause harm. That's when the meat lobby stepped up and declared the ridiculous—that nitrates were necessary! If bacon was made without it they predicted scores of people would die from botulism! As Guillaime Coudray explains in his recent expose on the meat industry, *Cochonneries,* that is utter bullshit. As reported in the Guardian, Coudray reveals "Any time someone eats bacon, ham or other processed meat, their gut receives a dose of nitrosamines, which damage the cells in the lining of the bowel, and can lead to cancer."[514] Yet despite all the trouble they cause, nitrates remain in use to this day. Unless we act, things won't change.

SOLUTIONS

- Protect your health by eating less processed foods
- Opt for homemade wholesome foods made with untainted ingredients.
- Cut back on bacon and packaged meats containing nitrates.
- Source uncured bacon, without nitrates. Canadian bacon is leaner & from pork loin.
- Mini Subnote: When I was writing an article about nitrosamines in cosmetics back in 2006, of course I wanted to quote Dr. Epstein's research. He invited me to visit him at his office at the University of Illinois. What an honor it was to meet him personally. He inspired me so much and strongly encouraged me to finish this book. I only wish he was still here to see it.

15. Refined Flour

Modern wheat: is this the source for many untold health issues? Though not genetically engineered, wheat in the U.S. has been bred to be different than wheat from the old country. It seems to be linked with an increasing surge of gastrointestinal and digestive troubles like celiac disease that have been occurring since 1950.[515]

Are these diseases related to wheat consumption occurring because of reactions to the plant itself, or is the process of growing wheat the source of the problem? Could it be related to soil health and fertilizers? It's common practice today for glyphosate to be applied to wheat as a preharvest treatment. Most wheat then, whether whole, or turned into white flour has been doused with glyphosate. Could this have something to do with it, after all it's well known that glyphosate disrupts the microorganisms in our stomach. Research indicates the presence of this herbicide contributes to and worsens gastrointestinal diseases, including gluten intolerance and celiac disease.[516] In celiac, the villi of the intestine are attacked when gluten is ingested[517], the villi are responsible for absorbing nutrients from foods being digested. Are the missing villi a result of the disturbance caused by glypohosate? In any case, without villi present, inflammation and havoc result when certain foods are eaten, preventing nutrient absorption—leading then to mineral and vitamin deficiencies.[518]

According to Dr. William Davis, author of *Wheat Belly,* wheat as we know it not only causes digestive disturbances but also more dramatic increases in blood sugar *than any other food,* including table sugar! It's also a major appetite stimulant making us continually hungry![519]

Diseases that can be associated with modern wheat include increased blood sugar and diabetes, Irritable bowel syndrome (IBD), Colitis, Crohn's Disease, Leaky Gut syndrome, Obesity, Gluten Intolerance, Symptoms can also include migraines.[520]

Since wheat is desiccated with glyphosate, lets add symptoms caused by exposure to glyphosate:

- "Glyphosate kills bacteria in the gut, and the gastrointestinal system is 80% of the immune system" (page 14)
- Disturbs good gut bacteria, enables bacteria to seep through intestinal wall
- Chelates and interferes with absorption of minerals,
- Causes anxiety, despair feelings, depression
- Glyphosate is an endocrine disruptor
- Glyphosate-based herbicides inhibit thyroid function
- Glyphosate impairs the liver's ability to detoxify xenobiotics
  (these points are outlined earlier page 13, 14, 32, 33)

As seen from the above list of symptoms caused by each, wheat when combined with glyphosate has the capacity to cause extraordinary debilitating symptoms. This surely calls for more in-depth studies and examination. If you are one who suffers with gastrointestinal problems, depression, anxiety, headaches, stress, diabetes, endocrine and thyroid issues you may want to avoid conventionally grown wheat and any food products containing it or glyphosate.

What is Refined Flour? Refined flour is the ghost of what remains of the wheat plant after its been stripped of all nutrients and wholeness. It offers our bodies no nutritional value. Only whole grains have nutrients in tact. This tale from *Sugar Blues* demonstrates the process and reveals what happened when whole rice suffered the same fate.

"Shortly after the perfection of machines for the ultimate refinement of sugar and flour, a German invention, the Engelberg machine, was patented. Each grain was stripped of its intermediate and inner shells. As with wheat grain and sugar cane, precious nutrients and minerals were removed; little was left but the pure white hydrate of carbon core. Suddenly, the food from the East had been made fit for the delicate palates and refined appetites of the West. Polished rice was introduced to the West as rice. The entire word was appropriated to describe what actually were the leavings. In French, white rice is *riz*. Unpolished, complete rice is *riz complêt*. Rice may have been an exotic delicacy in the West; in the East, it had been the principal food for centuries. The process of moving from whole grains through the various stages of ground meals had taken several centuries in the west, thus biological deterioration of the people was gradual. However, such deterioration was visited upon the Orient very rapidly. Polished white rice was new, modern, refined, and civilized. It was accepted wherever modernization was vogue. In its wake, it brought sudden outbreaks of new symptoms. Eventually these new symptoms were labeled *beriberi*, after the Senegalese word for weakness. When the outbreaks of beriberi followed the introduction of white rice into Japan, the common people frequently realized what the solution was. Traditional habits, fortunately still fresh in their memory, told them to go back to eating old-fashioned, complete rice. When they did, all was well. Eating whole rice, they became whole and healthy again."[521]

- **Bromated Flour:** This is refined flour with potassium bromate added. Bromated flour is banned in the EU, China, Canada and Brazil because it is causes cancer in the kidneys and thyroid cancer in animals[522]. In the US, however, it still exists no problem. It's used because of its quick performance that increases elasticity and rising capacity of bread dough and baked goods. Beware of bread, baked goods, crackers, dough, anything that contains it!
- **Bleached Flour:** This is refined flour exposed to chlorine. The EPA considers chlorine dioxide an EHS[523] (Extremely Hazardous Substance), yet allows its use for making flour whiter, as well as bleaching paper and for use in municipal water supplies. During the bleaching process, chlorine reacts with proteins in the flour to create Alloxan. Alloxan's only use is in medical research—to create diabetes in animals![524] Does alloxan in bleached wheat flour products help explain the surge in diabetes, heart disease, and strokes?[525]
- **Enriched Flour:** synthetic nutrients added to refined flour that was once whole grain.

SOLUTIONS

- Going off wheat, barley and rye—the gluten-containing grains can help your body heal. Avoiding anything containing glyphosate can help as well.
- Avoid consumption of refined, bromated or bleached flour
- Seek whole grains like brown rice, amaranth, millet, quinoa instead. If you like bread find a good baker or learn the art of baking your own bread. Sourdough can be tolerated better than other commercial breads.
- There are lots of delicious foods to eat besides those containing wheat: Eggs, brown rice, fresh smoothies made with kombucha and yogurt, flax seed bread with coconut flour.
- Avoid fried foods, margarine, and easy on the caffeine.[526]

16. Refined Sugar

Perhaps more than any other food, refined white sugar, sucrose, is public enemy #1—quite possibly the original source of many of our diseases. Perhaps now, high fructose corn syrup is as troublesome. Every good thing about the plant, sugar cane or sugar beet is refined out so nothing is left except high octane sugar. Glucose and sucrose are two very different types of sugar. Our bodies make glucose from natural foods we eat and then uses that sugar for energy.

Overuse of refined sugar leads to imbalance, particularly of the endocrine system—the control center for your body's hormones. The glands of the endocrine system include: the pituitary, thyroid, parathyroid, adrenal, pancreas, ovaries (females), and testicles (males).[527] If you eat a lot of refined sugar daily, you're setting yourself up for hormone imbalance,[528] moodiness, stress & irritability for starters. Double whammy if the foods you're eating also contain endocrine disrupting substances. As this book points out—Many foods today contain endocrine disruptors.

My own healing journey began nearly 30 years ago because of one book—the miraculous eye-opening *Sugar Blues* by William Dufty. This book provides a treasure chest of information that may be helpful to you, especially if you have any type of ailment or disease that's left you stumped. Here are a few highlights from the book:

"Refined sugar is lethal when ingested by humans because it provides only that which nutritionists describe as empty or naked calories. In addition, sugar is worse than nothing because it drains and leeches the body of precious vitamins and minerals through the demand its digestion, detoxification, and elimination make upon one's entire system. Sugar taken everyday produces a continuously over acid condition, and more & more minerals are required from deep in the body in the attempt to rectify the imbalance. In order to protect the blood, so much calcium is taken from the bones and teeth that decay and general weakening begin."

"People have been bamboozled into thinking of their bodies the way they think of their checking accounts. If they suspect they have low blood sugar, they are programmed to snack on candies and sodas in order to raise their blood sugar level. Get it up. Actually, this is the worst thing to do. The level of *glucose* in their blood is apt to be low because they are addicted to sucrose. People who kick sucrose addiction and stay off sucrose find that the glucose level of their blood returns to normal and stays there."[529]

Diseases caused by over consumption of refined white sugar include: stomach ulcers, diabetes mellitus, low blood glucose, hypoglycemia, mineral deficiency, poor digestion, gastrointestinal disorders, psychological disorders, memory disorders, pellagra, skin disorders, hyperactivity, delinquency, fatigue, nervousness, depression, apprehension, craving for sweets, inability to handle alcohol, inability to concentrate, allergies, cancer, low blood pressure, and may contribute to predisposition to drug addiction, alcoholism, schizophrenia, tuberculosis[530]

SOLUTIONS

- Keep away from refined white sugar and high fructose corn syrup—both are hidden in many processed foods, condiments, beverages. Sugar's also in many brands of cigarettes.[531]
- Refined sugar can be hidden under "carbohydrate" on food labels. To avoid it, make sure labels say, "no sugar added." Replace refined sugar with raw honey, molasses, or turbinado.

17. FOOD SAFETY

Over 95% of all farm animals in the US are raised on factory farms."[532] The conditions at factory farms are beyond despicable, animals are deprived of sunlight, exercise, fresh air, they're crowded and cooped up their entire lives in tiny cages not fit for any creature. They're fed gmos, manure, carcasses of dead and diseased animals;[533] you name it, as well as provided daily doses of synthetic hormones and antibiotics giving rise to ARB, antibiotic-resistant bacteria. These conditions surely give rise to contaminated meat products.

FOOD RECALLS: It's not just meat that we have to be concerned with, but many other foods have been the source of scandal: romaine lettuce, chicken strips, flour, tomatoes, eggs, cookies, ice cream, peanuts, ground beef, ground turkey, tahini, the list goes on and on[534]. What is happening to make these foods recall-worthy? Is manure and waste from factory farms contaminating food? Overwhelmingly we're importing more and more foods, yet "the U.S. Government Accountability Office, says the FDA is simply not up to the task of ensuring the safety of food imports."[535] That means we must be vigilant and do what we can to protect ourselves from food contaminants.

At a time when ARB and food recalls are spiking, the number of food inspectors should be increasing! Instead, President Trump as of May of 2019 cut the number of federal inspectors at pork facilities by 40%![536] Rather than inspectors, plant employees will bear the responsibility for ensuring the meat is safe and uncontaminated.

In 2018 the USDA decided to allow poultry slaughterhouses to speed up their lines from 140 birds per minute to 175 birds per minute.[537] That doesn't even allow 1 full second to inspect a bird. Along with the new changes for the pork industry, the USDA is permitting unlimited speeds for pork slaughter lines. In what world could such changes be a good idea?

According to PIRG (Public Interest Research Group) "between 2013 and 2017 there was an 83% increase in the most hazardous meat and poultry recalls known as Class 1. These recalls are most likely to cause a health hazard or death."[538] Was this a result of the HAACP (Hazard Analysis and Critical Control Point) integration that began in 1998? While HAACP should've improved the process, it actually shifted control away from inspectors and to the processing plants. Instead of inspecting meat first hand, the inspectors are generally pushed aside.[539]

At cattle slaughter houses, there's more troubling news. In 2004, Dr. Lester Friedlander, veterinarian and federal inspector got fed up with the system and spoke to the Winnipeg Free Press about what can end up in meat, "Hormones, antibiotics, hair, feces, cancers, tumors. My plant in Pennsylvania processed 1,800 cows a day, 220 per hour. It also processed the highest number of downed cows[540], 25 to 30 a day... There is no question. Some cancers end up in the human food source." Inspectors and handlers are encouraged to look the other way if they notice anything that should be flagged. The reason, stopping the line cost the plant $5000 per minute.[541] Friedlander and Dr. Kellosalmi, founder of The Responsible Animal Care Society predicted further danger related to factory farms, "They will be the breeding ground for the next global human pandemic. Already, the feeding of cattle offal to cattle has spiked an enormous increase in brain-wasting BSE in beef herds and Creutzfeldt-Jakob disease in humans. Even more worrying is that Nobel Prize winner Dr. Stanley Prussiner, who discovered prions, the aberrant protein that triggers BSE and CJD, now believes prions may also cause Alzheimer's disease. Dr. Kellosalmi says the number of Alzheimer's deaths in the U.S. has spiked from 800 in 1979-80 to 50,000 in 2002."[542] The prion link continues to gain evidence in 2019.[543]

From 1906 to 2019 we've nearly come full circle. Due to Upton Sinclair's *The Jungle* in 1904 and the increased public awareness of the unsanitary conditions at meat packing facilities, President Theodore Roosevelt created the country's national meat inspection system. "The Federal Meat Inspection Act of 1906 (P.L. 59-242) and the Wholesome Meat Act of 1967 (P.L. 90-201) were designed and implemented to provide the public with a safe, wholesome meat supply. Today's consumer relies on the Food Safety and Inspection Service (FSIS) inspectors to ensure this."[544]

Without sufficient meat inspections are we falling back to times reminiscent of *The Jungle*? The beforementioned PIRG Report points out, "The current, convoluted system splits primary responsibility for different foods between the USDA's Food Safety and Inspection Service and the FDA. This has caused inconsistent oversight, ineffective coordination and inefficient use of resources." If only Harvey Wiley[545] was here today to get the FDA and USDA in order!

PARASITES: These little buggers are more common than you might think.

- Vegetables and other foods can be contaminated with parasites from manure,
- Water-based plants like watercress can be contaminated with microscopic eggs & worms.[546]
- Food handled improperly due to unsanitary conditions can expose us to parasites.
- Contaminated water can also be a source of exposure.
- Raw fish: Fish can be infected with parasites and worms.[547] Unless the fish is frozen first at a deep enough temp for at least 7 days we can be affected by these critters. Some worms are resistant to freezing,[548] but cooking at high heat may do the trick.[549]

Washing and rinsing foods before eating is the best method for making sure your vegetables and fruits are clean. Perhaps the most thorough method is one I learned during my college internship. In preparing meals, we gave foods a long soak in a deep bowl of water before rinsing them. This allows dirt and other particles to release more easily.

SOLUTIONS Food Recall Chart at back of book, page 189-192.

- Be mindful of where your meat comes from.
- Wash off, rinse and soak your vegetables thoroughly before preparing
- Avoid Bacteria and Parasites by:
  1. Rinsing foods adequately
  2. Wash hands, surfaces, knives, cutting boards, utensils often with soap and water
  3. Don't cross contaminate—keep raw meats and other food items separated
  4. Freeze fish for at least 7 days at -4 degrees Fahrenheit[550]
  5. Cook meat to adequate temperatures:
     - Ground beef 160 degrees; poultry 165 degrees; hams 165 degrees
     - Seafood 145 degrees, shellfish til shell opens
     - Eggs 160 degrees; raw beef, lamb, pork, steaks, chops 145 degrees
     - Heat leftovers to 165 degrees

18. MOLDS in FOOD

Molds are a part of this world, but when we ingest them they can cause toxicity issues and problems for our liver. Continued exposure may set us up for more serious diseases down the road. The late Hulda Clark[551] explained molds in foods and how to combat them in her book, *The Cure for All Diseases*. Here is a brief summary of some of the information she shared:

- **Aflatoxin is a potent toxin, carcinogen and immune-suppressant:** It's very common in store bought bread wrapped in plastic. Don't salvage moldy foods or eat what you think may be safe parts; throw them away. Suggests removing any moldy fruit from the fridge, as these spores can spread. Get fresh baked bread or bake your own. To prevent mold add a little vitamin c powder to the dough when you're preparing it. Keep vitamin C powder in a salt shaker, put it in everything possible. When cooking pasta or rice, sprinkle some in the water. Put some in your honey jar. Maple syrup can also be affected. To cure, heat to almost boiling, add vitamin C. Then rebottle & keep in the fridge.
- **Ergot** is another food mold often contaminating grains, cereals, nuts and nut butters, wine and honey. Ergot can trigger abnormal behavior and anger, temper tantrums, cruelty, saying mean things, expressing irrational thoughts. To test whether ergot is causing issues, go off grains, cereals, soy sauce, and other grain-derived ingredients. Also avoid alcohol, which makes symptoms of ergot toxicity worse. Go off cold cereals, store bought bread, nut butters, anything that could be contaminated. Eat cooked cereals instead, but be sure to add vitamin c, fresh baked bread is safe, or make your own but don't put it in a plastic bag. Adding vitamin c powder to pasta and rice and everything you make will help nullify toxins.
- **T2 Toxin** is attributed to high blood pressure and kidney disease. It can be found on dried beans and peas, but easily removed by soaking beans in water with vitamin c powder for at least 5 minutes. Throw away any imperfect peas or beans.
- **Kojic Acid** is a mycotoxin, harms pancreas and disables body's ability to detoxify wood alcohol. It can be found in potatoes; peel potatoes and remove any gray parts.
- **Sorghum Molds** are present in sorghum and millet. Avoid sorghum syrup. Rinse millet in vitamin c water before cooking. These toxins cause inability to swallow, appetite loss, hemorrhaging can show up as strokes and purple blotches on skin.
- **Patulin, Fruit mold:** Present in bruised fruits. This mold is dangerous, it can grow in your intestine. Where it grows, shigella and E. Coli can pass through the colon wall to invade your body. Don't eat bruised or moldy fruit, avoid soft mushy fruits. Black walnut Hull will kill these fungi. Be meticulous and avoid getting reinfected.

SOLUTIONS

- Don't eat moldy foods. Add vitamin C powder when cooking grains or baking bread
- Soak foods in vitamin c water, add Vit C to honey and syrups, avoid bruised fruit
- Keep fresh bread stored in a cloth or paper bread bag & tightly sealed
- Cut out dark patches on fruits, veges and potatoes.

19. LABELING

We have some interesting food labeling rules in the U.S. GMO labeling was finally, *sort of* approved in 2016. The National Bioengineered Food Disclosure Law, passed by Congress in July of 2016, directed the USDA to establish a national mandatory standard for disclosing foods that are or may be GMO.

GMO LABELING: The Standard defines bioengineered foods as those that contain detectable genetic material that has been modified through certain lab techniques and cannot be created through conventional breeding or found in nature. The Standard requires food manufacturers, importers, and certain retailers to ensure bioengineered foods are appropriately disclosed.[552]

In 2019 the so-called labels were unveiled, and they're a bit vague:

- Labels state the food is bioengineered (BE), rather than GMO
- Some ingredients are exempt, such as sugar from GMO beets and GMO soybean oil.[553]
- Further, no disclosure is required for refined foods derived from GMO/bioengineered crops, if the food does not contain detectable modified genetic material![554]
- Foods that can go without a label, even though they're made from GMOs: **high fructose corn syrup, refined sugar, refined oils, foods from animals fed GMOs**[555].
- Labeling is not uniform and consistent.

The American Farm Bureau is perhaps the most powerful food organization. They more than any other group influence laws controlling our food supply, and they see nothing unsafe about GMOs.[556] If they did, it might not seem as if Biotech is calling the shots. "Biotech's concerns have always been that any mandated disclosures must not disparage biotechnology, impose undue regulatory burdens or create market discrimination when there are no material differences between conventional foods and foods derived from biotechnology."[557]

NON-GMO VERIFIED: this does not mean the food is organic, it more or less equates to food made with ingredients from conventionally-grown foods i.e. typically heavy pesticides, lots of harmful synthetic fertilizer.

COOL COUNTRY OF ORIGIN: Other labeling of importance that's disappeared was a result of Codex guidelines. In 2015 the US repealed Country of Origin Labeling (COOL) for meat, namely because the Codex Committee felt such labeling was biased toward American meat.[558] To avoid retaliation from Codex and the WTO, the Senate revoked meat labeling. As a result beef, pork and turkey no longer indicate country of origin, but chicken and lamb still must. If we want to know where our meat comes from we have to get labeling back. What future repeals or laws may they try to enforce we do not yet know.[559]

We've saturated our country and spread GMO farming far and wide across the globe. All this meddling with nature and transforming of foods, will this end up being our worst crime yet against nature, against our own health?

GENE EDITING + LABELING

Gene editing of food is a very new development that appears to be receiving the green light from the FDA. It's a process whereby existing genes in a plant or other life form are "edited." It's unlike bioengineering (GMOs) in that the process does not include inserting new genes from a different organism. With the FDA's approval, food manufacturers can develop foods containing gene-edited ingredients and sell them to us without testing or labeling.

The US and The European Union have vastly different views of gene-edited foods. In the US the government considers it not a risk because no new DNA is added. In Europe, on the other hand, since the DNA is altered/edited in an unnatural process, the courts ruled in 2018 that gene edited foods must be regulated with the same safety safeguards as genetically modified foods. As reported by the journal *Nature*, "Gene-edited crops should be subject to the same stringent regulations as conventional genetically modified (GM) organisms, Europe's highest court ruled on 25 July, 2018. It also called for all products made through gene editing to be regulated, assessed for their health and environmental impacts, and labeled."[560]

Sorting out the Differences

- **Gene Editing:** Existing genes are edited or deleted to achieve certain results
- **Gene Modification (GMOs, Bioengineering):** New genes not naturally present are added to a plant or animal, genes can be from same species or other life forms
- **Bioengineering, Genetic Engineering:** *See gene modification*
- **Traditional Plant Breeding:** Different plants are crossed together with the intent to produce offspring with desired characteristics as an outcome of blending their genes

These gene tinkering methods may share similarities, but they are different. With new technologies safety precautions are certainly warranted and logical. Isn't having absolute certainty of safety and harmlessness necessary before moving forward? The companies making them and agencies responsible for safeguarding the food supply must do the best job possible to keep us safe, keep our health and earth protected. Unlike Europe, why does the US choose to ignore the precautionary principle? Is the FDA American approach in our best interest?

As the Merck Manual explains, "Genes are segments of deoxyribonucleic acid (DNA) that contain the code for a specific protein that functions in one or more types of cells in the body. Chromosomes are structures within cells that contain a person's genes.

- Genes are contained in chromosomes, which are mainly in the cell nucleus.
- A chromosome contains hundreds to thousands of genes.
- Every human cell contains 23 pairs of chromosomes, for a total of 46 chromosomes.
- A trait is any gene-determined characteristic, often determined by more than one gene.
- Some traits are caused by abnormal genes that are inherited or from a new mutation."[561]

As of this spring of 2019, the first gene edited food, a soybean oil designed to produce more 'heart-healthy fat' is already being used in select restaurants in the Midwest. As AP News reports, other gene edited foods currently in development include: "Mushrooms that don't brown, wheat with more fiber, better-producing tomatoes, herbicide-tolerant canola and rice that doesn't absorb soil pollution as it grows."[562] Sounds a lot like GMOs to me.

IRRADIATION + LABELING

Food Irradiation has been allowed as an acceptable process under GRAS (*Generally Recognized as Safe*) since the 1990s. It's where the Department of Energy and the USDA coincide. Many question irradiation's effect on food, whether there are changes to the molecular structure, and if it's safe to eat food that's been exposed to radiation? There is also concern irradiation diminishes nutrient content of food.

What is food irradiation? Food irradiation is a technology for controlling spoilage and eliminating foodborne pathogens. The fundamental difference between food irradiation and pasteurization is the source of the energy. While conventional pasteurization relies on heat, irradiation relies on ionizing radiation.[563]

Foods Approved for Irradiation: Beef and pork, poultry, crustaceans and shellfish, fresh fruits and vegetables, lettuce, spinach, seeds for sprouting, shell eggs, spices and seasonings.[564]

Is it Safe? One study demonstrated that irradiation of dietary fats produces compounds that 'promote colon carcinogenesis.'[565] The Organic Consumers Association states, "Studies on animals fed irradiated foods have shown increased tumors, reproductive failures and kidney damage. Some possible causes are: irradiation-induced vitamin deficiencies, the inactivity of enzymes in the food, DNA damage, and toxic radiolytic products in the food."[566] Other concerns raised by the Food Commission in Britain are as follows:

- "Food irradiation can result in loss of nutrients, for example vitamin E levels can be reduced by 25% after irradiation and vitamin C by 5-10%. This is compounded by the longer storage times of irradiated foods, and by loss of nutrients during cooking, which can result in the food finally eaten by the consumer to contain little more than 'empty calories'. This is potentially damaging to the long and short-term health of consumers, particularly for (those) already failing to obtain adequate nutrition.
- When food is exposed to high doses of ionizing radiation, the chemical composition and nutritional content of food can change. Radiolytic by-products are often formed in irradiated food. Very few of these chemicals have been adequately studied for toxicity. One such chemical - 2-DCB - can cause DNA damage in rat colon cells at high doses.
- Food irradiation does not inactivate dangerous toxins which have already been produced by bacteria prior to irradiation. In some cases, such as C. botulinum, it is the toxin produced by the bacteria, rather than the bacteria itself, which poses the hazard.
- Irradiation can cause mutations in bacteria and viruses leading to resistant strains.
- Irradiation can be used to maintain or even worsen poor standards of animal husbandry. Overcrowding of animals whist rearing and prior to slaughter, as well as the use of cheap but inappropriate feeds, all contribute to contamination of animal products such as meat, poultry and eggs. Cleaning up these products at the end of the production line removes the incentive to improve animal welfare." [567]

When John Mackey's Whole Foods first opened its doors, it pledged to never sell irradiated food[568]. I'm not sure that Amazon is keeping that promise or what others store do. Perhaps Food irradiation can be useful to keep food safe, or perhaps it needs more thorough safety testing.

20. PESTICIDE RESIDUES

Will residues ever be on the label? "Over 1 billion pounds of pesticides are used in the United State (US) each year and approximately 5.6 billion pounds are used worldwide."[15] If that many chemicals are used to grow foods we eat, our food and beverages very likely contain residues of those pesticides. See pages 20-21 for a sampling of residues found on foods. Residue levels are regulated by the EPA, and then enforced by the USDA and FDA. Often manufacturers petition to raise their pesticide tolerances and succeed. You can find all the allowed residue levels under the Code of Federal Regulations, but be warned it's a little tricky to navigate: https://www.epa.gov/pesticide-tolerances. See page 143 for a look at allowed glyphosate residues.

85% OF FOOD TESTED CONTAINS PESTICIDES!

As reported by US Right to Know in 2016, data released by the USDA shows "Residues of many types of insecticides, fungicides and weed killing chemicals have been found in roughly 85 percent of thousands of foods tested."[569] In April 2018, through Freedom of Information Requests the Guardian obtained information related to glyphosate residues on food--not disclosed by the FDA or USDA. As the newspaper uncovers, glyphosate is so prevalent in the food supply that "the FDA has had trouble finding any food that does not carry traces of the pesticide."[570]

Back in 2017 California made quite a declaration. As reported by Eco Watch, "the State's proposed safe level (for glyphosate) is more than 100 times lower than the U.S. Environmental Protection Agency's legal allowance for the average-sized American."[571] This begs the question, are the EPA and FDA too lenient when it comes to setting pesticide tolerances and maximum contaminant levels in water? What levels are truly safe? We'll have to see if the glyphosate tolerance levels are lowered closer to zero since the Courts have determined its link with cancer to humans, and Monsanto's deceptive behavior. Can we really trust any company with a history of misleading the public? How can we count on safety testing information companies like that supply when we know that they knowingly withheld vital information related to the safety of their products? "By law, EPA is responsible for regulating the pesticides that are used by growers to protect crops grown for human food and animal feed and for setting limits on the amount of pesticides that may remain in or on foods marketed in the USA. The U.S. Department of Agriculture (USDA) and the Food and Drug Administration (FDA) enforce tolerances to ensure that the nation's food supply is maintained safely at all times"[572]

If pesticides were harmless, residues wouldn't matter so much. However, pesticides are not harmless, they're actually the exact opposite. Residue regulations currently are further flawed in that each pesticide is measured individually, as if only one pesticide is usually used on food, or that we are only ever exposed to one pesticide at a time. Food tests reveal numerous types of pesticide residue levels present in food samples. No one knows yet what cumulative or long-term health risk such wild combinations might pose to us.

RESIDUES IN BEVERAGES

It's not just foods that can be contaminated with pesticides. Many of our favorite beverages can have residues of pesticides, fungicides, GMOs, and unlabeled ingredients. In fact, nearly all foods and beverages can contain residues in connection with one of its ingredients. Tea, juices, coffee, alcohol, beer and wine come from plants that are treated with fungicides and pesticides while growing. The organic label provides some assurance that a beverage does not contain synthetic pesticides or fertilizer residues, yet due to pesticide drift and water pollution even organic farms can encounter contamination. However, organic farms will differ in that they will not be applying the dangerous pesticides directly. Those that do use pesticides will be using substances of natural origin and usually less amounts than the typical conventional or gmo outfit. As such organic and biodynamic remain the better choice for less toxic exposure. Keep in mind that many smaller farms and vintners may indeed be utilizing no pesticide, organic methods, but may not yet have invested in the organic certification of their product. The USDA doesn't make certification cheap! What this means is don't rule out the small guys--even if their label doesn't specifically say "organic." Look into their product, it could very well be as close to pesticide free as you can get.

HEALTH EFFECTS

As reported by the US Right to Know, "We don't know if you eat an apple that has multiple residues every day what will be the consequences 20 years down the road," said Chensheng Lu, associate professor of environmental exposure biology at the Harvard School of Public Health. "They want to assure everybody that this is safe but the science is quite inadequate. This is a big issue. The USDA said in its latest report that 441 of the samples it found were considered worrisome as "presumptive tolerance violations," because the residues found either exceeded what is set as safe by the Environmental Protection Agency (EPA) or they were found in foods that are not expected to contain the pesticide residues at all and for which there is no legal tolerance level. Those samples contained residues of 496 different pesticides, the USDA said. Spinach, strawberries, grapes, green beans, tomatoes, cucumbers and watermelon were among the foods found with illegal pesticide residue levels. Even residues of chemicals long banned in the United States were found, including residues of DDT or its metabolites found in spinach and potatoes. DDT was banned in 1972 because of health and environmental concerns about the insecticide."[573]

SOLUTIONS

- By sourcing foods grown with less or no pesticides, you will reduce your exposure to residues. Opt for organic and locally grown food at your nearest farmer's market.
- If you're interested in searching for specific pesticide residue level allowances, one of the most thorough databases is provided by Oregon State University in collaboration with the EPA, known as the National Pesticide Information Center (NPIC): http://npic.orst.edu/reg/tolerance.html, **1-800-858-7378** or email npic@ace.orst.edu.

21. ENDOCRINE DISRUPTORS

Endocrine disruptors are perhaps the most insidious and harmful chemicals on earth. These little monsters can be found everywhere, in food, in water, and beyond. The most harmful come from chemicals and plastic. One little tiny miniscule amount is capable of causing great harm. These little beasts affect our bodies in numerous ways, mimicking hormones, disrupting body cycles, causing chemical imbalance, disrupting enzyme function, triggering mood swings, behavioral changes, aggression, causing birth defects, cancer, etc.

WHAT ARE ENDOCRINE DISRUPTING CHEMICALS?

Endocrine disrupting chemicals are chemicals that interfere with normal hormone action. For example, they can mimic or block hormones, and/or affect their production, their movement throughout the body, or their metabolism.

HOW DO HORMONES WORK IN THE BODY?

Hormones are chemicals such as insulin, thyroxin (thyroid hormone), estrogen, and testosterone. There are upwards of 50 different known hormones in the human body. Hormones send messages through the body by traveling to receptors in and on different cells, resulting in biological actions, such as ovulation or changes in blood sugar. The endocrine system is so finely tuned that it depends upon changes in hormones concentrations comparable to one drop in 20 Olympic swimming pools.

WHAT IS THE ENDOCRINE SYSTEM?

The endocrine system is the body's exquisitely balanced system of glands, organs, and hormones that regulates such vital functions as body growth, response to stress, sexual development, production of insulin and utilization of glucose, metabolism, neurodevelopment intelligence, behavior, sleep patterns, blood pressure, and the ability to reproduce.

HOW DO ENDOCRINE DISRUPTING CHEMICALS AFFECT OUR HEALTH?

Endocrine disrupting chemicals have been implicated in numerous adverse health outcomes, including those of the endocrine, reproductive, neurological, and metabolic systems. Examples include infertility, endometriosis, early puberty, breast and prostate cancer, thyroid disorders, Alzheimer's and Parkinson's disease, attention-deficit hyperactivity disorder, obesity, diabetes, asthma, immune disorders, and more.

Effects can occur from a very small amount of a chemical, and these 'low dose effects' can be different than the effects of higher doses. This makes the outcomes difficult to predict. Further, health effects may not show up until many years after exposure occurred, making it hard to connect cause and effect. We may even inherit susceptibilities from chemicals to which our parents, grandparents, or great-grandparents were exposed.

WHERE DO ENDOCRINE DISRUPTING CHEMICALS COME FROM?

Endocrine disruptors are in our everyday products: from the personal care products and cosmetics we apply, to the chemicals we use to clean our homes, to the materials our homes, schools, and offices are built from. Most synthetic endocrine disrupting chemicals are derived from chemicals associated with fossil fuel extraction, processing, and/or burning. These include chemicals used as food additives, pesticides, plastics, dyes and more. Others are naturally occurring, such as phytoestrogens produced by plants.

HOW DO ENDOCRINE DISRUPTING CHEMICALS GET INTO OUR BODIES?

Endocrine disrupting chemicals can be found in common products like canned food, perfume, plastic food containers, cosmetics, and furniture. They get into our bodies through food, water and dust, directly through our skin, from hand to mouth contact, and from the air we breathe.

HOW ARE ENDOCRINE DISRUPTING CHEMICALS MEASURED IN PEOPLE?

Scientists and doctors can detect endocrine disrupting chemicals in blood, urine, stool, saliva, tears, perspiration, placental tissue, umbilical cord blood and the meconium of newborn babies. Endocrine disruptors have been found in every person tested, across world populations. Some endocrine disruptors remain in the body for years and others are excreted relatively quickly.

WHO IS MOST AT RISK FROM THE HARMFUL EFFECTS?

The age at which a person is exposed to endocrine disruptors is a primary factor in the level of risk. Exposure can be particularly harmful during times when the body undergoes a great deal of change, including during prenatal and early postnatal development, puberty, pregnancy, and menopause/andropause. Further, infants and children are more susceptible to exposure because they spend more time closer to the ground where chemicals settle, have more hand to mouth behavior than adults, have greater food and water intake per unit of body weight, and their immune and metabolic systems are immature so they don't process chemicals as well as adults. Exposure risk is also elevated in lower income areas, among minority populations, and in areas with fewer resources to reduce exposure.[574] www.tedx.org

The preceding was presented courtesy of TEDX, the Endocrine Disruptor Exchange www.tedx.org

Remembering Theo Colborn

"Hormone disrupting synthetic chemicals are today an inescapable fact of life. They are in our food and water. They reach us through the air and through consumer goods we bring into our homes. They have spread across the face of the Earth and insinuated themselves into virtually every nook and cranny of the food web. There is no way to recall them. That is the dilemma we face. We can, though, as suggested above, reduce the risks of exposure by personal choice and through government action." Theo Colborn, *Our Stolen Future*. Theo Colborn (1927-2014) was one of the first scientists to ultimately identify and describe the harming effects of endocrine disruptors. She wrote the books to awaken us. *Our Stolen Future* and *Great Lakes, Great Legacy* shed light on the destruction caused from exposure to endocrine disruptors.

POPs: PERSISTENT ORGANIC POLLUTANTS

When the environmental classic "Silent Spring" was first published in 1962, the public became aware of the risks and harmful effects of chemicals, and hope for the future was born. People, animals, birds, trees and nature now had an advocate seeking to protect them. No longer were they without a voice. Through her exquisite writing and observations, Carson shed light on the chemical industry and toxins amongst us. She was especially important in raising awareness of persistent chemicals that caused harm. Her work led to the banning of DDT, which carved the way for the ban on persistent organic pollutants years later.

Today, the chemical industry has grown into the almighty bioengineering syndicate, the chemical cartel. We are no longer protected by the likes of Carson or the Delaney Amendment; and instead we are assaulted by exposure to new toxins on a daily basis. We need more pioneers, warriors and heroes like Rachel Carson and Theo Colborn to help wake the world, protect our health and save our planet. Do you have the courage to stand up and help change it?

Persistent Organic Pollutants: POPs are especially sinister as these are endocrine disruptors, they don't break down, they travel far by water and air, and once ingested they bioaccumulate in fatty tissue. They affect people and animals at the top of the food chain most. The Stockholm Convention was embraced worldwide to ban these substances. Because of their persistent nature, however, they still can be found in our environment, waterways, fish, animals, and people.

In Honor of Rachel Carson 1907-1964: "The task is by no means a hopeless one. In one important respect the outlook is more encouraging than the situations regarding infectious diseases at the turn of the century. The world was then full of disease germs, as today it is full of carcinogens. But man did not put the germs into the environment and his role in spreading them was involuntary. In contrast, man has put the vast majority of carcinogens into the environment, and he can, if he wishes, eliminate many of them. The chemical agents of cancer have become entrenched in our world in two ways: first, and ironically, through man's search for a better and easier way of life; second, because the manufacture and sale of such chemicals has become an accepted part of our economy and our way of life.

It would be unrealistic to suppose that all chemical carcinogens can or will be eliminated from the modern world. But a very large proportion are by no means necessities of life. By their elimination the total load of carcinogens would be enormously lightened, and the threat that one in every four will develop cancer would at least be greatly mitigated. The most determined effort should be made to eliminate those carcinogens that now contaminate our food, our water supplies, and our atmosphere, because these provide the most dangerous type of contact—minute exposures, repeated over and over throughout the years."[575] Rachel Carson, *Silent Spring*

Today, 1 out of 3 could get cancer in their lifetimes.

576

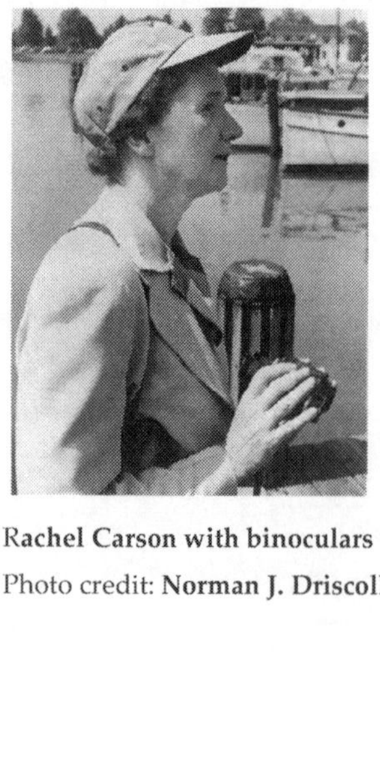

Rachel Carson with binoculars on the pier at Woods Hole, MA. 1951.

Photo credit: **Norman J. Driscoll,** used with PERMISSION OF RACHEL CARSON COUNCIL, INC.

22. FOOD PACKAGING

After all the toxins we face from growing food today, we can't rest yet. Our health can also be affected by substances lurking in food packaging. When it comes to food and beverages, the bulk of it is packaged in earth damaging health-harming materials. Most everything comes in plastic or Styrofoam, especially take-out food. You wouldn't know it, but even most pizza boxes are laced with grease-proofing PFAS toxins that stay in the environment for a thousand years.

The chemicals allowed in food packaging can and do seep into foods and beverages, which means we not only handle them, we ingest them. What makes it worse is that most packaging is excessive and sucking up earth's resources. Double jeopardy is the fact that chemical-tainted packaging restricts recycling ability. We already have an urgent problem on our hands today due to littering and because so much that could be recycled just isn't being recycled.

WHAT TOXIC CHEMICALS ARE IN FOOD CONTAINERS:

BPA: water bottles, receipt paper, sippy cups, can lining (soup can), pacifiers

PFASs: food wrappers, pizza boxes, microwave popcorn bags, sandwich wrappers

STYRENE: Styrofoam cups, plates, bowls, containers, packing peanuts

PHTHALATES: straws, plastic cups, plastic wrap

PERCHLORATE: plastic bags containing dry cereal, dry foods

FLAME RETARDANTS: food containers made from recycled plastic

BPA: A wretched endocrine-disrupting chemical allowed in food packaging. BPA (bisphenol A) is found in plastic containers, water bottles, linings of cans containing beverages and food, sippy cups, pacifiers, plastic toys, even most receipts you get from stores today contain BPA! BPA mimics estrogen in our bodies, and it's quite likely, as reported by Newsweek in March of 2015 that "the chemical plays a role in a litany of health concerns: obesity, diabetes, problems with fertility and reproductive organs, susceptibility to various cancers and cognitive/behavioral deficits like ADHD."[577]

Receipt Paper is loaded with BPA! Next time they ask if you want the receipt, have them email it. Studies show handling one receipt can leave residues of BPA in your system for a week or more![578] Thermal paper is used in many modern cash registers and ATM machines—it has a BPA coating—Some companies have switched to non-BPA paper, which means they all can do it!

How do I know if a receipt is thermal paper?

A receipt is probably thermal paper if it discolors easily when scratched with a coin or paperclip. Thermal receipt papers are quite thin, and often have a slick feel or sheen finish. They are run through thermal printers and the printing develops from the heat; ink is not physically printed onto the paper. Note that plain "bond" paper used as receipts, where ink is actually applied to the paper, is not of concern and doesn't use chemical developers.[579] Source: *Minnesota Pollution Control Agency*

TABLE 1:
Evidence of PFC wrappers, bags and boxes from popular fast food chains

Restaurant	Food contact paper items tested[1]	Percentage of items testing positive for fluorine, likely indication of PFCs[2]
Arby's	16	19%
Burger King	37	27%
Carl's Jr.	5	0%
Checkers	2	0%
Chick-fil-A	5	80%
Chipotle	17	65%
Church's Chicken	2	50%
Culver's	2	0%
Dairy Queen	5	20%
Domino's	2	0%
Dunkin' Donuts	12	33%
Five Guys	1	0%
Jack in the Box	7	14%
Jimmy John's	9	100%
KFC	20	25%
Krispy Kreme	4	50%
Local restaurants	7	43%
McDonald's	31	19%
Panera	23	43%
Pizza Hut	3	33%
Quiznos	9	100%
Round Table Pizza	1	0%
Starbucks	21	76%
Steak 'n Shake	3	67%
Subway	19	42%
Taco Bell	28	43%
Taco Time	5	100%
Wendy's	31	23%
TOTAL	**327**	**40%**

PFASs: Did you know many take out containers and food wrappers are covered in polyfluoroalkyl substances (PFASs) sometimes also called perfluorochemicals (PFCs). These grease-proofing and nonstick chemicals are used despite the fact they leach into foods, especially hot foods and beverages. These chemicals don't break down easily, once consumed can linger in our bodies and the environment for an extremely long time. PFOA (perfluorooctanoic acid or C8, commonly known as *Teflon*) was the most used, yet due to health concerns it's been phased out of food packaging since 2011. However, it is still detected in some packaging along with replacement chemicals that were supposed to be less harmful. "PFCs are linked with kidney and testicular cancer, abnormal thyroid levels, high cholesterol, pregnancy induced hypertension and pre-eclampsia, obesity."[581]

PFAS REPLACEMENT CHEMICALS: February 2017, "Because there's still little known about this next generation of chemicals, manufacturers can put them out into the market through an FDA loophole that allows them to claim a product is "generally recognized as safe" without actually testing its safety."[582] Source: *Mother Jones*

Gen X: one of the replacement chemicals could be an environmental time bomb. It's been produced for years near Fayetteville, North Carolina. Only recently have they begun to notice the dramatic contamination of GenX in the Cape Fear River and private drinking wells. March 2018: "After the discovery of GenX in drinking water, the level found in the Cape Fear River measured as high as 39,000 parts per trillion."[583] The EWG reports the EPA had information from Dupont admitting that "GenX, could pose a "substantial risk of injury," including cancerous tumors in the pancreas, testicles, liver damage, kidney disease and reproductive harm."[584]

FLAME RETARDANTS: People are trying to do good and recycle plastic. Yet some plastic comes with more than we anticipated. Scientists have recently found some recycled food packaging containing flame retardants. This is because the food packaging used to be part of some type of electronic equipment, which is often treated with brominated flame retardants.[585] Stay clear of black plastic food containers & you should be safe. Brominated vegetable oil (BVO) is also classified as a flame retardant, used on foam furniture. Beware though amounts legally allowed have been reduced, it can be found in different brands of soda pop. Use of BVO is beverages is banned in other countries.

PHTHALATES: are chemicals that soften plastic, used in food containers, plastic wrap and plastic straws, cups and containers, vinyl, PVC, fragrance, air freshener, oils, nail polish, pharmaceuticals, toys. Phthalates are not health promoters. As reported by EWG, "Phthalates trigger what's known as "death-inducing signaling" in testicular cells, making them die earlier than they should," and "studies have linked phthalates to hormone changes, lower sperm count, less mobile sperm, birth defects in the male reproductive system, obesity, diabetes and thyroid irregularities."[586] Check out TEDX.org to get the full lowdown on endocrine disruptors.

PERCHLORATE: Perchlorate is known as rocket fuel. It's also a health harming substance that for no good reason is lining plastic food packaging containing dry cereals and other dry foods. Approved by the FDA in 2005, perchlorate was selected for use in food packaging for its anti-static abilities. "Perchlorate disrupts the thyroid gland's normal function and reduces production of the thyroid hormone needed for healthy fetal and child brain development." Between 2008 and 2012, Perchlorate levels in humans have been increasing specifically in children under 6 years of age. Based on data collected by the FDA in its Total Health Study, "levels increased 34% for children 6 to 11 months; 23% for 2-year-olds; and 12% for 6-year-olds. Older children and adults did not show an increase, indicating that foods eaten by children six or younger had higher concentrations of perchlorate than foods favored by adults."[587]

Since originally approved, test results provided by the manufacturer were found to be inaccurate; perchlorate does migrate to food afterall. Yet the FDA has not recalled perchlorate from food packaging! Perchlorate is an endocrine disruptor, thyroid toxin, and can impair brain health and development. A 2006 CDC study found perchlorate in the urine of every one of a nationally representative group of 2,820 people they tested.[588] Clearly we must get this substance out of food packaging. Why are toxic substances allowed in food or beverage packaging? By banning them we can improve water quality and make food safer for all.

STYRENE: 100% of people tested have styrene in their bodies.[589] Source: EPA Styrofoam cups and containers contain styrene. Styrene is carcinogenic. Avoid using Styrofoam, (technically, called single-use polystyrene), especially do not use for hot beverages or soups! "In China most styrofoam had been made from trash—much of it imported from Western countries—rather than from new materials. There are currently no official standards regulating inputs such as the number of whitening products or other additives. Styrofoam is unsafe under high temperatures."[590]

HEALTH EFFECTS: These chemicals—PFCs, BPA, Flame Retardants & Phthalates-- are all endocrine disruptors that affect hormones, which affect us in big ways! Hormones control everything about our bodies, our brain, our development, our mood, our glands, our nervous system, reproductive organs, heart, energy, sleep. Hormones are so fragile and so dependent on a very particular balance. The slightest bit off balance can trigger massive problems. In addition to harming the health of people around the world, plastic and endocrine disruptors pollute water everywhere and damage the planet in catastrophic ways.

PACKAGE WASTE: As if these chemicals aren't bad enough, think of all the excess wasteful packaging that comes with our foods and beverages. Almost none of these things are recyclable and they all cause harm to us and the planet: plastic wrappers, plastic straws, styrofoam cups, plastic lids, plastic utensils wrapped in plastic. Sadly much of what can be recycled just isn't going that direction right now; instead most recyclable items end up in landfills and waterways. Items that are typically not recyclable include:

- Styrofoam: Not Recyclable
- Plastic Bags: Can be reused but not recycled
- Chip bags (aluminum laminated with polypropylene): recycled only by *Terracycle*
- Pizza boxes: Not Recyclable because of PFASs

SOLUTIONS: REDUCE CONTACT

- **AVOID PLASTIC FOOD & STYROFOAM PACKAGING**
- Use reusable materials like cloth, glass, steel, ceramic, or paper
- **AVOID HANDLING RECEIPT PAPER CONTAINING BPA!**
- We need to prevent chemicals from contact with our food supply
- Laws in the US can & must do a better job of protecting people + animals from chemicals that cause disease and chemical imbalance. The chemicals found in these plastics are not just causing cancer and disease, but they could very well also be the primary drivers fueling rising trends of gun violence and aggression.
- We need to work on this on a big scale, as in worldwide. Eventually most toxins, especially plastic and food packaging toxins become water contaminants. The EPA regulates water contaminant levels for some chemicals, not all chemicals.

23. PLASTIC

PLASTIC, STRAWS, STYROFOAM

Plastic and pesticides must be the greatest curse humans have placed upon this planet. Like pesticides, plastic is made from petrochemicals. These chemicals have a tendency to leach from packaging into foods and beverages, so ultimately, they become substances we ingest. Most plastic is not recyclable and that which is, seldom gets recycled but rather ends up littering the earth and polluting waterways. This pollution is harming animals, the oceans and ecosystems the world over. Isn't it time to kick our plastic dependence?

> **"I don't want any plastics!"**
> George Bailey,
> *It's a Wonderful Life*

"The world produces about 400 million metric tons of plastic a year, the equivalent of 882 billion pounds, and 80 percent ends up deposited in landfills and other parts of the environment. The smallest particles, the microplastics, range from 10 nanometers — so tiny they are invisible to the human eye — up to 5 millimeters in diameter. Microplastics — including microfibers from clothing — are floating in the air and are found in most of our bottled and tap water, our beer, our sea, rock and lake salt, and our soil."[591] Plastic harms people, animals, oceans, waterways, the whole planet. We're surrounded, it's everywhere and it's wreaking havoc on not just the planet but on our health as well. As of 2018 researchers discovered microplastics are making their way into people's bodies. Up to 9 plastics were found in every person tested, including polypropylene and polyethylene.[592] If only we could bundle it all together and ship it off to the edge of the galaxy.

The worst and most notorious plastics littering the planet include:

- **Styrofoam (Styrene):** It may be cheap, but styrofoam is not nice. The Chemicals in styrofoam seep into food and beverages, they're neurotoxins, endocrine disruptors, can harm the liver, stomach, reproduction; they're linked with many, many health maladies including leukemia and cancers.[593] Don't heat or microwave any foods or beverages in Styrofoam. When a Styrofoam cup is filled with a cold or hot beverage, the chemicals in the Styrofoam meld into your drink. These are not ordinary chemicals, these are benzene and styrene--potent carcinogenic chemicals that shouldn't be entering your body. Anytime a food or beverage is in contact with polystyrene, contamination can occur--increasingly so the warmer the food or drink. Styrene does not biodegrade, nor is it recyclable, so anything made from this nasty substance will still be around in 500 or more years.
- **Straws:** Plastic straws are a menace—made from polypropylene, the plastic can leach into our body, straws harm animals and pollute waterways worldwide. They do not biodegrade.
- **Plastic Bags and Plastic Wrap:** Plastic wrap may be helpful in storing food, but do not heat or cook food with plastic wrap on it, or in plastic containers of any kind. Plastic is notorious for leaching into food and beverages especially when foods and liquids are hot.

- **Water Bottles:** made of PET, polyethylene, can leach into human body as well.
- **Six Pack Rings:** we have to start making these out of something else that biodegrades and doesn't cause harm to animals. Soda and beverage companies please help.

Microplastics

"Plastic is the most prevalent type of marine debris found in our ocean and Great Lakes. Plastic debris can come in all shapes and sizes, but those that are less than five millimeters in length (or about the size of a sesame seed) are called 'microplastics.'"[594] Is there any escape from plastics? We've developed these substances that in reality will remain on earth until the end of time. They don't biodegrade, they don't disappear, they may get smaller and become micro-sized, but they're persistently a problem—relentlessly contaminating every crevice of earth, compromising every living creature that makes contact. A new subcategory of plastics has been identified: microfibers. These are teeny plastic bits shredding off clothing when we do laundry.

Plastic is a problem for everyone, especially sea creatures where plastic pollution has become so problematic. Once ingested plastic does unmeasurable harm to animals. Because of the minute size of microplastics we unknowningly absorb much more of them than other plastic. Tiny particles are even drifting through the air in dust. The only viable solution humanity has is to reduce production of plastics so we can cease polluting the planet with them.

REDUCE, REUSE, RECYCLE PLASTIC.

Which plastics can we recycle?

NOT RECYCLABLE, NOT SAFE:

Beware, all of these plastics leach harmful endocrine disrupting chemicals:

#3 **PVC, Polyvinyl Chloride**
Leaches phthalates, p-nonylphenols, Toxic, NOT recyclable, used in plastic wrap teething rings, plumbing pipes, baby toys, pet toys, shower curtains

#6 **PS, Polystyrene, Styrofoam**
Leaches styrene and p-nonylphenols, NOT Recyclable, major oceanic pollutant, used in Cups, food & drink **containers**, packaging, egg cartons, **don't microwave!**

#7 **Polycarbonate**
Toxic, leaches BPA (bisphenol-A), NOT Recyclable,
Found in sippy cups, jugs, **don't heat or microwave, don't reuse**

MOST OF THESE PLASTICS CAN BE RECYCLED:

Beware, these plastics still can leach endocrine disruptors:

#1 PET: Polyethylene Terephthalate, **Recyclable** used in water, soda, honey bottles

#2 HDPE: High-Density Polyethylene, **Recyclable,** used in milk, water jugs

#4 LDPE: Low-Density Polyethylene, **Recyclable**, used in squeeze bottles, shrinkwrap

#5 PP: Polypropylene, **Recyclable,** used in food packaging, yogurt containers, straws

#7 PLA (corn-based) Safer, **Not Recyclable**, **Compostable**, made from corn (GMO)

ENDOCRINE DISRUPTORS

"Endocrine disrupting chemicals (EDCs) are chemicals made outside of the body that can block, mimic or otherwise disrupt normal hormone signals. This can result in misinformation that leads to diseases and poor health conditions. Importantly, because small amounts of hormones play a role in so many of life's functions, exposures to EDCs even at very low levels during certain times of life can have substantial and sometimes permanent impacts on health.

EDCs interact with the endocrine system, which is a complex chemical messaging system that is involved in every stage of life, from conception through gestation, birth, puberty, adulthood, and senescence. The endocrine system sends hormone signals such as estrogen, testosterone, thyroid hormone, and insulin from one organ to another and in turn controls cell function in the target organ. Thus it orchestrates vital functions including metabolism, immune function, reproduction, intelligence and a variety of behaviors."[595] Source: TEDX.org,

SOLUTIONS

Thank you Maine!
As of May, 2019, Maine became the first State to ban single-use Styrofoam (aka single use polystyrene)!
The law takes effect Jan 1, 2021.

REDUCE PLASTIC USE.

By reducing use of plastic and products wrapped in plastic, and instead buying products packaged in zero or natural packaging materials we help the earth and help protect our health and our family's health.

- Can we ween ourselves off plastic? Can food companies stop using it?
- Avoid plastic, Styrofoam & other toxins containing endocrine disrupting substances.
- When you store food at home, use safe materials like glass, ceramic, stainless steel, put leftovers in a bowl and cover it with a plate.
- Don't use or buy any products containing microplastics
- Don't heat or cook in plastic, plastic wrap, or Styrofoam.
- Don't let plastic litter our world anymore, join the crusade and help clean it up.
- Prevent microfibers, filter your washing machine drainage water: www.filtrol.net.
- Can anyone deny the time has come to separate plastic from the food supply?
- Let's be like NYC and get the packing peanuts banned as well.

DON'T COOK, MICROWAVE, or HEAT FOOD IN PLASTIC!

Remove food from plastic packaging before microwaving or defrosting. Do not use foam trays and plastic wraps because they are not heat stable at high temperatures. Melting or warping may cause harmful chemicals to migrate into food.[596]

Collectively we must come up with better solutions for product containers—ones that are plastic-free & free of BPA, phthalates, endocrine disruptors & other health harmers. We must come up with better end solutions for the containers that already exist—how else can we recycle or dispose of them that causes harm to none?

24. FISH + WATER

Our water friends are challenged everyday with an endless assortment of toxins and human interference: plastic, oil spills, pollution, overfishing, algae blooms, fertilizer, chemicals, red tide, on and on the list goes. It's time to reverse this course and help marine life and waterways recover.

- **Help Fish Populations Rebound: Say No to Overfishing:** Overfishing causes major devastation to fish populations and marine ecosystems. Many fish numbers are so low that we must avoid catching them, so they can recover and not go extinct. The worst possible fishing method is bottom-trawling. This involves dragging large heavy nets over the seafloor catching and harming everything in its path. From Oceana, "Trawling can cause irreversible damage to sensitive habitats like deep-sea coral reefs, gorgonian gardens and sponge grounds. It rips up coral and sponge bed habitats that fish and shellfish depend on for breeding, spawning and nurseries. This significantly hampers the recovery of depleted fish stocks. Trawling is also wasteful. Scientists estimate that it generates as much as half of all discarded fish and marine life globally."[597]
- **Microplastics (MP):** Plastic is contaminating and killing our planet & oceans. Plastic microbeads are already tiny, but all other plastics break down into teeny tiny pieces, never fully biodegrading. Many aquatic animals and birds mistake plastic for food; once swallowed it accumulates and clog animals' stomachs. It's not digestible. The smaller pieces migrate through the animal's body and transfer to animals or us when we partake. The endocrine disruptors & such come too. Microplastics have been found in all people tested.[598]
- **Ocean Acidification (OA):** caused by excessive carbon dioxide, OA is changing the pH balance of the oceans. Agricultural runoff tainted with pesticides, fertilizer and other farming toxins cause algae blooms & eutrophication. When algae die, bacteria eat them releasing CO2.[599]
- **POPs and Heavy Metal Contamination:** Many chemicals and heavy metals like mercury, dioxin, and dieldrin are persistent pollutants that linger perpetually in water, soil and the environment. These substances are easily absorbed and ingested by marine animals and aquatic organisms. They bioaccumulate as they move up the food chain. In order to reduce exposure, avoid fishing in the most polluted lakes, rivers, and waterways. Some seafood should be consumed only moderately. "Exposure to POPs can lead to serious health effects including certain cancers, birth defects, dysfunctional immune and reproductive systems, greater susceptibility to disease & damages to the central and peripheral nervous systems."[600] Are contaminants from the Fukishima spill affecting the ocean life too?
- **Fish Advisories:** Due to the presence of pesticides like dieldrin, dioxin, mercury, and PCBs many fish and the bodies of water they live in are off limits for fishing. Unless we clean up these water sources and stop the pollution, eventually we may have no more fish left to eat. "TWO Federal studies have confirmed fears that many paper mills are discharging dioxin into rivers and that the toxic chemical is accumulating in fish downstream."[601]

RED TIDE ALERT!

Red tides have been occurring for hundreds, perhaps thousands of years. Yet today's pollution stemming from agricultural runoff and fertilizer facilities could be the reason they're worse and more frequent.[602] Like factory farms have manure ponds, phosphate fertilizer facilities stretching from the Louisiana Gulf Coast to Florida have radioactive gypsum ponds[603]. This stuff is so unsafe the EPA won't allow disposal anywhere![604] "Because the wastes are concentrated, phosphogypsum is more radioactive than the original phosphate rock."[605]

How might all this affect the Gulf of Mexico? The world's largest dead zone already exists along the Gulf Coast where the Mississippi meets the ocean, and it's expected to be bigger than ever in 2019. All the agricultural runoff from the center of the country flows into rivers that eventually flow here. "While this year's zone will be larger than usual because of the flooding, the long-term trend is still not changing. The bottom line is that we will never reach the dead zone reduction target of 1,900 square miles until more serious actions are taken to reduce the loss of Midwest fertilizers into the Mississippi River system. *Don Scavia, professor emeritus at the School for Environment and Sustainability*."[606]

Add to that all the runoff from Florida's sugar cane and citrus farming. Much of this runoff is diverted away from the wetlands that would naturally filter out pollutants, and sent instead directly to the sea. [607] Toxic pollution from Florida's phosphate fertilizer facilities frequently escapes into waterways[608] and ocean water.[609] Is this mix of contaminants exacerbating the blooms? Then of course bad storms and hurricanes cause more toxic water and dust from the radioactive gypsum mounds to get into the sea. National Geographic pointed out that the recent especially prolonged red tides of 2004, 2005 and 2017 all followed massive hurricane seasons. "Recent exceptional red tide years seem to follow massive storms."[610]

Mote Marine Laboratory can't state with certainty that there is a link between the Florida red tide, Karenia brevis, and fertilizer pollution but admits when the algae moves toward shore it can feed off the nutrients produced from human sources. "Florida red tides develop 10-40 miles offshore, away from human-contributed nutrient sources. Red tides occurred in Florida long before human settlement, and severe red tides were observed in the mid-1900s before the state's coastlines were heavily developed. However, once red tides are transported to shore, they are capable of using human-contributed nutrients for their growth."[611]

The Loop Current: The water in the Gulf flows up from Mexico and then east and south along the Florida coast. "This forms the Gulf Loop Current, which curves east and south along Florida's coast and exits through the Straits of Florida."[612]

SOLUTIONS

- By reducing & avoiding use of synthetic fertilizers we reduce toxins in runoff, and we'll use less pesticides too! This reduces total toxic contaminants getting into water.
- We need to discontinue business as usual at fertilizer manufacturing facilities—these places are capable of killing us all! Where's the EPA? No more gypsum mounds!
- Help Strengthen regulations at fertilizer facilities under RCRA, the reclamation law!
- Keep our waterways clean, don't pollute. Please help keep plastic out of the water!
- Abide by the Safe Fish List from Monterey Bay Aquarium: www.seafoodwatch.org.

25. DRINKING WATER

Water is essential for life, we couldn't live without it. Most of our foods are grown with water, cooked with water, made with the help of water; and most of our beverages are derived and made with the help of water. Without water we would have no food, without water we could not live. Water is essential for farming and growing food. Logically cleaner water is healthier for us, for plants and animals.

What happens to our health when most of the water we drink or cook with is tainted? Everyday, water sources around the world get polluted with chemicals, plastic, heavy metals, polystyrene, industrial pollution, persistent organic pollutants and health harmers of all kinds. These contaminants contribute to both physical and mental disease—are they not endocrine disruptors, carcinogens, neurotoxins, and reproductive toxins capable of causing a wide range of diseases? In relation to agriculture, the primary offenders include: pesticides, fertilizer, fungicides, fumigants, agricultural runoff, factory farm waste. There are countless sources of pollution, many directly or indirectly related to food, farming, food production, food packaging, and manufacturing.

> "Indeed one of the most alarming aspects of the chemical pollution of water is the fact that here—in river or lake or reservoir, or for that matter in the glass of water served at your dinner table—are mingled chemicals that no responsible chemist would think of combining in his laboratory." Rachel Carson *Silent Spring*

Throughout the world we're drowning in chemicals that we don't truly need. Agricultural pollutants are some of the most harmful. If you live in a rural area near farms, be sure to have your water tested for toxins, herbicides, and nitrates. Private water wells are not tested and maintained by anyone but the well owner. However, please keep in mind these substances can also be found in urban water systems.

We've been trained to rely upon so many toxic substances whose benefits are quite outnumbered by risks and consequences. For what reasons must we continue using them? The only benefits are to the industries and corporations producing them and profiting off their use. Every time someone uses synthetic fertilizer or sprays pesticides, our entire world is assaulted—from the air to the water, from people to animals and pollinators the cycle continues. The cunning innate nature of these substances ensures they contaminate the groundwater and waterways wherever they are applied, seeping into every corner of this precious planet. It is of utmost importance that we ween ourselves off these toxic substances at once.

Agriculture and Water Pollution

The damage caused from chemical agriculture is extensive. In most of the country glyphosate is used in such abundance that it inevitably contaminates water resources. As reported by *Reuters*, "It is out there in significant levels. It is out there consistently." Glyphosate, the key ingredient in "Roundup" herbicide, was found in every stream sample examined in Mississippi in a two-year period and in most air samples taken.[613] Glyphosate is not alone, many other troubling herbicides also present problems. "Atrazine was found in a majority of water samples from Midwestern homes and farms. Atrazine is found more often than any other pesticide in groundwater – 94% of drinking water tested by USDA contains the chemical. The weed killer is the second most widely used pesticides in the U.S., with more than 76 million pounds used last year, mostly on Midwestern corn fields. Atrazine is applied most heavily in Illinois, where applications exceed 85 pounds per square mile."[614]

Dieldrin, a persistent pesticide toxic to the brain and linked with Parkinson's, is readily being found in fish, wildlife, and human blood, breast milk, and umbilical cord tissue. Contamination is significant in the Midwest, especially Illinois, where it was applied most extensively. Even though it's been banned since 1987 it's still here.

- "During 2008-2009, the EPA analyzed concentrations of contaminants in fish from rivers and streams of the U.S. Dieldrin was detected in 71 percent of samples.
- Dieldrin is "water-phobic," attracted to fat. It's bound to soil that's washed into aquatic environments. Small organisms ingest the contaminated sediment. Each time a fish eats a contaminated organism, most of the dieldrin transfers to the fish's fat. The same thing happens when a predator, whether otter or human, eats a dieldrin-contaminated fish. It takes the human body one year to excrete just half the dieldrin absorbed from a meal."[615]

Even the wondrous great lakes, one of the world's largest fresh water ecosystems[616] is in trouble due to agriculture. The Food and Agriculture Organization reports, "there are more than 200 chemicals of concern in water and sediments of the Great Lakes ecosystem. Because the environmental burden of toxic chemicals includes both agriculture and non-agricultural compounds, it is difficult to separate the ecological and human health effects of pesticides from those of industrial compounds that are intentionally or accidentally released into the environment. However, there is overwhelming evidence that agricultural use of pesticides has a major impact on water quality and leads to serious environmental consequences."[617]

Synthetic Fertilizer & Water Pollution

Overuse of synthetic fertilizer causes exaggerated levels of nitrates in drinking water that in turn cause cancer. Additionally this garbage causes toxic algae, algae blooms, dead zones, and though debatable, there's lots of evidence it contributes to more frequent and deadly red tides.

- "Studies have shown increased risks of colon, kidney, and stomach cancer among people with higher ingestion of water nitrate and higher meat intake compared with low intakes of both, a dietary pattern that results in increased NOC (N-nitroso compounds) formation. Other studies have shown modest evidence that higher nitrate intake can increase the risk of thyroid cancer and ovarian cancer among women."[618]
- "Water pollution caused by nitrogen and phosphorus fertilizers causes the rapid growth of toxic algae. This uncontrolled algae bloom can lead to dangerously low levels of oxygen, or hypoxia, and the spread of a toxin known as cyanobacteria. People exposed to cyanobacteria while swimming or fishing can experience abdominal pain, nausea, vomiting, diarrhea, sore throat, dry cough, headache, blistering of the mouth, and sometimes even liver failure.
- Scientists report more than 350 cases of hypoxia, or dead zones, around the world.

- Nitrates in Mississippi River water make their way into the drinking water of millions of Americans. Studies have found that drinking water high in nitrates could double a person's chances of getting bladder, thyroid and ovarian cancer."[619]

Fertilizer & Fluoridated Water

While fluoride is touted as the ultimate cavity fighter, fluoridated water is very suspect. Looking at the source for the fluoride will make it easy to see why many consider it unsafe. The fluoride added to much of the public water supplies is hydrofluorosilicic acid.[620] This substance is derived from waste produced at phosphate fertilizer manufacturing facilities[621].

In the1940s and 50s before wet scrubbers—pollution control devices—were installed, fertilizer facilities emitted this fluoriosilicic gas into the air. The gas killed vast amounts of animals, livestock and vegetation nearby[622]. This toxic substance contains not just fluoride but also mercury, lead and arsenic. Somehow in a double coup, the phosphate facilities captured the gas with the wet scrubbers and then resold it to municipalities throughout the country to fluoridate our water. Dumping their toxic waste in water supplies throughout the country became a convenient remedy for industry to avoid costly disposal expenses and turn a profit instead.

Simply put, applying fluoride to the surface of teeth may be safe, but even your toothpaste tube alerts you to contact the poison control center *if you swallow it*. If it's poisonous to swallow fluoride, how can swallowing fluoridated water be beneficial for us? There's no way to modify the amount of fluoride any of us ingest from water, we're all getting the same dose unless your filter can remove it. Common water filtration systems though do not have the capability to filter fluoride out. Considering all the substances and foods made with unfiltered water, how much fluoride are we ingesting daily?

Fluorine & chlorine (and bromine) all affect the thyroid and prevent iodine absorption. So, tap water containing chlorine disinfection byproducts and fluoride must definitely have a negative effect on our endocrine system health. Keep in mind, there's no history of fluoride deficiency disease in humans.[623] What does a lifetime of drinking this water do?

> This is against all principles of modern pharmacology. It's really **obsolete**. No doubt about that. I mean, I think those nations that are using it should feel ashamed of themselves. It's against science—anti-scientific.
> Dr. Arvid Carlsson Nobel Laureate in Medicine, www.fluoridealert.org

HEALTH EFFECTS: Fluoride accumulates in the pineal and thyroid glands, it's a known enzyme disruptor[624], it prevents iodine absorption and disrupts thyroid function, it causes bone disease, bone changes, cancer, notably bone cancer in young men under 20, painful skeletal and dental fluorosis, gene mutations, reproductive effects, discolored teeth, depression, hyperactivity, hip fractures, osteoporosis, arthritis, hypothyroidism, and it lowers IQ. [625]

Note: If you have kidney disease or are undergoing dialysis you must avoid fluoridated water, or you could develop osteomalacia, a bone softening disease that causes extreme pain.[626]

When you consider all the beverages and food made with *unfiltered* fluoridated water, like soft drinks, soups, coffee, and tea—we're consuming a lot of fluoride! If it's so harmful we're not supposed to swallow it in toothpaste, how can all this fluoride consumption be good for us? Wouldn't it make more sense if vitamin c was added to our water? While fluoridated water has been mandated in the U.S. since the 1960s, most of the world opposes fluoridated water. It's banned in 97% of Europe and most civilized countries[627]: Germany, Austria, China, Denmark, Italy, Sweden, Norway, Finland, Belgium, The Netherlands, Hungary, Japan, Israel, Czech Republic, Estonia, France, Greece, Iceland, Mexico, Luxembourg, Poland, Portugal, Russia, Slovakia, Switzerland, Turkey.

Chromium 6, Hexavalent Chromium: Many thanks to Erin Brockovich who raised awareness about this toxic carcinogenic chemical in drinking water supplies. Because of her work polluters in California were forced to clean up their pollution and compensate people they had harmed. California went to work to establish a safe threshold in water supplies. However, further studies have revealed this contaminant in higher concentrations in drinking water all across the country, serving 218 million Americans![628] The worst levels are in Norman Oklahoma. The top suspected causes for the pollution: toxic wastewater from fracking[629] and unlined coal ash ponds. In a complete about face, in 2017 California tossed the previous established water threshold ruling due to it being economically unfeasible.[630]

Fracking Wastewater, Spills and Pipelines: So many threats exist for our water, and so little precaution is used. How can we continue to let fracking wastewater go unregulated? We must forbid further dumping of toxic wastewater and reselling of untreated wastewater. Time to end the loopholes allowing such devastating pollution into the earth, into water sources (refer to the Halliburton loophole, page 61).

Between oil spills, air pollution emissions, toxic wastewater, pipeline leaks, and earthquakes, what is this so-called energy independence costing us? Aren't we smart enough to develop systems that don't pollute, that don't compromise our drinking water, that don't endanger the planet? Anytime a waterway is compromised, be it surface water or underground, we all, in one way or another are affected. Currently the Ogallala Aquifer is in Danger. It is the largest underground aquifer in this country and could be forever contaminated if the construction of the Keystone XL Pipeline goes on as planned. If the energy companies were using their senses, they would build it in a way that poses no threat at all to anyone. It can be done; it may take a few extra dollars, but it's so worth it!

Flint: Aging Plumbing Pipes, Heavy Metals & Road Salt

The water catastrophe that crippled Flint could have been avoided. It's certainly a wake-up call to all cities where older water pipes remain in use. Aged pipes can leach toxic heavy metals like lead into the water, especially if the water is at all corrosive. The situation in Flint, Michigan was caused mostly by older corroded pipes leaching lead. How did that happen? If they hadn't switched water sources it may never have happened, but they diverted to the river water and the tragedy unfolded. In Flint's case what ultimately caused the river water to be so caustic came down they believe to road salt usage in the winter months. When salt melts off it seeps into water ways, and in this case caused spiked chloride levels in the Flint River. As revealed by the National Resources Defense Council, "The cheapest and most common way to de-ice a road is by applying ordinary salt. Road salt is 40 percent sodium ions and 60 percent chloride ions. When the snow and ice melt, the salt applied to roads eventually washes its way into both groundwater and nearby rivers and streams, where the ions dissociate from each other. Water from the Flint River has an unusually high concentration of chloride ions—eight times higher than the tap water in Detroit, which supplied Flint with drinking water until April 2014, when the city made the switch. According to the Virginia Tech water experts who helped blow the lid off the public health scandal, those high chloride levels are likely responsible for the corrosiveness of Flint River water. Without an aggressive corrosion-inhibiting treatment, like the one Detroit uses, the water readily dissolved lead from the city's pipes."[631]

The Unmentionables: Pharmaceutical and Personal Care Products

(PPCPs) are an ever-growing body of new pollutants literally flushing into our waterways. Composed of the many substances we ingest and use on our bodies, or throw into the toilet, PPCPs are becoming a global water crisis. Because of the resilient nature of these compounds, they are found in both untreated and *treated* water. Water treatment facilities throughout the world are simply not advanced enough to filter them out. Most prevalent chemicals found include: pharmaceuticals, antibiotics, anti-inflammatory drugs, sex hormones from oral contraceptives, anticonvulsants, beta-blockers, antidepressants, bronchodilators, antibiotics, hypnotics, sunscreen products and synthetic fragrance. This is a dire problem, just the accumulated presence of antibiotics can lead to an escalated situation with antibiotic resistance. According to the Office of National Drug Policy, you should take unused, unneeded or expired prescription drugs out of their original containers and throw them in the trash. They suggest mixing prescription drugs with used coffee grounds or kitty litter and putting them in sealed bags to ensure the drugs are not diverted.

Methods of Decontaminating Water Pose a Risk Also!

Houston, we have a problem. For the past 100 years, most cities throughout the country have relied on chlorine to disinfect water. Now many cities use chloramines, a crazy combination of chlorine and ammonia to "purify" water. While chlorine has curbed illnesses from water-borne diseases, chlorine and ammonia together create dangerous disinfection byproducts (DBPs).

When chlorine is mixed with water that contains any type of organic matter like leaves or dirt, cancer-causing halocetic acids, MX,[632] and trihalomethanes like chloroform are created. Trihalomethanes are released through hot chlorinated water vapors. This means that the everyday tasks of taking showers and doing dishes can be hazardous to your health. Scientists have learned that the gene-mutator MX is 170 more potent and dangerous than chloroform.

Using ammonia to prepare water for drinking is equally troubling. Though recently approved by the EPA, this method creates iodoacids. Michael Plewa, a genetic toxicologist at the University of Illinois' Urbana campus, along with fellow scientists, identified iodoacids as the most toxic disinfection byproduct yet discovered. His studies show that iodoacids severely damage DNA.[633] When combined, all these disinfection byproducts contribute to cancer, aggravate allergies, stimulate production of free radicals, weaken normal blood vessels and cause plaque build-up. They can also contribute to heart attacks and strokes and anemia, as well as cause nervous system disorders, birth defects and miscarriages.

DRINKING WATER CONTAMINANTS

The below charts are courtesy of the EPA[634]

Disinfection Byproducts

Contaminant	MCLG[1] (mg/L)[2]	MCL or TT[1] (mg/L)[2]	Potential Health Effects from Ingestion of Water	Sources of Contaminant in Drinking Water
Bromate	Zero	0.010	Increased risk of cancer	Byproduct of drinking water disinfection
Chlorite	0.8	1.0	Anemia; infants & young children: nervous system effects	Byproduct of drinking water disinfection
Haloacetic acids (HAA5)	n/a[6]	0.060	Increased risk of cancer	Byproduct of drinking water disinfection
Total **Trihalomethanes** (TTHMs)	None[7] ---------- n/a[6]	0.10 --------- -0.080	Liver, kidney or central nervous system problems; increased risk of cancer	Byproduct of drinking water disinfection

Disinfectants

Contaminant	MRDLG[1] (mg/L)[2]	MRDL[1] (mg/L)[2]	Potential Health Effects from Ingestion of Water	Sources of Contaminant in Drinking Water
Chloramines (as Cl_2)	MRDLG=4[1]	MRDL=4.0[1]	Eye/nose irritation; stomach discomfort, anemia, DNA damage	Water additive used to control microbes
Chlorine (as Cl_2)	MRDLG=4[1]	MRDL=4.0[1]	Eye/nose irritation; stomach discomfort	Water additive used to control microbes
Chlorine dioxide (as ClO_2)	MRDLG=0.8[1]	MRDL=0.8[1]	Anemia; infants & young children: nervous system effects	Water additive used to control microbes

Inorganic Chemicals

Contaminant	MCLG[1] (mg/L)[2]	MCL or TT[1] (mg/L)[2]	Potential Health Effects from Ingestion of Water	Sources of Contaminant in Drinking Water
Antimony	0.006	0.006	Increase in blood cholesterol; decrease in blood sugar	Discharge from petroleum refineries; fire retardants; ceramics; electronics; solder
Arsenic	0[7]	0.010 as of 01/23/06	Skin damage or problems with circulatory systems, and may have increased risk of getting cancer	Erosion of natural deposits; runoff from orchards, runoff from glass & electronics production wastes
Asbestos (fiber >10 micrometers)	7 million fibers	7 MFL	Increased risk of developing benign intestinal polyps	Decay of asbestos cement in water mains; erosion of natural deposits
Barium	2	2	Increase in blood pressure	Discharge of drilling wastes; discharge from metal refineries; erosion of natural deposits
Beryllium	0.004	0.004	Intestinal lesions	Discharge from metal refineries and coal-burning factories; discharge from electrical, aerospace, and defense industries
Cadmium	0.005	0.005	Kidney damage	Corrosion of galvanized pipes; erosion of natural deposits; discharge from metal refineries; runoff from waste batteries and paints
Chromium (total)	0.1	0.1	Allergic dermatitis	Discharge from steel and pulp mills; erosion of natural deposits

Copper	1.3	TT[8]; Action Level=1.3	Short term exposure: Gastrointestinal distress Long term exposure: Liver or kidney damage. People with Wilson's Disease should consult their doctor if the amount of copper in their water exceeds the action level	Corrosion of household plumbing systems; erosion of natural deposits
Cyanide (as free cyanide)	0.2	0.2	Nerve damage or thyroid problems	Discharge from steel/metal factories; discharge from plastic and fertilizer factories
Fluoride	4.0	4.0	Bone disease (pain and tenderness of the bones); Children may get mottled teeth	Water additive which promotes strong teeth; erosion of natural deposits; discharge from fertilizer and aluminum factories
Lead	Zero	TT[8]; Action Level=0.01 5	Infants and children: Delays in physical or mental development; deficits in attention span and learning abilities. Adults: Kidney problems; high blood pressure	Corrosion of household plumbing systems; erosion of natural deposits
Mercury (inorganic)	0.00 2	0.002	Kidney damage	Erosion of natural deposits; discharge from refineries and factories; runoff from landfills and croplands
Nitrate (measured as Nitrogen)	10	10	Infants below the age of six months who drink water containing nitrate in excess of the MCL could become seriously ill and, if untreated, may die. Symptoms include shortness of breath and blue-baby syndrome.	Runoff from fertilizer use; leaching from septic tanks, sewage; erosion of natural deposits

Nitrite (measured as Nitrogen)	1	1	Infants below the age of six months who drink water containing nitrite in excess of the MCL could become seriously ill and, if untreated, may die. Symptoms include shortness of breath and blue-baby syndrome.	Runoff from fertilizer use; leaching from septic tanks, sewage; erosion of natural deposits
Selenium	0.05	0.05	Hair or fingernail loss; numbness in fingers or toes; circulatory problems	Discharge from petroleum refineries; erosion of natural deposits; discharge from mines
Thallium	0.00 05	0.002	Hair loss; changes in blood; kidney, intestine, or liver problems	Leaching from ore-processing sites; discharge from electronics, glass, and drug factories

Volatile Organic Chemicals (including Pesticides)

Contaminant	**MC LG[1] (mg /L)[2]**	**MCL or TT[1] (mg/L)[2]**	**Potential Health Effects from Ingestion of Water**	**Sources of Contaminant in Drinking Water**
Acrylamide	Zer o	TT[9]	Nervous system or blood problems; increased risk of cancer	Added to water during sewage/wastewater treatment
Alachlor	Zer o	0.002	Eye, liver, kidney or spleen problems; anemia; increased risk of cancer	Runoff from herbicide used on row crops
Atrazine	0.00 3	0.003	Cardiovascular system or reproductive problems	Runoff from herbicide used on row crops
Benzene	Zer o	0.005	Anemia; decrease in blood platelets; increased risk of cancer	Discharge from factories; leaching from gas storage tanks and landfills
Benzo(a)pyre ne (PAHs)	Zer o	0.0002	Reproductive difficulties; increased risk of cancer	Leaching from linings of water storage tanks and distribution lines

Carbofuran	0.04	0.04	Problems with blood, nervous system, or reproductive system	Leaching of soil fumigant used on rice and alfalfa
Carbon tetrachloride	Zero	0.005	Liver problems; increased risk of cancer	Discharge from chemical plants and other industrial activities
Chlordane	Zero	0.002	Liver or nervous system problems; increased risk of cancer	Residue of banned termiticide
Chlorobenzene	0.1	0.1	Liver or kidney problems	Discharge from chemical and agricultural chemical factories
2,4-D	0.07	0.07	Kidney, liver, or adrenal gland problems	Runoff from herbicide used on row crops
Dalapon	0.2	0.2	Minor kidney changes	Runoff from herbicide used on rights of way
1,2-Dibromo-3-chloropropane (DBCP)	Zero	0.0002	Reproductive difficulties; increased risk of cancer	Runoff/leaching from soil fumigant used on soybeans, cotton, pineapples, and orchards
o-Dichlorobenzene	0.6	0.6	Liver, kidney, or circulatory system problems	Discharge from industrial chemical factories
p-Dichlorobenzene	0.075	0.075	Anemia; liver, kidney or spleen damage; changes in blood	Discharge from industrial chemical factories
1,2-Dichloroethane	Zero	0.005	Increased risk of cancer	Discharge from industrial chemical factories
1,1-Dichloroethylene	0.007	0.007	Liver problems	Discharge from industrial chemical factories

cis-1,2-Dichloroethylene	0.07	0.07	Liver problems	Discharge from industrial chemical factories
trans-1,2-Dichloroethylene	0.1	0.1	Liver problems	Discharge from industrial chemical factories
Dichloromethane	Zero	0.005	Liver problems; increased risk of cancer	Discharge from drug and chemical factories
1,2-Dichloropropane	Zero	0.005	Increased risk of cancer	Discharge from industrial chemical factories
Di(2-ethylhexyl) adipate	0.4	0.4	Weight loss, liver problems, or possible reproductive difficulties.	Discharge from chemical factories
Di(2-ethylhexyl) phthalate	Zero	0.006	Reproductive difficulties; liver problems; increased risk of cancer	Discharge from rubber and chemical factories
Dinoseb	0.007	0.007	Reproductive difficulties	Runoff from herbicide used on soybeans and vegetables
Dioxin (2,3,7,8-TCDD)	Zero	0.00000003	Reproductive difficulties; increased risk of cancer	Emissions from waste incineration and combustion; discharge from chemical factories
Diquat	0.02	0.02	Cataracts	Runoff from herbicide use
Endothall	0.1	0.1	Stomach and intestinal problems	Runoff from herbicide use
Endrin	0.002	0.002	Liver problems	Residue of banned insecticide
Epichlorohydrin	Zero	TT[9]	Increased cancer risk, and over a long period of time, stomach problems	Discharge from chemical factories; impure water treatment chemicals

Ethylbenzene	0.7	0.7	Liver or kidneys problems	Discharge from petroleum refineries
Ethylene dibromide	Zero	0.00005	Problems with liver, stomach, reproductive system, or kidneys; increased risk of cancer	Discharge from petroleum refineries
Glyphosate	0.7	0.7	Kidney problems; reproductive difficulties	Runoff from herbicide use
Heptachlor	Zero	0.0004	Liver damage; increased risk of cancer	Residue of banned termiticide
Heptachlor epoxide	Zero	0.0002	Liver damage; increased risk of cancer	Breakdown of heptachlor
Hexachlorobenzene	Zero	0.001	Liver or kidney problems; reproductive difficulties; increased risk of cancer	Discharge from metal refineries and agricultural chemical factories
Hexachlorocyclopentadiene	0.05	0.05	Kidney or stomach problems	Discharge from chemical factories
Lindane	0.0002	0.0002	Liver or kidney problems	Runoff/leaching from insecticide used on cattle, lumber, gardens
Methoxychlor	0.04	0.04	Reproductive difficulties	Runoff/leaching from insecticide used on fruits, vegetables, alfalfa, livestock
Oxamyl (Vydate)	0.2	0.2	Slight nervous system effects	Runoff/leaching from insecticide used on apples, potatoes, and tomatoes
Polychlorinated biphenyls (PCBs)	Zero	0.0005	Skin changes; thymus gland problems; immune deficiencies; reproductive or nervous system difficulties; cancer risk	Runoff from landfills; discharge of waste chemicals

Pentachlorophenol	Zero	0.001	Liver or kidney problems; increased cancer risk	Discharge from wood preserving factories
Picloram	0.5	0.5	Liver problems	Herbicide runoff
Simazine	0.004	0.004	Problems with blood	Herbicide runoff
Styrene	0.1	0.1	Liver, kidney, or circulatory system problems	Discharge from rubber and plastic factories; leaching from landfills
Tetrachloroethylene	Zero	0.005	Liver problems; increased risk of cancer	Discharge from factories and dry cleaners
Toluene	1	1	Nervous system, kidney, or liver problems	Discharge from petroleum factories
Toxaphene	Zero	0.003	Kidney, liver, or thyroid problems; increased risk of cancer	Runoff/leaching from insecticide used on cotton and cattle
2,4,5-TP (Silvex)	0.05	0.05	Liver problems	Residue of banned herbicide
1,2,4-Trichlorobenzene	0.07	0.07	Changes in adrenal glands	Discharge from textile finishing factories
1,1,1-Trichloroethane	0.20	0.2	Liver, nervous system, or circulatory problems	Discharge from metal degreasing sites and other factories
1,1,2-Trichloroethane	0.003	0.005	Liver, kidney, or immune system problems	Discharge from industrial chemical factories
Trichloroethylene	Zero	0.005	Liver problems; increased risk of cancer	Discharge from metal degreasing sites and other factories
Vinyl chloride	Zero	0.002	Increased risk of cancer	Leaching from PVC pipes; discharge from plastic factories

Xylenes (total)	10	10	Nervous system damage	Discharge from petroleum factories; discharge from chemical factories

SOLUTIONS DRINK CLEAN WATER

"Filtering home tap or well water can decrease exposure to numerous known or suspected carcinogens and endocrine-disrupting chemicals. Unless the home water source is known to be contaminated, it is preferable to use filtered tap water instead of commercially bottled water."

The President's Cancer Panel [635]

Water is the earth's most precious resource. All life depends on clean water. For our health and this amazing planet, we must do all we can to keep contaminants out of water supplies. You mustn't drink or cook with contaminated water. Use filtered water, spring water, any water source that is known to be free of contaminants.

- **Filter filter filter**! To make your tap water safe for drinking and cooking, get a filter today. The Berkey filter is a stainless-steel gravity-fed filter--easy to set up, it sits on your counter--make sure to get the additional fluoride filters that come with it. Reverse osmosis and carbon filtering systems are really good. Make sure whatever you use it removes the toxins.
- Use filtered water for all drinking and cooking purposes
- If you have a private well be sure to have it tested for nitrate and pesticides!
- Look up your water for contaminants here by zipcode: www.ewg.org/tapwater/
- Be a water guardian and help the planet by not polluting it.
- Industry must not pollute waterways, their wastewater must be filtered and cleaned before recycling or dumping back into our water resources.
- We must enforce the Clean Water Act Only through reduced toxic runoff, can waterways, plant and animal populations begin healing.
- The EPA must set stricter limits and boundaries on toxins while monitoring water pollution more seriously. Too many toxic farm chemicals are infiltrating waterways. Until these chemicals are cutback or no longer in use, we must insist on careful regulation.
- Let's get the fluoride out of our water!
- We must get water pipes upgraded in this country.
- We must develop stronger and more effective water filtration methods that remove all toxins, not most, but all.
- If we use less toxins, it'll be easier to keep our drinking water clean
- For more info on water filters, visit www.ewg.org/tapwater/water-filter-technology.php
- The Water Issue is so complex and will be more thoroughly exposed in the next book.

The Precautionary Principle

On January 15, 1998 the precautionary principle was defined at a weekend meeting at Wingspread, headquarters of the Johnson Foundation in Racine, Wisconsin. Subsequently known as the Wingspread Statement, the precautionary principle was defined as follows: "When an activity raises threats of harm to human health or the environment, precautionary measures should be taken even if some cause and effect relationships are not fully established scientifically."[636]

> **Precautionary Principle, a working definition**
>
> When human activities may lead to morally unacceptable harm that is scientifically plausible but uncertain, actions shall be taken to avoid or diminish that harm.
> Morally unacceptable harm refers to harm to humans or the environment that is:
>
> - threatening to human life or health, or
> - serious and effectively irreversible, or
> - inequitable to present or future generations, or
> - imposed without adequate consideration of the human rights of those affected.
>
> The judgement of plausibility should be grounded in scientific analysis. Analysis should be ongoing so that chosen actions are subject to review. Uncertainty may apply to, but need not be limited to, causality or the bounds of the possible harm. Actions are interventions that are undertaken before harm occurs that seek to avoid or diminish the harm. Actions should be chosen that are proportional to the seriousness of the potential harm, with consideration of their positive and negative consequences, and with an assessment of the moral implications of both action and inaction. The choice of action should be the result of a participatory process.
>
> www.unesco.org
> United Nations Educational, Scientific, and Cultural Organization

FOUR

Trends + Remedies

The shifts in food production and control are nothing short of significant. As Michael Pollan states in the *Omnivore's Dilemma*, "Corn is present in nearly every processed food that you will find in the supermarket, and even fed to the animals we eat, from cows to farmed salmon."[637] This is affecting biodiversity across the spectrum of the food supply, plant and animal world. Overuse of pesticides is decimating pollinators and wild habitats. Most corn grown today is bt corn that contains the bt toxin--capable of poking holes in cell walls and turning your stomach into a pesticide factory.[638] We must remember, without synthetic fertilizer, soil would be far healthier, plants would be healthier, and we wouldn't need so many pesticides and chemicals! In case you were wondering, corn requires more nitrogen per acre than any other crop.[639] Is it just coincidence that we grow so much of it? Our entire food system has been shifting to accommodate the profit margins of the chemical cartel. Are we taking notice?

26. TRENDS + DISEASE

Everyday we're exposed to numerous toxins. As far as food's concerned, major routes of exposure include the foods we eat, the water we drink, tools we cook with, containers and packaging—there's countless ways health harming substances make contact with us. The best we can do is to be aware and protect ourselves as best we can.

We do have a right to know what ingredients are in foods and in products. Currently, there's little regulation and there's way too many dangerous substances used not just to grow food but also to package food, and to get food to our tables. Where's the disclosure? We used to have a law in this country that prevented carcinogens from being added to any food substance, be it for humans or animals. It was called the Delaney Amendment, but alas it was quietly expired in the mid 1990s. Interesting, the same time GMOs were approved.

People are inherently trusting, when we shop it's like we're kids again and we don't question the safety of food on the shelves. But alas, today's world is not like it used to be. Now we have to question, especially since many ingredients are absent from labels. We definitely need better rules, and labels that inform us, so we then can make informed decisions when we're shopping. The only alternative is that all the dangerous substances and questionable ingredients need to be forbidden. If they don't want to label their products accordingly, what other option is there?

Toxins vary greatly, some far more dangerous than others. They come in large and small amounts, and exposure can be minute or it can be long-term. Certainly chronic exposure, *daily* exposure through food and beverages cannot be without some risk. [640]

Due to modern chemical agriculture, food is different now than when our grandparents were growing up. Today, many foods come from seeds that are modified with toxins in a lab before even hitting the field. When planted these seeds develop into plants containing new and unusual proteins that our bodies aren't accustomed to. Our bodies perceive these proteins as unnatural, as invaders. Does this explain the boom in food allergies? Inflammation, cancer, autoimmune diseases have all escalated wildly over the past 30 or so years. With GMO foods, people and animals are exposed to exceptionally high levels of glyphosate. Are these new food production methods creating toxins responsible for the rise of diseases like gluten intolerance, allergies, celiac disease? Could they be involved somehow with the increased incidence of disease and cancer in people and in animals also? If these chemicals are harming bees and pollinators, frogs, and lab animals, to what extent is our health impacted?

XENOBIOTICS

"Foreign to Life," synthetic chemicals, not found in nature, can be stored in various body organs and tissues

The World Health Organization Cancer Report 2014 states:

- Cancers figure among the leading causes of morbidity and mortality worldwide, with approximately 14 million new cases and 8.2 million cancer-related deaths in 2012.[641]
- The number of new cancer cases is expected to rise by 70% over the next 2 decades.[642]
- "Inherited genetic factors make a minor contribution to susceptibility to most types of neoplasms. This finding indicates that the environment has the principal role in causing sporadic cancer."[643]

"The good news is that a large number of cancers can be prevented. It is estimated that as many as two-thirds of all cancer cases are linked to environmental causes. This number may even be higher. Many of these are linked to lifestyle factors that can be modified."[644]

National Institutes of Health

"Throughout the world more toxins are used today to grow food than ever before.
As reported by the Soil Association, "In 2016, over 16,600 tonnes of pesticides were used on British farms to kill weeds, insects and control crop diseases.

Many people don't realize almost 300 pesticides can be routinely used in non-organic farming and these are often present in non-organic food we eat despite washing and cooking.

Glyphosate—the active ingredient in Monsanto's Roundup—is the most widely sold weedkiller in the world. Government figures show its use in UK farming has increased by a shocking 400% in the last 20 years.

Glyphosate is one of three pesticides regularly found in routine testing of British bread, appearing in over 60% of wholemeal bread samples tested by the Defra committee on Pesticide Residues in Food." SOURCE: SOIL ASSOCIATION UK[645]

President's Cancer Panel Report 2008-2009

"The entire U.S. population is exposed on a daily basis to numerous agricultural chemicals, some of which also are used in residential and commercial landscaping. Many of these chemicals have known or suspected carcinogenic or endocrine-disrupting properties. Pesticides (insecticides, herbicides, and fungicides) approved for use by the U.S. Environmental Protection Agency (EPA) contain nearly 900 active ingredients, many of which are toxic. Many of the solvents, fillers, and other chemicals listed as inert ingredients on pesticide labels also are toxic, but are not required to be tested for their potential to cause chronic diseases such as cancer. In addition to pesticides, agricultural fertilizers and veterinary pharmaceuticals are major contributors to water pollution, both directly and as a result of chemical processes that form toxic by-products when these substances enter the water supply. Farmers and their families, including migrant workers, are at highest risk from agricultural exposures. Because agricultural chemicals often are applied as mixtures, it has been difficult to clearly distinguish cancer risks associated with individual agents."

From the National Institutes of Health Report, *Cancer and the Environment*

"Studies of people with high exposures to pesticides, such as farmers, pesticide applicators, crop duster pilots, and manufacturers, have found high rates of blood and lymphatic system cancers, cancers of the lip, stomach, lung, brain, and prostate, as well as melanoma and other skin cancers. So far, human studies do not allow researchers to sort out exactly which pesticides are linked to which cancers. Therefore, most of these pesticides are still listed in the *Report on Carcinogens* as likely to be cancer-causing, rather than as known carcinogens."[646]

Agriculture, the growing of food and domestication of animals is over 10,000 years old. Little by little, planting and growing techniques were cultivated; tools and machinery were developed to speed along the seed-to-plate process. In the beginning, farmers planted by seasons and moon phases, and they learned how to care gently for the land. Chemicals were only introduced into this process in the mid to late 1800s. The upward growth and extent to which chemicals are now involved with farming and food is quite significant—and even more significant is the correlating rise of disease and cancer, and depression, anxiety, aggressiveness and violence. Could these foods—the chemicals they're grown with—be affecting not just our physical, but our mental wellbeing as well?

If glyphosate can in fact reduce our levels of dopamine, tryptophan, melatonin and serotonin and others (see page 32-33), then that automatically interferes with our ability to be happy, to relax, to sleep. Such effects surely can't help us feel good or peaceful. If the chemicals used to grow food have such ill effects on us, are they in fact also having similar ill effects on the planet? Of course they're polluting waterways and soil but does the earth have a biochemical balance like ours that's disrupted and corrupted from these chemicals? When the earth is off, everything on the earth—dependent on the earth surely will be off as well. Imbalance begets imbalance. In any case reducing the amount of chemicals that contact our food and water and soil will help our physical and mental health improve, and quite likely help the earth in more ways than we can possibly currently understand.

The President's Cancer Panel Report 2008-2009[647]

"A precautionary, prevention-oriented approach should replace current reactionary approaches to environmental contaminants in which human harm must be proven before action is taken to reduce or eliminate exposure. Though not applicable in every instance, this approach should be the cornerstone of a new national cancer prevention strategy that emphasizes primary prevention, redirects accordingly both research and policy agendas, and sets tangible goals for reducing or eliminating toxic environmental exposures implicated in cancer causation."

CAUSE and EFFECT

Before GMOs existed, there was already plenty of research documenting the environmental differences between conventional and organic farming. I became involved in organics in 1991, five years before GMOs ever appeared. I was truly dedicated to organics for not just my own health, but to keep the world, the water, and the whole earth well. The benefit of eating foods with less pesticides and without toxic fertilizers was gaining traction. Then, suddenly a new player came to town and with it, more powerful chemicals. Between industry and government, far too many secrets are concealed from us concerning the safety of these substances.

There's a great deal of evidence from all over the world that toxic chemicals cause health problems as well as water issues, air, wildlife, and biodiversity disasters. Everyday it seems we hear about another devastating situation somewhere in the world. People are suffering everywhere, the whole planet needs band aids and nurturing. These tragedies aren't stopping or slowing down, they're growing in number and intensity. If the overuse of chemicals, of pesticides, of agricultural chemicals in anyway contributes, causes or worsens these devastating health and environmental problems, do we continue letting these chemicals, these corporations conduct business as usual? If we move away from using so many toxic substances, do we start getting better? Is there less stress, imbalance, less violence? Does the world start recovering, mending its wounds and becoming friendly again?

DISEASE TRENDS

The following graphs are the result of an extensive research project that examined GMOs and glyphosate in the U.S. food supply since 1996. GMOs were permitted without safety testing for human consumption, and now glyphosate is the most commonly used herbicide. Usage has increased from 27 million pounds in 1996 to nearly 300 million pounds by 2016 (see USGS chart below). Curiously its deployment runs nearly parallel with spikes in several diseases.

"In the US, glyphosate residues allowed in food are some of the highest in the world. In July of 2013 the Environmental Protection Agency (EPA, 2013) raised the maximum allowable residues of glyphosate', particularly for animal feed.[648] In studies, "chronically ill humans had significantly higher glyphosate residues in urine than healthy humans." Cows had glyphosate in their urine as well as in their kidneys, liver, lung, spleen, and muscles indicating 'meat and dairy are an additional route of exposure for humans'.[649]

The highest allowed residue levels for glyphosate include these foods[650]:

Commodity	Parts per million
Animal feed, nongrass	400
Cotton	210
Grain, cereal, forage, fodder and straw	100
Grass, forage, fodder and hay	300
Kenaf, forage	200
Leucaena, forage	200
Peppermint and spearmint tops	200
Teff, hay and forage	100
Canola seed	20
Corn, field forage	100
Grain, aspirated fractions	300
Soybean, hay	200
Soybean, forage	100
Soybean hulls	120

The authors don't claim that GMOs and glyphosate are the only reason for the diseases they examined, but since the spikes in all the diseases correlate such with the timing and onset of GMO expansion in our food supply, the connection should be explored in greater depth. Could it merely be coincidence? The graphs that follow were published in *Genetically engineered crops, glyphosate and the deterioration of health in the United States* found in the Journal of Organic Systems, Vol 9(2) 2014.[651] Authored by *Nancy Swanson, Abacus Enterprises, Lummi Island, WA, USA Andre Leu, International Federation of Organic Agricultural Movements, Bonn, Germany Jon Abrahamson, Abacus Enterprises, Lummi Island, WA, USA, Bradley Wallet, Crustal Imaging Facility, Conoco Phillips School of Geology and Geophysics, University of Oklahoma, USA.

Escalation of GMO foods and Disease, U.S. since 1996

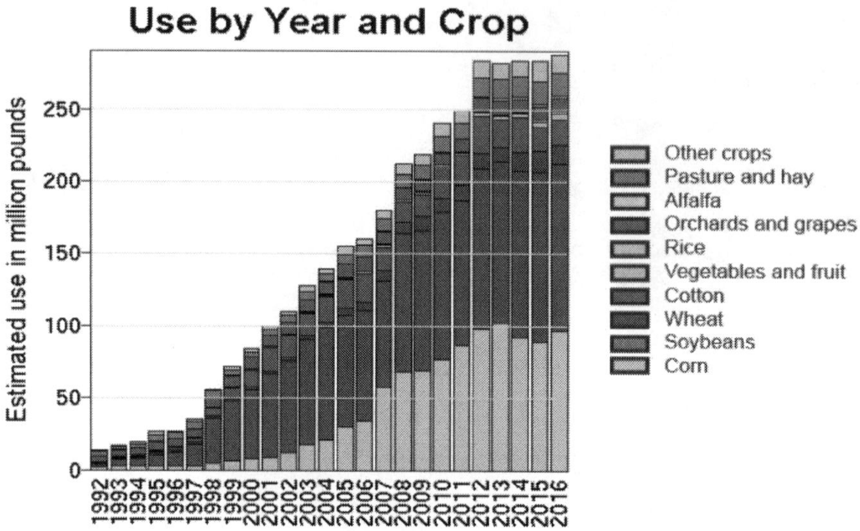

Graph Source USGS National Water Quality Assessment Project[652]

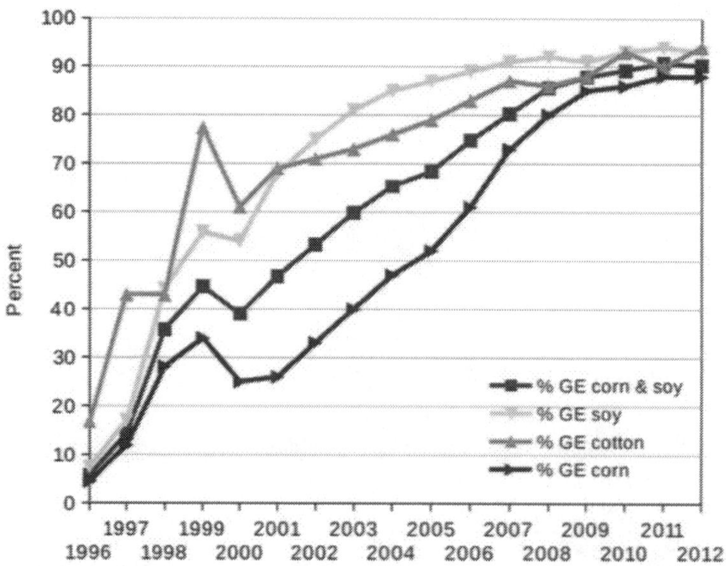

Figure 1. Adoption of GE crops in US.

DISEASE TRENDS SINCE 1996

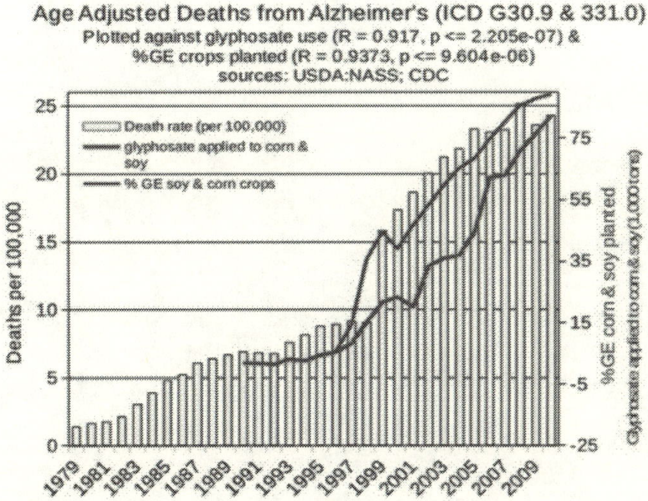

Figure 25. Correlation between age-adjusted Alzheimer's disease deaths and glyphosate applications and percentage of US corn and soy crops that are GE.

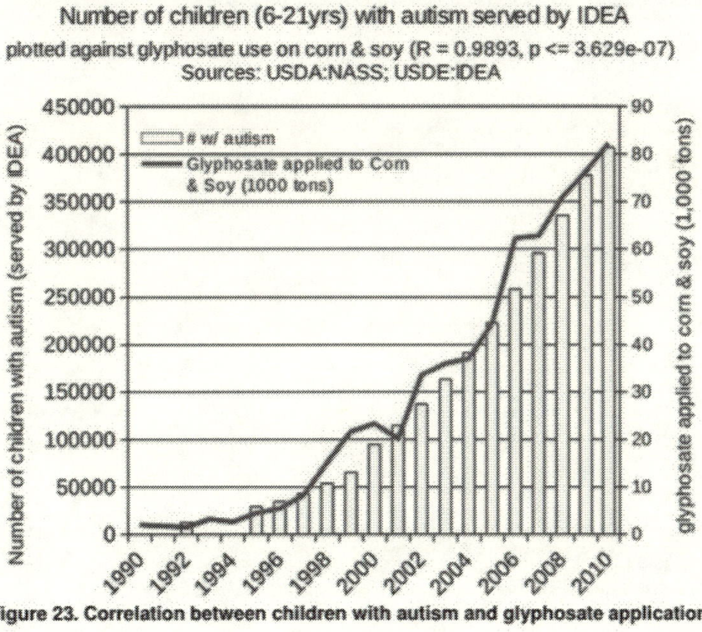

Figure 23. Correlation between children with autism and glyphosate applications.

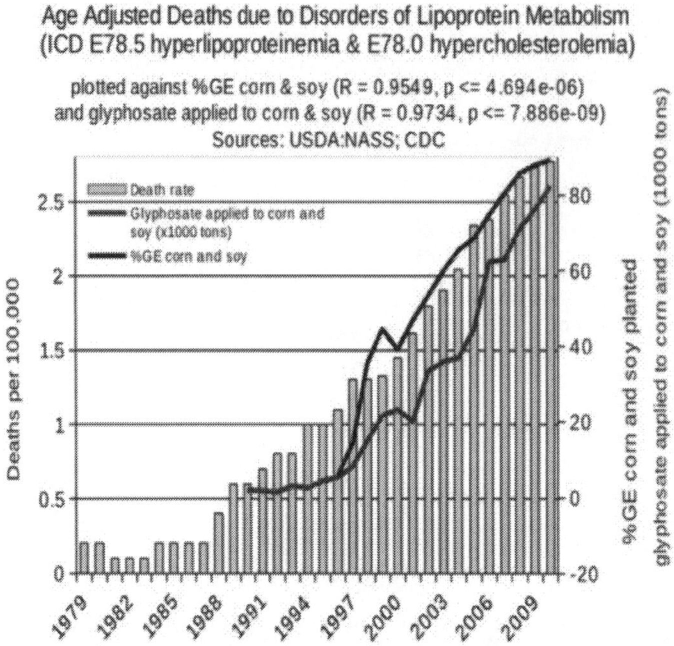

Figure 16. Correlation between age-adjusted lipoprotein disorder deaths and glyphosate applications and percentage of US corn and soy crops that are GE.

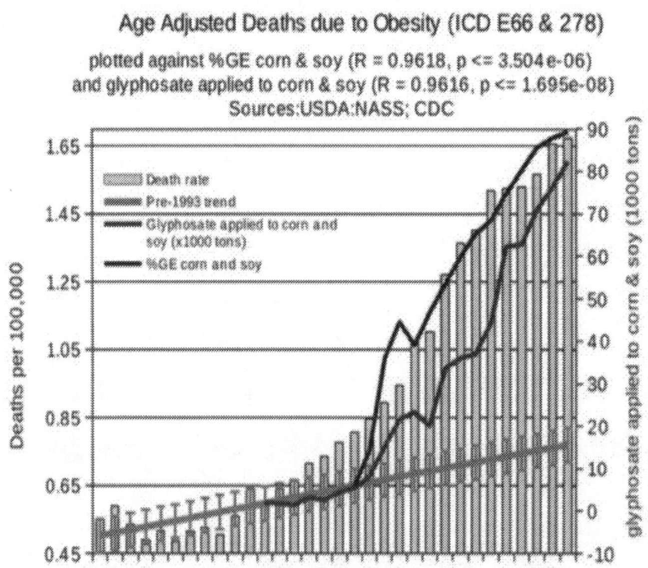

Figure 13. Correlation between age-adjusted obesity deaths and glyphosate applications and percentage of US corn and soy crops that are GE.

Figure 11. Correlation between age-adjusted hypertension deaths and glyphosate applications and percentage of US corn and soy crops that are GE.

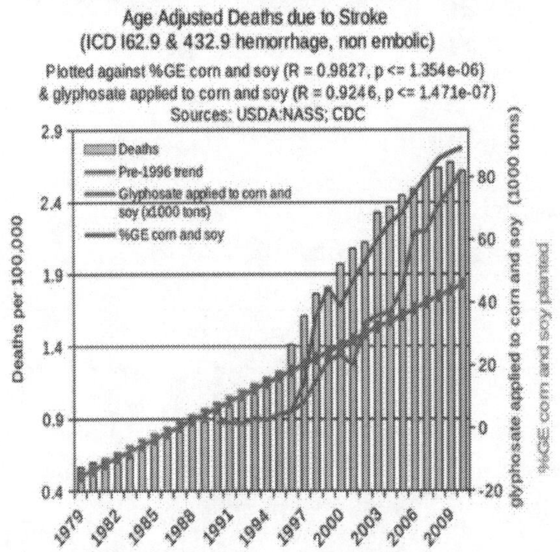

Figure 12. Correlation between age-adjusted hemorrhagic stroke deaths and glyphosate applications and percentage of US corn and soy crops that are GE.

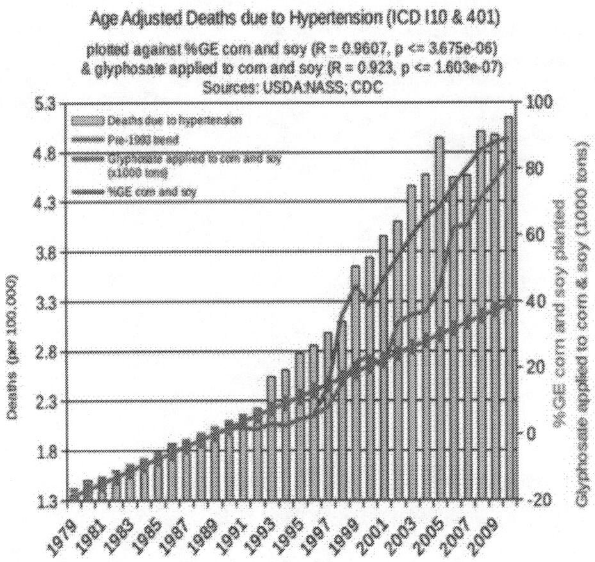

Figure 11. Correlation between age-adjusted hypertension deaths and glyphosate applications and percentage of US corn and soy crops that are GE.

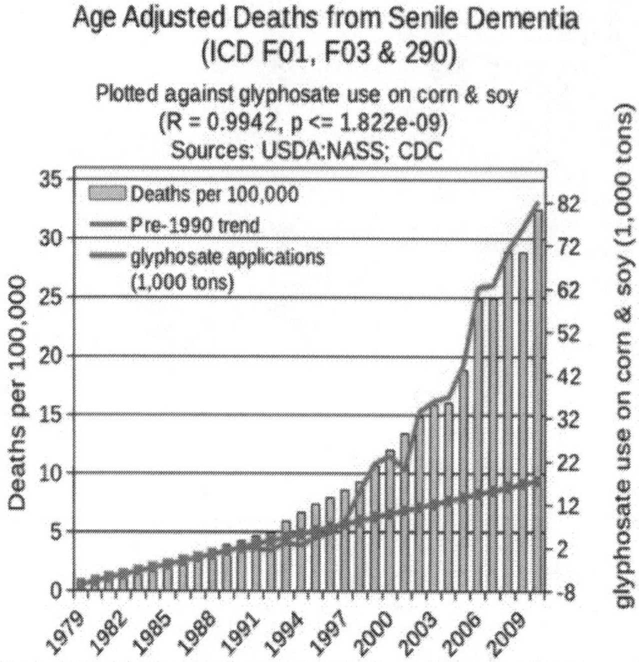

Figure 24. Correlation between age-adjusted dementia deaths and glyphosate applications.

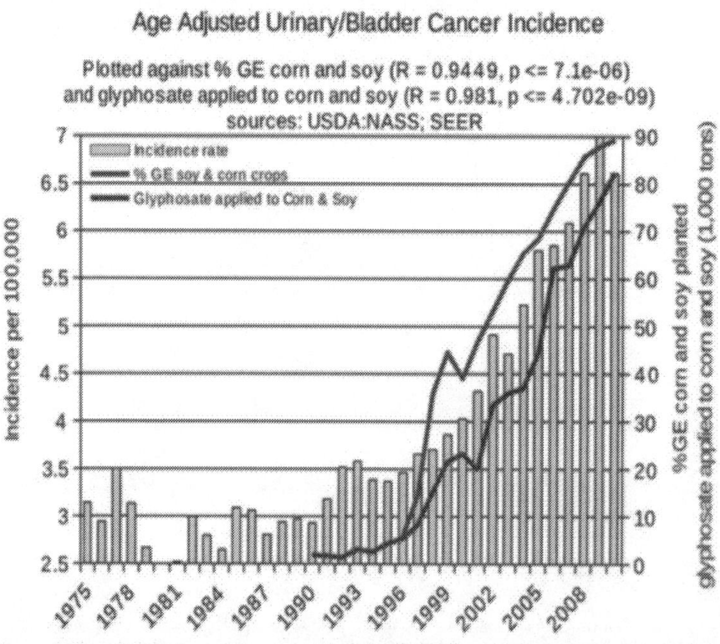

Figure 9. Correlation between age-adjusted bladder/urinary tract cancer and glyphosate applications and percentage of US corn and soy crops that are GE.

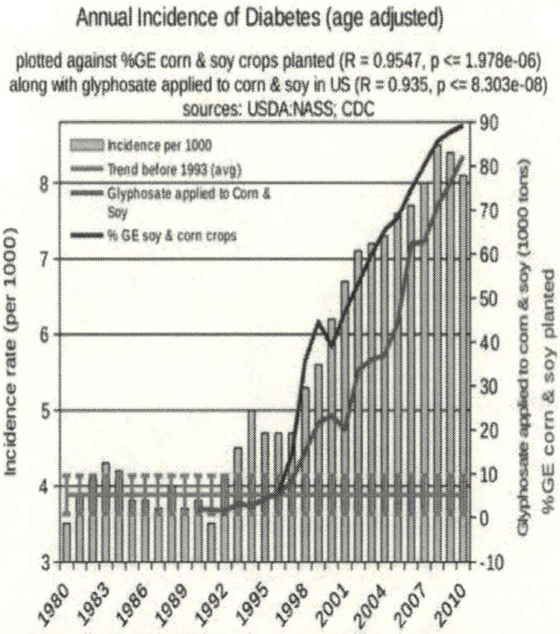

Figure 14. Correlation between age-adjusted diabetes incidence and glyphosate applications and percentage of US corn and soy crops that are GE.

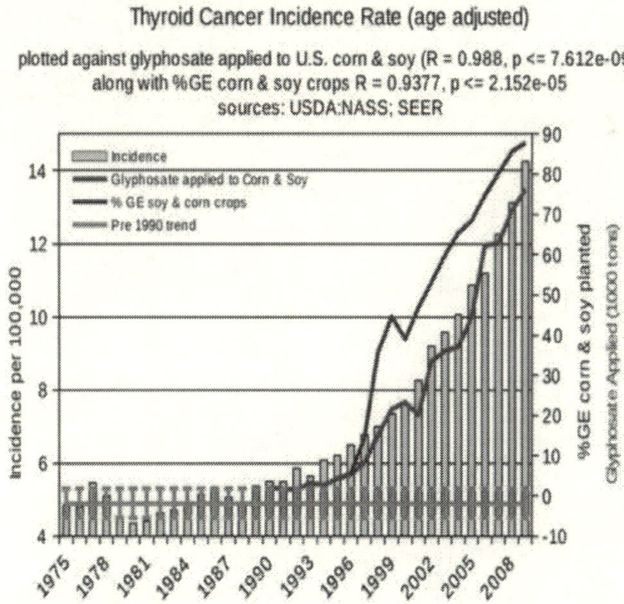

Figure 10. Correlation between age-adjusted thyroid cancer incidence and glyphosate applications and percentage of US corn and soy crops that are GE.

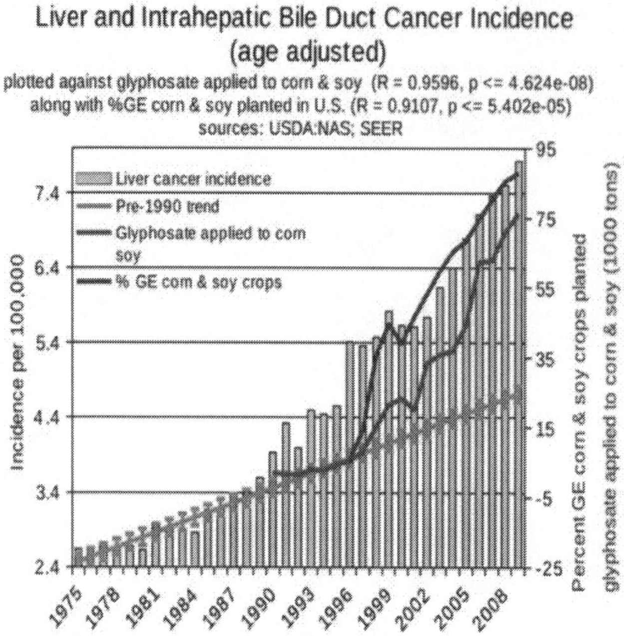

Figure 7. Correlation between age-adjusted liver cancer incidence and glyphosate applications and percentage of US corn and soy crops that are GE.

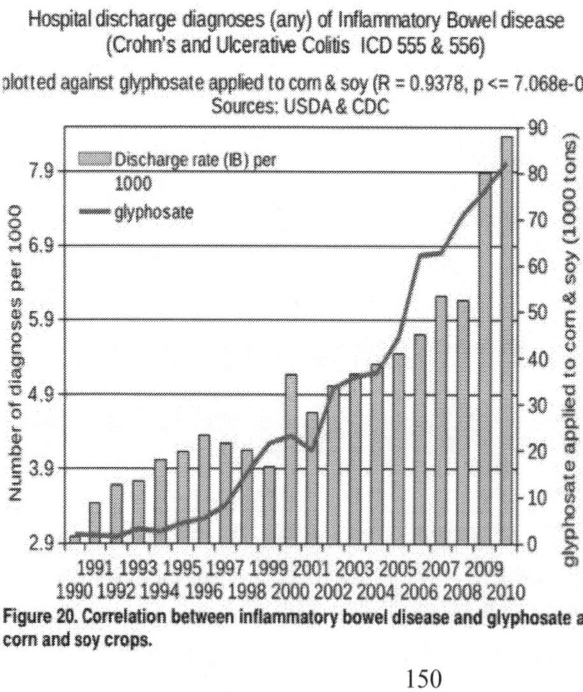

Figure 20. Correlation between inflammatory bowel disease and glyphosate applications to US corn and soy crops.

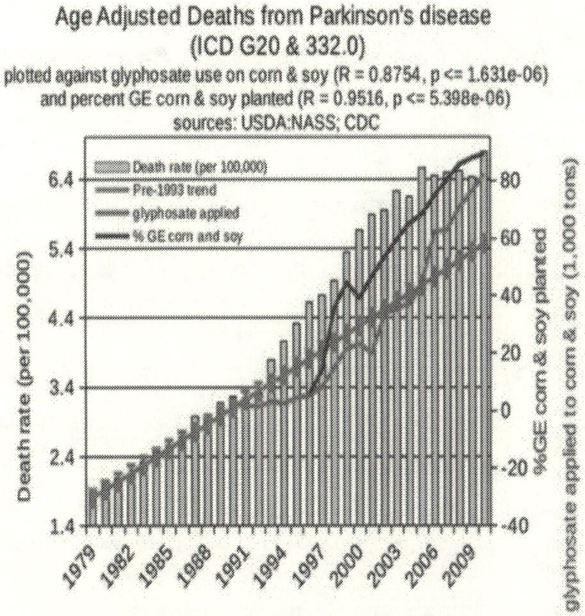

Figure 26. Correlation between age-adjusted Parkinson's disease deaths and glyphosate applications and percentage of US corn and soy crops that are GE.

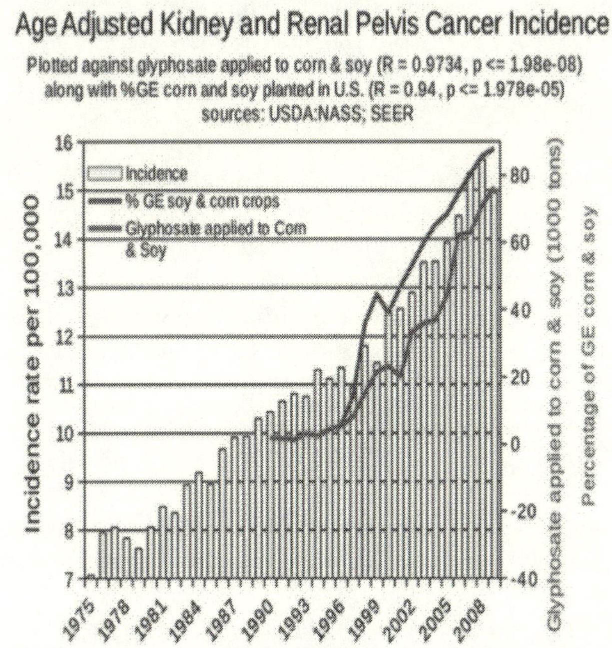

Figure 8. Correlation between age-adjusted kidney cancer incidence and glyphosate applications and percentage of US corn and soy crops that are GE.

SOLUTIONS PROTECTION

To protect yourself and your family as much as possible, avoid disease-causing substances in your food and beverages. Ask farmers to move away from using synthetic fertilizer! Once that is used, many more chemicals and pesticides are needed that wouldn't be otherwise. If you choose organic natural food, you can reduce your exposure to many toxins. Local small farmers, even if not technically "certified organic," in many cases may be organic or IPM and not using the big harmful pesticides or harmful fertilizer. If so they can be a super safe choice! Ask them what farm chemicals, if any they use to be sure. Before preparing foods, make sure to rinse and soak fruits and veges well. Cut out bad spots and bruises, peel root vegetables if too much dirt remains.

SUMMARY of HARMERS in FOOD and WATER

Health Harmers: Endocrine Disruptors, Reproductive Toxins, Neurotoxins, Carcinogens, PFCs/PFASs, Phthalates, Flame Retardants, BPA, Plastic, Styrene, Pesticides

Herbicides and Pesticides all conventional and GMO grown fruits and vegetables

- Glyphosate (mainly GMO crops: corn, soy, rice, alfalfa, canola, sugar beets, squash, potato, apple, cotton. Desiccation crops include: oats, lentils, peas, flax, wheat
- Atrazine (main crops: Corn, Soy, and Sugar)
- Neonicotinoids (mainly corn, canola, cotton, sorghum, sugar beets)
- Organophosphates (mainly bell peppers, snap beans, watermelon, tomatoes, potatoes, pears, cucumbers, grapes, raisins, lettuce, apple)[653]
- Chlorpyrifos (mainly apples, broccoli, strawberries, oranges, citrus, corn, wheat)
- 2,4-D, (mainly sugar cane, corn, wheat, rye, millet, rice, pears, soy, soybeans,
- Enlist Duo (mainly corn, soy, soybeans)
- Dicamba (mainly soy, soybeans)

Factory Farm Residues Synthetic Hormones, Drugs, Antibiotics, Manure, Bacteria

Fertilizer, Synthetic: (all GMO and conventionally grown crops, fruits, vegetable, grains), mixtures can include additional baggage: heavy metals, biosludge, hazardous waste & other. Synthetic fertilizer is so overused—we must get off it and get our soil healthy again!

Fumigants (mainly strawberries, potatoes, other fruits, vegs grown in or near the ground)

Fungicides (mainly corn, grapes, cabbage, spinach, kale, tomatoes, lettuce, apples, pears)

GMOs (mainly corn, soy, canola, cotton, sugar, alfalfa, apple, squash…)

- Glyphosate (corn, soy, rice, potato, sugar, apple, squash…)
- Glufosinate (GMO corn, soy, rice, alfalfa, canola, sugarbeets, squash, potato…)
- rBGH (milk and dairy products)

GRAS: Additives and Preservatives, Nanoparticles, Fats, Artificial Flavors & Sweeteners

Processed food: nearly always contain pesticide residues & lots of other harmers including additives & endocrine disruptors, not everything is written on the label.

Antibiotic Resistant Bacteria, Fungus, Pathogens Causing Food Recalls: We must seek and demand a cleaner food supply that's not prone to recalls.

Food Packaging: Time to get the chemicals and dangerous substances out of food packaging!

27. REMEDIES: Nourish

"Health is variously defined as 'soundness of body,' 'state of bodily or mental well-being', 'freedom from disease, disorder, pain or weakness.' It is, in fact, a variable condition of body as in good, bad, poor or ill health. At its best it is 'that state of being in which all the parts and organs are sound and in proper condition; that condition of the body and its various parts and functions which conduces to efficient and prolonged life. This optimum state of being can be attained when-but only when-the animal organism is adequately nourished. Further, it is possible to produce at will in animals under experimental conditions every grade of health—good, bad or indifferent—by alterations in the composition of their diets." Sir Robert McCarrison, 1936

The body is amazing at keeping healthy when its properly nourished and not assaulted with toxins. Further, the body is capable of recovering itself when it's provided the nutrients it needs and all substances interfering with its health are removed. If the majority of farming systems would start bending toward less chemical usage, amazing things could happen for the earth and ourselves. If we want health, we must select foods and beverages that contain less toxins. Although our world is crippled at this time with a slew of pollutants, and we all endure exposure just by living in this modern world, we can make strides toward health by protecting ourselves. First, reduce exposure to pollutants found in food and water. Then protect yourself with nourishing food and supplements. All of us, every single one of us on this planet may be experiencing some deficiency of minerals and nutrients our bodies need. This is due mostly to the current condition of soil around the world. Especially if we've had disease, we most likely have some level of mineral and vitamin deficiencies. You may wish to consult your physician to find out which ones specifically you need to start supplementing. In any state of health though, all of us can benefit from a full spectrum supplement containing all the minerals, micronutrients, vitamins, as well as omega oils. When we're getting all necessary nutrients and nourishing our bodies, amazing things can unfold.

Personally it was my own experience that convinced me of the relationship between our health and what we eat. After my parents passed away, I was of course in grief, but I felt stuck with some serious skin problems and other health stuff that had developed and wouldn't go away no matter what I tried. At the time my friend Dianna gave me a copy of *Sugar Blues,* and I can tell you that book really started a new life for me. I started examining my food for the first time, what was I eating? What was in my food? I ate normal foods or so I thought, but I hadn't realized how much was processed and full of hidden sugar. Immediately I changed what I ate. Giving up refined sugar and any foods containing sugar was number one on the list. Then I started eating wholesome foods—going out trying to locate these strange new foods like organic brown rice—that was an adventure in itself. By the end of the first week though, it was incredible—my skin was clear. I felt energized and amazed. I was so intrigued that I started working at the little organic food store where I found the brown rice—it became my training lab. These were the days before Whole Foods, little health food stores were quaint and exciting places.

On the wall of the store was a plaque that read, "Let food be thy medicine and medicine be thy food," Hippocrates, the Father of Medicine. Those words were my inspiration. I started experimenting with other natural foods—I became a vegetarian for a while, then vegan. I ate a lot of vegetables I had never heard of before, and whole grains like amaranth and quinoa that I couldn't pronounce. For a while I was macrobiotic and ate tons of seaweed, and also experimented with fasting and juicing. On top of that I started learning about herbs and tea, homeopathic medicine, Bach flower remedies and essential oils. I even started making my own medicinal herbal tea recipes, which really boosted my health. I had felt so depleted, but this new knowledge about food and how it can restore health gave me new life. In fact the vision for this book came at that time, the summer of 1991. A mystical series of events occurred that involved my late mom. It was as if I was receiving a message, a bittersweet one at that. The jist of it was, had we been aware and known any of this information earlier, it seemed very possible that my parents could've lived longer, and recovered their health for a period of time. This was how it occurred to me that this information might be helpful for other people.

Disease and cancer can be such a mystery, there are so many factors that play a role. But when facing any disease, I do believe that nourishing, real food can be of great help to our bodies when we need it most. And if Hippocrates based all his cures on that premise, well that makes it even more convincing. That was the first summer the Bulls—the amazing Michael Jordan and John Paxon & his shot from downtown won the NBA title. It was an incredibly exciting time in Chicago! My life truly changed forever that summer & it all began with the no-sugar experiment.

To be Nourished: Epigenetics

We don't need to live forever, but let's have health while we're here. Today there's a branch of science called Epigenetics. Basically, it means we're not doomed to disease, genes aren't everything. Our bodies can and do react to nutrients in certain foods and substances to alter gene expression. Scientists are discovering that many cancers and diseases can be healed or reversed with the proper nutrients and healing foods. In seeking health, nourishment truly is of utmost importance along with avoidance of substances that trigger disturbance within us.

In general, the more natural the food we eat the more easily our bodies can digest and absorb the nutrients in the food. For many people just making minor modifications to your diet can resolve a lot of suffering. For instance, if for two weeks you eliminate sugar, processed foods and alcohol you'll shift toward rebalancing your health. By adding more fresh vegetables and wholesome foods, you could be on your way toward health freedom. Adding sufficient supplements to your regime can further improve and protect your health as well. Everyone's body is different so what you may need specifically depends on many factors, you'll have to consult with your doctor for that. However, all of us can benefit from abstaining from refined sugar as well as artificial sugars—of this I have no doubt.

Healing foods by and large are natural and have no harmful toxins. We can prepare foods in countless ways. A few key points:

- Use good filtered water for drinking and cooking, preparing coffee and tea
- When shopping and cooking source clean, fresh, unpolluted ingredients
- As much as you can avoid factory farm dairy, eggs, or meat with synthetic hormones
- Use good cookware, avoid nonstick pans
- Avoid plastic and Styrofoam, especially in food packaging
- Limit contact with pesticides, nitrates, endocrine disruptors, health harming substances

To uncover the most wholesome diets that promote health without virtually any sign of, if that's possible, we'll first look to Sir Robert McCarrison's research dating back to 1927. Dr. McCarrison was a medical doctor as well as founder of the Nutritional Research Laboratories in Canoor, India. He is best known for the nutrition research he conducted on animals using varying diets. The results proved again and again that through a most wholesome diet, superior health could be maintained. Whereas, withholding or deficiency of even one essential nutrient led to multiple health maladies. When animals were fed a diet mostly of sweets and carbohydrates lacking essential minerals and protein, they exhibited aggression, violence and even cannibalism. As interesting, malnourished animals exhibiting behavioral and physical defects could often be corrected when proper nutrition was provided consistently.

McCarrison ultimately found the foods consumed by the Sikhs in northern India promoted ideal health. These people were outstanding farmers and caretakers of earth, their soil was made rich with glacial minerals. He duplicated their diet and fed it to animals. What he observed was made possible firstly with food grown and derived from healthy soil. From this type of soil plants grow in vibrance and animals (as well as people) eating those plants also grow vibrantly. "Their food consisted of chapattis lightly smeared with fresh butter, sprouted Bengal gram (pulse), raw, fresh vegetables (cabbage and carrots) *ad libitum*, milk, the hard crusts of bread (to keep their teeth in order), a small ration of meat with bone once a week, and water."[654] Here are the basic foods involved in the diet Dr. McCarrison claimed promotes health:

- Milk and butter: Whole milk and dairy products without rBGH
- Chapattis, Bread: Fresh ground whole grain bread
- Pulses: chickpeas, lentils sprouted
- Vegetables fresh and raw: carrots and cabbage unlimited amounts
- Meat with bone sometimes
- Clean water

It's important to note his experiments and observations were carried out in the 1920s-1940s, well before chemical pesticides and synthetic fertilizer were used widely; and for that matter, well before the existence of genetically modified foods (GMOs). It's more than likely that only the above foods grown without toxic substances or containing residues of pesticides could have such health bearing benefits. Would his experiments hold true today if the animals were provided food and water containing pesticide residues? Containing GMOs? Very doubtful.

Further, of extreme importance in wielding healthy food is not just the quality of the soil in which food is grown, but also the methods of preparing foods. To peel or not to peel the vegetables, leaving foods whole with the skin on can increase nutrient density. Peels are packed with nourishment as long as food is rinsed sufficiently and bad parts are cut out. If cooking food, use good, filtered water and save the water from cooking for drinking or cooking other foods, for it's full of nutrients that you don't want to pour down the drain. If you're eating GMOs or conventional foods, especially those grown in the ground, you can't necessarily wash the pesticides off the food. So, for these foods and those grown with conventional methods, it may be best to peel them to avoid as many toxic chemicals as possible.

In addition to Dr. McCarrison, Dr. G.T. Wrench also was on a quest to uncover the healthiest people on earth in the 1930s. The people he observed to be the healthiest also tended the land and took care of the soil. Mostly they were simple and didn't use chemicals at all to grow food. Like McCarrison he put the Hunza (Sikhs) at the top. However, he found 4 other groups of people, with slightly different diets, all of optimum health. These groups included: Islanders off Iceland, Greenland and the Arctic who mostly ate meat and whole carcasses; secondly people in the South Atlantic whose diet was particularly dependent on the sea and on eggs. Next was the North American Indian from pioneer times who ate mostly wild game from pristine habitats uncompromised by today's modern chemicals. Lastly, he chose the people of modern China who relied on a diet similar to the Hunza but also included rice rather than wheat, meat, birds, fish, eggs and sprouted grain.

The common factors amongst all these people boiled down to a few factors: fresh nourishing foods from the sea or soil, wild animals, fresh air, nature. All in all they were getting all the nutrients their bodies needed. In contemplating Wrench's observations, Eva Balfour pointed out, "there is a complete and continuous transference of health from a fertile soil, through plant and/or animal to man, and back to the soil again. The whole carcass, the whole grain, the whole fruit or vegetable, these things fresh from their source, and that source a fertile soil. Herein appears to lie the secret. If this be true, then it would appear to be that any diet is a health-promoting diet so long as it conforms to these three rules, and the first of these is a fertile soil."

Jumping forward 90 years to modern day, the areas of the world noted for healthy happy people often living to a hundred years old are regions interestingly that lie near the sea: Japan, Sardinia, Costa Rica, Greece and a small community in California.[655] In addition to eating naturally grown foods, could their closeness to the sea translate to healthier life, healthier soil? Is their good health due to the seawater and ocean breezes and a healthy thyroid? It has been noted that women in Okinawa, Japan who consume seaweed daily—up to 45mg of iodine daily have a far less probability of contracting breast cancer than women in the U.S.[656] (Perhaps they don't have a lot of contact with substances contradicting iodine absorption either.) Sardinia is noted for having more centenarians per capita than any other country. Their food is simple, the sea air is fresh, and they walk a lot. All these factors contribute to their health no doubt, but it's likely that the root of their health emanates from good plants grown in healthy soil.

Whatever you're seeking, may you have good health while you're here. Our bodies and minds, our spirits need more than just clean food and good water to be our best. Getting back to nature can often be the best remedy. Do you give yourself any quiet time? In this noisy chaotic world, moments of quietness can instill rejuvenation, new life. Even a few minutes a day can transform you. I like to meditate and end the day with a quiet soak in the ofuro, or a deep soak in a hot bath with lavender will do. Prayer and meditation are life enhancing, helping you get in touch with the life force and your inner power. Computer screens, cell phones and harsh lighting can strain us and drain us, causing downgrade and stress—making us even more in need for restoration. I went for years without a television; if you don't remember what it's like to have the tv off, give it a try. You might rediscover yourself. Over the years I've spent lots of time at retreats in the wilderness. Do you ever walk in nature, go to the forest, or walk beside the water? Go to the woods when you can, sing and say hello to the trees, the wildflowers, to the birds, and breathe. Run, walk, bicycle, stretch, dance, feel your energy and reconnect to the planet. Yoga and stretching will awaken you, get you back in touch with your body, with the universe. Do yoga in a quiet space so you can engage and really reflect on this thing called life. Breathing is so important—do you take time to take deep breaths daily? It helps keep us grounded. Practice. If you really want to learn how to breathe fully like you've never done before, find an Art of Living Class near you and go. You'll discover a new you. I like to begin the mornings connecting with nature, stretching, and classical music whenever possible. This is me, find out what works for you and make your own rituals so your life and time on this planet will be supernatural.

PREPARE TO RISE

"For this country is moving and it must not stop. It cannot stop. For this is a time for courage and a time for challenge. Neither conformity nor complacency will do. Neither the fanatics nor the faint-hearted are needed. And our duty as a party is not to our party alone, but to the Nation, and indeed, to all mankind. Our duty is not merely the preservation of political power but the preservation of peace and freedom. So let us not be petty when our cause is so great. Let us not quarrel amongst ourselves when our Nation's future is at stake. Let us stand together with renewed confidence in our cause—united in our heritage of the past and our hopes for the future—and determined that this land we love shall lead all mankind into new frontiers of peace and abundance." JFK

President John Fitzgerald Kennedy

November 22, 1963 Speech for Austin, TX, not delivered[657]

SOLUTIONS PLANET

Reducing Disease: By significantly reducing the widespread use of toxic chemicals in the environment, we may see significant declines in cancer and diseases of all kinds.

Climate Crisis: We can seriously slow it down by controlling Big Agriculture: reduce use of pesticides, fumigants, fungicides and above all, synthetic fertilizer! This will improve water health and soil health, reduce greenhouse gas emissions, dead zones, algae blooms, red tides. Redesign factory farms, reduce monocropping and land used for growing GMOs. This will further reduce toxic emissions as well as food recalls, contamination, antibiotic resistance, fungus resistance, acid rain and smog. Think how much healthier our environment would become and how much this will help us live healthier lives.

Save Wildlife and People from Extinction!

Bees, Birds, Bats: Help them by not using synthetic fertilizers, pesticides or fungicides!

Pesticides: Reduce use of pesticides, toxic chemicals, fungicides, neonicotinoids

Fertilizer: Avoid using any synthetic fertilizers (SF)! SF increases the need for pesticides

Factory Farms: All animals must be included in the Animal Welfare Act

GMOs: Protect your health, avoid GMO meat, milk and dairy

GMO Feed: Free factory farm animals of GMOs, let them eat grass & roam in pasture

GMO Alfalfa: Help ban it before it's too late

Palm Oil: Avoid products containing palm oil sourced from deforested areas

Planet Health: Don't support farms that pollute our planet

Soil: Protect it, nurture it, feed it, help it thrive, return nature to the soil

Food Packaging: Why are toxins in food containers? If it's not edible it doesn't belong.

Plastic and Styrofoam: ban single use & disposable plastics, nationwide, worldwide

WILDLIFE: "Through 'transformative change', nature can still be conserved, restored and used sustainably – this is also key to meeting most other global goals. By transformative change, we mean a fundamental, system-wide reorganization across technological, economic and social factors, including paradigms, goals and values." IPBES Global Assessment[658] United Nations, International Panel Biodiversity and Ecosystem Services

TRENDS AND FIGURES RELATED TO AGROBIODIVERSITY[659]

- Since the 1900s, some 75% of plant genetic diversity has been lost as farmers worldwide have left their multiple local varieties & landraces for genetically uniform, high-yielding varieties.
- 30 percent of livestock breeds are at risk of extinction; six breeds are lost each month.
- Today, 75%of the world's food is generated from only 12 plants and five animal species.
- Of the 4 percent of the 250,000 to 300,000 known edible plant species, only 150 to 200 are used by humans. Only three - rice, maize and wheat - contribute nearly 60 percent of calories and proteins obtained by humans from plants.
- Animals provide some 30 percent of human requirements for food and agriculture and 12 percent of the world's population live almost entirely on products from ruminants.

100 YEARS OF AGRICULTURAL CHANGE Source: FAO

SOLUTIONS HELP THE PLANET

What we can do personally to lessen the damage to planet and ourselves:

- Filter your water! Use filtered water for drinking and cooking.
- Don't use toxic pesticides or synthetic fertilizer in your lawn or garden.
- Replace pesticides with safe substances that do the job, see recipes page 45.
- Support the earth. Choose food grown with sustainable methods & least pesticides.
- Best food options: locally grown, farmers markets, organic, biodynamic, IPM.

1. **Source foods grown with sustainable methods**. That means avoiding foods grown with pesticides, synthetic fertilizer, and monocropping methods. The easiest way to do this is to opt for foods grown organically and biodynamically. Industrial, corporate, and GMO farms use the most toxins on their farmland and practice monocropping almost exclusively. The use of synthetic fertilizer has a dire effect on our atmosphere, our land, and our water.
2. **Protect Pollinators**. Without bees & pollinators most of our cherished fruits and vegetables will no longer exist. The simplest way to protect pollinators is to not use pesticides, herbicides, fungicides in your yard or garden. As important is to not purchase foods grown with these substances.
3. **Avoid foods and products containing *unsustainable* palm oil**. This translates to avoiding oil involved with deforestation and animal extinction. Many processed and fast foods companies making donuts, cereal, snacks and cookies use palm oil from sensitive deforested areas. To help reverse the impact palm oil farming is having on the planet, we must avoid companies that irresponsibly contribute to the problem. Show those companies you won't continue eating their products no matter how much you love them. Think how quick they'd make the switch if everyone did the same til they switched.
4. **Avoid meat and milk products from factory farms**. Factory farms are notorious for food recalls, causing the increase in antibiotic resistant bacteria as well as severe air and water pollution. The animals are confined their entire lives in massive warehouse-type barns that offer no sunlight, no exercise, no fresh air, no comfort. Animals are injected with antibiotics and growth hormones, and only fed GMO feed that is grown of course with surreal amounts of pesticides and synthetic fertilizer. These substances contribute to climate change and transfer to our bodies when we consume such products. Factory farm products repeatedly are implicated in outbreaks of food-borne disease & antibiotic resistance. If we can be more selective about what we put in our bodies, soon these farms will not exist. No animal should have to endure life at a factory farm. We can demand that all confined animals be included in the Animal Welfare Act.
5. When you eat meat, especially when you cook at home opt for that grown on smaller farms that not just protect and nourish animals but also protect and nourish the planet.
6. **Avoid GMO foods**. GMO farming uses more pesticides[660] than any type of farm. These pesticides linger on foods, many are grown within the foods so you can't wash them off.
7. If you don't garden at home, consider donating your food scraps to a community garden or compost pick-up service. Learn more about composting at www.nyccompost.org.

SOLUTIONS HELP THE PLANET

PROTECT YOURSELF AND YOUR FAMILY

8. **Help children** and their health by getting the toxins, corn syrup and junk ingredients out of school lunches and food packaging! Similarly, we must help those in hospitals and nursing homes—only nourishing toxin free food and beverages should be allowed.
9. **Food Packaging**-Let's get toxic chemicals removed from food packaging! Be especially vigilant with baby food packaging and dried cereals, try to source foods for your kids and family packaged in eco-friendly, human-health friendly materials.
10. **Reduce use of single use plastic, Styrofoam**, polystyrene, bleached & nonrecycled paper products.
10. **Use recycled toilet paper**, not bleached. You'll help keep forests standing.
11. **Grow your own food using natural methods**, not chemicals. Learn about the soil and land and how to care for it. DIY pesticide recipes page 45!
12. **Compost food waste**
13. **Help end littering**. when you see garbage on the sidewalk or in the park please help put it in the trash so it doesn't get in the waterways.
14. **Help the Water, don't litter, don't pollute.**
15. **Don't use Synthetic Fertilizers**—they make soil sick, makes plants sick, makes us sick
16. **Filter Your Water** Get a Berkey filter, or reverse osmosis at your sink. If you're lucky your home already has filtered water, but if not, consider installing a whole house filter
17. **Eat well**
18. **Supplement** with high quality minerals, micronutrients, vitamins & fish oil
19. **Avoid toxins** as much as possible
20. **Eat Fish,** rotate and avoid fish that are on not on the Safe Fish list: seafoodwatch.org
21. **Use nontoxic cleaning products at home**

> New York City
> Thank You!
> As of June 30, 2019, Styrofoam is banned!
> (aka single use polystyrene)
> Bye Bye packing peanuts!

22. Protect children's health: Protect your children from food that could harm them down the road. Foods like high fructose corn syrup and refined sugar can interfere with their well being. Many reports have reflected on the connection between obesity in America and government subsidies. Subsidies are implicated in the spread of non-nourishing food. "Childhood obesity rates have more than tripled in the past 30 years, almost one in five children aged six to eleven are seriously overweight, making them highly vulnerable to heart disease, diabetes and other serious illnesses. At the same time, Congress and the Department of Agriculture are spending more than $1.28 billion annually to subsidize the crops that are used as additives in manufacturing cookies, candies, soda pop and other highly popular junk food that arguably are among the primary contributors to childhood obesity."[661]

SOLUTIONS SCHOOL LUNCHES

What do kids in US schools eat during the day? Eating right can set us up for a lifetime of health. Providing nourishing foods to children, food without toxins would make sense, as school is designed to encourage learning. Anything we can do to improve brain health has to be encouraged. When I was teaching at Chicago Public Schools I was happy seeing good foods on the students' trays. But all too often, whether breakfast or lunch the food supplied appeared pretty processed and loaded with sugar.

Many additives and so-called GRAS substances in foods can trigger allergies and other maladies that disrupt a child's learning potential. Any substance with potent neurotoxins must be removed from our foods, especially foods provided to children. There's already reports out now regarding public school water fountains distributing water laced with lead, something that must be corrected ASAP. Is it not absolutely essential we do what we can to reduce the toxic burden on these young folks?

Food affects our health, wellbeing and learning ability. Wholesome food nourishes and sustains us. School is hard enough, making friends, taking tests, spending time away from home, sitting at a desk all day—through food we can give them the strength they need to be successful and feel good inside and out. Perhaps this can encourage an environment for learning, peace, and patience without threat of bullying, violence and rage.

One group, Turning Green launched an organic lunch program in the Bay City area in 2015. As reported by EcoWatch, "In two years, the program saw a steep decrease in disciplinary cases, increased attendance and a greater sense of community. Students everywhere are vulnerable to pesticide residues and unsafe environmental toxins," says Judi Shils, founder and executive director of Turning Green. "Not only does this program far exceed USDA nutritional standards, but it ties the health of our children to the health of our planet. It's the first program to say fundamentally, you cannot have one without the other."

In Japan, school children are provided nourishing lunches as well as an education in food and nutrition. This gives them a better understanding of where food comes from as well as what foods are nourishing and what aren't. This is helpful for young people to know and what better way to help them maintain their own health. As reported by City Lab, "Japan's school lunch program has also no doubt contributed to the country's low global rate of obesity. And Japan's life expectancy, at 85 is one of the world's highest. In contrast, the U.S. has a high obesity rate and a lower life expectancy of 79.8."

By serving food without toxins, without additives that are known to contribute to disease, by providing meat and dairy free from artificial hormones, drug and antibiotic residues, we can help children feel whole and feel good about themselves. The substances in foods can cause attention disorders and other maladies. Perhaps we can eliminate discipline issues and bullying through good food. If we can create an environment for health, learning, and peace then that is what we must do.

Through the Farm Bill we can help get more natural wholesome foods with less pesticides and less additives into schools. See page 166 for Farm Bill highlights and contact the USDA.

SOLUTIONS FARMERS MARKETS

Good health starts with healthy plants. Healthy plants start with good soil. Healthy soil is voided when synthetic fertilizers are used. Synthetic fertilizer kills soil and weakens plants, making pesticides necessary. If that's all we eat, our immune systems will be weak and we'll be prone to disease. If we stop using synthetic fertilizer, soil gets healthier, plants get healthier, we don't need so many pesticides! Isn't it time to say bye bye to the chemicals so soil, plants, people and animals can get healthier and happier? Food grown at smaller farms tends to be exposed to less chemicals. Local markets give us an opportunity to support farmers using sustainable methods.

Farmers Markets

Your local farmer's market is a great place to shop! These foods tend to be fresher than what you find at the grocery store. Chances are the farmers harvested the foods the morning of the market or the night before. Plus you'll be cutting down on all the transport and emissions involved with shipping food long distances. Abby Mandel was a champion for locally grown foods and back in the late 1990s created the historic Green City Market in Chicago. In the early days I was one of their regular volunteers. These days most communities have their own weekly market. Go and explore, take your own bags, meet the farmers and make your own farm to table delights tonight!

Local Growers

Support local farmers, support your community, save on transport, get fresher foods! Many local small farms use natural earth-friendly methods of farming that don't require heaps of chemicals.

Farm to Table, Local Chefs & Restaurants

Support chefs who source foods grown locally and strive to abide by the safe fish list. Ask your favorite restaurants to source more locally grown foods. One of my favorite chefs with eco-minded tendencies is Chicago's Rick Bayless.

Join the fun, grow sustainable food yourself!

You can grow food in planters, on your deck or rooftop. If you don't have space you can build a vertical indoor garden. If you're lucky and have a yard you can get your soil up to speed naturally and start growing your own organic foods! Soil tests can often be done for free by your local university extension service. Look here: https://www.gardeningknowhow.com/extension-search

Volunteer at a Sustainable Farm: They're all over the world. See Worldwide Organization of Organic Farmers WWOOF: www.wwoofer.net. This is a fun way to travel and learn more about farming, or you can always look into volunteering at a local farm near you.

Shopping at the Farmers Markets

- Bring your own cloth bags if you have them, reuse and recycle
- Avoid wasting food, freeze food before it goes bad, only buy what you need.

SOLUTIONS ACTION

"While much is known about the science of cancer, its prevention depends largely on political action." Dr. Samuel Epstein[662]

If you want to go further and really get involved in making changes to protect your health and the food supply, consider writing letters and making phone calls. By significantly reducing the widespread use of toxic substances we may cause widespread reductions of cancer and disease.

1. Let's create a big new law to protect the planet, the people, the waterways, and the environment from toxins. By keeping these substances out of the environment, we protect all people and animals. Just say no to synthetic fertilizer & pesticides. Perhaps we can keep trying to strengthen the Toxic Substances Control Act, or is it more effective to start over?
2. Bring Back THE DELANEY Amendment or something better. Delaney had been part of the U.S. Food, Drug and Cosmetic law since 1958. It stated that "no cancer-causing agent, as demonstrated in humans or animals, shall be deliberately added to or found as a contaminant in food." The FDA and the EPA worked together with one goal: to prevent cancer. The law was extinguished in 1996.[663]
3. Pollinator Protection Law: We can no longer allow the use of pesticides that kill pollinators! We need the bees, the birds and the bats and butterflies!
4. Ban neonicotinoids & GMOs from our National Parks and Wildlife Refuges.
5. Let's help farmers break free from the chemical industry and regain their livelihoods.
6. Help reverse the Climate Crisis by instilling new rules for Big Agriculture!
   Maybe we can't get full outright bans, but significant reductions will help tremendously:
   - Cut use of synthetic fertilizer
   - Cut use or ban toxic pesticides (includes herbicides, fungicides, fumigants)
   - Redesign factory farms to be climate compliant:
     Implement sewage regulations, Clean Water act, Clean Air Act regulations, bring farm animals and all confined animals under the laws of the Animal Welfare Act
   - Reduce amount of land used for growing GMO crops
   - Eliminate monocropping farming methods
   - Eliminate GMO alfalfa
7. Stop the rollback of crucial environmental protection laws. Let's reinvent the EPA, FDA, and USDA so they can do their job of protecting us and protecting the planet.
8. We have to eliminate the Fracking Provision (p. 61) and protect water & our health!

6. Eliminate farm subsidies and clean up farming
   - No subsidies for farmers that cause water and air pollution or climate crisis toxins.
   - Keep water clean, protecting our water sources from dangerous contaminants
   - Avoid toxic additions to soil and reduce agricultural runoff

What is the future for America, for a country relying on GMOs? Unlike the U.S., Russia has banned GMOs and is intent to become the world's leading producer of organic food.[664] This could prove to be the one factor in the future that saves or elevates one country over another.

SOLUTIONS POLITICS

> **"Politics is too important to be left to the politicians."**
> **John Fitzgerald Kennedy Jr, 1999**

PRESIDENT

The Honorable ___________
The White House
1600 Pennsylvania Avenue NW
Washington, D. C. 20500
Voice: 1-202-456-1414
TTY/TDD: 1-202-456-6213
Fax: 1-202-456-2461
president@whitehouse.gov
White House Comment Desk: 202.456.1111

VICE PRESIDENT

The Honorable ___________
Old Executive Office Building
Washington, D.C. 20501
(202) 456-1414
Fax: (202) 456-2461
vice.president@whitehouse.gov

> **Remembering Ethics**
> "Politics is not just about power and money games. Politics can be about the improvement of peoples' lives, about lessening human suffering in our world and bringing about more peace and more justice."
> The late Senator Paul Wellstone

CONGRESS

Find Your Representatives and Senators:
www.capwiz.com/awc/dbq/officials/ or
www.info.gov/phone.htm

SENATORS & REPRESENTATIVES

Locate your Senators:
www.senate.gov

Locate your Representatives:
www.house.gov

When writing, address your Senators and Representatives as follows:

The Honorable __________
U.S. Senate
Washington, D.C. 20510

The Honorable___________
U.S. House of Representatives
Washington, D.C. 20515

> **Toll Free Government Directory:**
> **800-FED-INFO**

YOUR GOVERNOR

www.nga.org

RESEARCH

The Stacks at the Library of Congress:
www.loc.gov

Keep Track of Activity in D.C.

The government's daily journal
www.federalregister.gov

SOLUTIONS US GOV

ETIQUETTE GUIDELINES

The letter remains a very powerful way to send a message. My dad always told me, you have to send letters to get letters. Done properly, politely, and respectfully, a letter will be welcomed. Stay true and nice. Remember the Golden Rule, say what you like but do it as a good neighbor. Let's be encouraging and hopeful, not judgmental or mean. Kindness is the key to opening doors and hearts.

WRITE A LETTER TO YOUR NEWSPAPER
Find your paper at: http://www.usnpl.com/

THE EPA www.epa.gov
U.S. Environmental Protection Agency
Administrator
1200 Pennsylvania Avenue, NW
Washington, DC 20004
(202) 272-0167
(202) 564-4700
www.epa.gov

The ATSDR
1600 Clifton Rd F-32
Atlanta, GA. 30333
(404) 639-3534,
FAX: (770)-488-4178
Email: ATSDRIC@cdc.gov

THE FDA fda.gov
U.S. Food and Drug Administration
10903 New Hampshire Ave
Silver Spring MD 20993-0002
(202)566-1729, 1-888-INFO-FDA

GAO Government Accountability Office
www.gao.gov
441 G Street, NW
Washington, D.C. 20548
(202) 512.3000

The USDA www.usda.gov
U.S. Department of Agriculture
Secretary of Agriculture
1400 Independence Avenue, S.W.
Washington, D.C. 20250
(202) 720-3631, (202) 720-2791
Agsec@usda.gov
(301)734-8660

The CDC cdc.gov
1600 Clifton Road NE, Mailstop
Atlanta, GA 30333
(404) 639-3311
(800) 311-3435
www.cdc.gov

EPA Water Resource Center
(800) 832-7828

Interior Dept www.doi.gov
1849 C Street, N.W.
Washington DC 20240
(202) 208-3100

PEER www.peer.org
Great Resource! Public Employees for Environmental Responsibility!

SOLUTIONS ACTION

Create a Farm Bill that Makes Sense and Helps People and Planet

Every 5 years a new farm bill is enacted. Here are some the highlights from the Farm Bill of 2018 (Source: Farm Aid)[665]:

- Not good: Continues subsidies for Big Ag, wealthy farmers and their relatives
- Tax dollars still subsidizing dirty factory farms
- Funding limited for USDA farm to school grant program, limits access to local and organic foods for school children

Good Stuff:

- Supports urban agriculture, community compost and reducing food waste
- SNAP, supplemental nutrition assistance program (food stamps) reinforced
- Reinstates Undersecretary of Rural Redevelopment
- LAMP, Local Agriculture Market Program
- Smaller dairy farms have access to safety net
- Stress Assistance program and access for farmers
- Crop insurance expanded to include smaller farmers Read more @ farmaid.org

> **THE USDA**
> Founded by President Abraham Lincoln in 1862, the *United States Department of Agriculture* was originally called the "**People's Department**."

USDA: The USDA controls much about our food, but lobbyists and corporate interests have a lot of sway with the agency, especially when former lobbyists are appointed government roles.

FOOD, NUTRITION, AND CONSUMER SERVICES, USDA

This department oversees school meal programs, dietary guidelines, and SNAP (food stamps). There's a lot of controversy since they put a former lobbyist from the corn syrup association[666] in charge of decisions that affect the whole country's health. It's time to set things right. Until the USDA is functionally ethically, use your best judgement in selecting foods.

GROCERY MANUFACTURER'S ASSOCIATION

The GMA is one of the strongest lobbyist organizations in the country.
1001 19th Street North, 7th Floor, Arlington, VA 22209

NATIONAL GROCERS ASSOCIATION

1005 N Glebe Rd #250, Arlington, VA 22201, (703) 516-0700

AMERICAN FARM BUREAU FEDERATION

Through the American Farm Bureau, we should be able to improve the Farm Bill: Help small farms survive, instill animal rights for farm animals, and help farmers adopt more sustainable soil enhancement methods so use of synthetic fertilizer and pesticides can be greatly reduced.
600 Maryland Avenue, Suite 1000W, Washington D.C. 20024

SOLUTIONS US GOV

Your Government Phone List		
Office	**Phone**	**Email**
President	202.456.6213	president@whitehouse.gov
Vice President	202.456.1414	vice.president@whitehouse.gov
Congress	1.800.FED.INFO	www.info.gov/phone.htm
Senators	find your senator	www.senate.gov
Representatives	find your rep	www.house.gov
Governor	find your governor	www.nga.org
EPA	800-832-7828	www.epa.gov
Hotline	800-426-4791	
FDA	888-463-6332	www.fda.gov
USDA	800-414-1226	www.usda.gov
USDA Secretary	202-720-6361	
Forest Service	800-832-1355	
Dept of the Interior		www.doi.gov
Fish and Wildlife	800-344-WILD	
Bureau of Land Mngmt	202-208-4896	
BLM Arctic Drilling	202-208-4201	
Oceans & Great Lakes	202-208-3100	
HHS	202-619-0257	
Health and Human Services	877-696-6775	
CDC	800-311-3435	www.cdc.gov
Center for Food Safety	888.723.3366	
OSHA Occupational Safety		www.osha.gov
Agricultural Health Study	800.424.7883	https://aghealth.nih.gov
POISON CONTROL	800-222-1222	
GOV ACCT OFFICE	202.512.3000	contact@gao.gov
Freedom Information Req	301.796.3900	

PREPARE TO RISE

Adore Yourself

Nourish Nourish Nourish

Let Food be thy Medicine
and Medicine be thy food.
Hippocrates, the Father of Medicine

"Western medicine, while excelling at acute care and surgery, puts great emphasis on the chronic use of drugs to suppress the symptoms of illnesses. What is forgotten is that our bodies have a natural wisdom and intelligence; they have an intrinsic knowledge of how to grow, heal, maintain balance, restore homeostasis, and regenerate. Our bodies have evolved over aeons with these capabilities, but when they are suppressed, for example, when nutrition, exercise, and diet are not given adequate attention, or people ingest toxins, then "lifestyle-related" diseases including obesity, diabetes, cancer, and heart disease are much more likely to arise."[667]

Deepak Chopra and fellow doctors, "Evidence-Based Complementary and Alternative Medicine"

ADOREYOURSELF

PROTECT YOURSELF, YOUR KIDS, YOUR FAMILY

"Although a small proportion of tumors can be inherited, it is believed that majority of cancers result from changes that accumulate throughout the life because of exposure to various endogenous factors such as nutrients, infections, physical activity, social behavior and other environmental factors. Even when cancer initiation and progression is driven by acquired genetic alterations, epigenetic disruption of gene expression plays an equally important role in development of disease, and arguably diet and environment-mediated epigenetic perturbations play a crucial role in cancer progression in humans." National Institutes of Health[668]

WHAT'S IN YOUR FOOD?

- is your water pure and filtered?
- Are hidden ingredients lurking in your food?

SIMPLE THINGS YOU CAN DO

- Eat nutritious foods, green vegetables, probiotics
- Drink enough pure clean water everyday
- Reduce consumption of factory farm eggs, meat and dairy
- Supplement your diet with good quality, full-spectrum minerals + vitamins
- Lessen food waste by composting food scraps, freezing food, donating food
- Grow your own food or buy food from local and organic farmers
- Protect your family, pets and animals from lawn chemicals
- Love our planet, don't poison it, don't litter, don't use synthetic fertilizer

FOOD QUALITY AND NUTRITION

Nutritive value of food can vary widely depending to a great extent on the quality of soil in which the plants were grown. Many factors have a bearing on food quality such as:

- Time between harvest and delivery to our table
- Has the food has been pre-peeled and cut? If so, how long ago?
- Has it been stored in plastic or Styrofoam?
- How much has the food been processed?
- Is the food product from a factory farm?
- What additives have been added to the food?
- Are pesticide residues present?

GROW FOODS WITH NONTOXIC METHODS

- Use natural growing methods and nontoxic methods of pest removal
- Choose plants that were designed to grow in your area.
- Prevent weeds by keeping your soil healthy so your plants will be strong.
- Use mulch to cover bare areas of soil.
- Use composting and natural fertilizers like wood ash to replenish the soil.
- Make your own nontoxic fungicide and pesticide remedies (page 45.)

ADORE YOURSELF

If you're ready to feel your best, then it's time to Adore Yourself. For those who want to feel their healthiest, or haven't been as well as can be, or have been diagnosed with a serious disease-- no matter the reason for your present condition, slowing down and giving your body, yourself an opportunity to access your healing forces may bring you stunning relief and recovery.

Let's live well while we're here. Get in the habit of examining your food and beverages:

- Is your glass of water pure fresh water, or is it unfiltered with hidden chemicals?
- Are those apples you're buying clean, or do they contain pesticides?
- Is the meat you're cooking tonight free from phony hormones and drug residues?
- Is your milk and butter free of rBGH/rBST?

The goal is to nourish your body, mind and spirit, to feel healthy and vibrant. To do that we have to aim to get all our nutrients while consuming the least amount of toxins as possible. This is an ideal scenario, of course in our day-to-day lives it's not always as easy. However, if we persist we may surprise ourselves. At least we can control what groceries we bring home, eating out can be a little tricky but do your best. Keep your food and beverages as close to nature as possible, with moderate processing and chemicals. Real food is wholesome, makes us feel good, may make us need less medicine, helps keep our heads clear, cleanses our body, can help prevent ailments or rid us of any ailments we may have been suffering with. Keep the chemicals, the pesticides, the sweeteners & synthetic hormones out of your food and body and see for yourself. No foods are disallowed, well ok, just some corrupted versions of foods like high fructose corn syrup— that's off limits. It's found in so many foods, lets hope food makers put our health first & begin removing it. Rule of thumb: opt for best options available. Ice cream for instance, go for organic because it's rBGH free and the cows aren't at factory farms. Also, organic varieties tend to use real sugar, not refined sugars or artificial flavorings. If you want to get real hip, make your own organic ice cream with the best ingredients you can source.

You, your body, your mind, you're one of a kind! Don't let anything in that can harm you. Feel love and appreciation for this gift called life, be good to yourself, forgiving and understanding for all your body has endured and overcome while carrying you through this world. Life isn't easy. Likewise, try to have understanding and compassion for those around you. Get in the habit: nourish your body with good food, good water, and nourish your mind, nourish your spirit, & your speech with healthy positive loving thoughts. Keep practicing 'til it becomes habit. Strive for peace every day.

Through methods we choose, how we prepare and eat food, words we choose, how we treat others, we contribute to our physical, mental and spiritual health. We are all so rushed and hurried throughout the day thinking of tasks and work we have to do, it's important to give yourself time to slow down and breathe. You may not need to radically change your diet, sometimes it's our thoughts that need more changing. For some, just sourcing food and ingredients that are free-er of toxins and pesticides will have a profound impact. Experiment and try your best, be good to yourself, to others, and to the planet.

ADOREYOURSELF KITCHEN

Good Water

It all starts with good clean water. Is the water you drink and cook with clean and pure, without contaminants? It's common to not know, in that case you can have your water tested or you can filter it to be on the safe side. You want to avoid chlorine, fluoride, and any pesticides, nitrates, chemicals, pharmaceuticals or disinfection byproducts hidden in the water. There's a wide range of filters out there, some are better than others. One of the most effective and affordable is the Berkey gravity filter, it's pretty simple to set up and it really does a fabulous job filtering tap water. You must get the fluoride filters that go with it to do the most effective cleaning. If you want to get technical, you can install a reverse osmosis filter or something as capable of removing impurities and chemicals. Good quality water is essential for your health! Only if you filter your tap water can you drink or cook with it without worry. To go full out you can get a whole house filter, but it's pretty pricey. A lot of new green homes have this type of filtration system installed. The filter that goes through your fridge can be ok, as long as you change it out when needed. Other less expensive filter pitchers can get some of the bad stuff out, but not all.

Quality Cookware

Cookware is important. Stainless steel, cast iron, ceramic, glass and copper are good. Wood, metal, and rubber spoons and spatulas are all good options. Avoid Teflon and nonstick pans. They scratch easily leaching chemicals into the food you're cooking and can also release VOCs. PFAS chemicals like GenX and PFOA are also implicated in disastrous water pollution issues. Avoid plastic utensils, these melt and leach into foods as well. Even plastic dishes and plastic silverware are troublesome for the planet as they tend to end up polluting our waterways and harming animals. Also avoid plastic toothpicks, try to use real wood or get a metal reusable one.

Food Storage

Opt for glass, metal, ceramic and sustainable containers whenever possible. Using dishes for leftovers works too, just cover with another dish or bowl. Plastic and Styrofoam are the least desirable as these can leach into foods and beverages. Especially avoid Styrofoam (polystyrene) as much as possible. Polystyrene chemicals seep into hot beverages and foods. Never heat or microwave food in Styrofoam containers or in plastic wrap or plastic. Save food by freezing leftovers and food before it spoils so you can use it later when you have time.

Cleaning Your Kitchen and Home

Use effective and safe cleaning products. Avoid using products with chlorine bleach and toxins. Using nontoxic cleaning products reduces the strain on water and on You by reducing the contaminant load. This also helps keep water sources cleaner in the long run. Look for dishwashing liquids, detergents and cleaning materials that are phosphate free, chlorine free, and without: petroleum derivatives, ammonia, microbeads, VOCs, nitrosamines, palm oil, etc.

Giving Your Greens and Vegetables a Water Bath

One of the best ways to thoroughly clean your fruit and veges is to give them a long soak in a big bowl of water. Let them sit for 5 minutes or longer. Drain water and rinse once more.

ADOREYOURSELF FOOD

Real Food and Nutrition, the Keys to Health

When it comes to our health, food and nutrition play a critical role. As illustrated throughout this book, there are many things occurring within the food supply and the environment that result in contamination. No doubt natural foods keep us healthier than food loaded with sugar, pesticides, and random badness. However, to maintain wellness and to recover from disease you also need all the essential nutrients. If you are under a doctor's care, make sure to consult with your physician.

WHAT TO EAT

Organic foods: fewer pesticides, no synthetic fertilizer and no GMOS
Veges: Fresh and organic is best, with least pesticides, eat abundantly
Dark leafy Greens: Organic, fresh, rinse well before eating, eat abundantly
Lemons and Herbs: Organic and fresh, season and flavor foods and beverages
Fruits: Organic, fresh and vibrant is best, eat abundantly
Fish: Wild when possible, rotate varieties to help fish and reduce exposures
Lentils & Beans, Pulses: Organic, eat often, use in soups, side dishes, sprout
Soups and Broths: Organic, homemade when possible, eat abundantly
Grains: Organic brown rice, amaranth, quinoa, buckwheat, millet are good for you
Fats: Unrefined Coconut Oil, Virgin Olive oil, ghee, butter (rBGH free), lard, tallow
Seeds, Nuts, Olives, Dried Fruit: Buy organic (others may be treated with fumigants)
Salt: Sea salt, Himalayan salt or Kosher
Eggs & Meat: Choose those free of antibiotics, steroids, hormones, antibiotics, nitrates
Milk & Dairy: Select products from good farms, not factory farms, free of rBGH
Deli Meats: Only those free of nitrates, sulfites, antibiotics, hormones, steroids
Frozen Lemons: Keep in freezer, grate whole lemon into dishes and treats

WHAT TO DRINK

- Water: fresh & filtered: no chlorine, fluoride, pesticides, nitrates, heavy metals
- Fresh & fresh vegetable juices (juices sitting over a day lose vitality)
- Fresh squeezed lemon juice with water
- Fresh fruit juice
- Vegetable broth and bone broth (very high in minerals and nutrients!)
- Organic Tea, herbal or caffeinated (made with good water)
- Kombucha, organic
- Coffee (made with good water)
- Natural sodas (without sugar, fake flavors, artificial sugar, HFCS, or BVO)
- Mineral Water
- Smoothies and juices: choose organic to reduce pesticide exposure

ADOREYOURSELF PREP

PREPARING and CLEANING FOOD

1. Wash your hands with soap and hot water before handling food.

2. Soaking fruits and vegetables helps reduce pesticide exposure

- Wash your hands with hot water and soap, under fingernails too before handling food
- Clean surfaces, cutting boards, utensils with soap & water before and after food prep
- Soak vegetables, greens, lettuce in clean, cool water for 5 minutes at least before rinsing;
- Soak grains, rice and raw beans in water (add pinch of vitamin c powder if you have it)
- Rinse and peel root vegetables like carrots and potatoes, cut out bruised and dark spots
- Use a clean knife and cutting board when cutting fruits and vegetables

3. To Peel or Not?: In addition to soaking, peeling vegetables grown in the ground reduces dirt, though if rinsed well and bad sections are cut away, peeling may not be necessary especially if you're cooking the vegetables in good water—(reuse it or drink it after--its full of nutrients!)

4. Cutting Board: use a clean wooden cutting board. Plastic isn't preferred as it's more easily nicked giving bacteria more hiding places. Keep cutting board clean with soap & hot water.

4. Reduce pesticide toxicity: opt for fruits and veges grown pesticide-free; eat and grow organic; don't use toxic fertilizer or pesticides at your home, in your garden or farm

5. Reduce heavy metals toxicity: Keep your body happy as much as possible; drink lots of pure water; eat + drink cultured foods that bind and discharge toxins such as yogurt, kefir, sauerkraut, kimchi, kombucha, pickles, cilantro, drink alfalfa and dandelion root tea.

6. Warding off disease: eat and drink foods high in antioxidants, fight free radical scavengers; boost your immune system with nourishing food; reduce your intake and exposure to chemicals and known carcinogens; use filtered clean water for drinking & cooking

7. Out there you may not know how many chemicals are on your food, here's a mini snapshot:

MOST PESTICIDES	Less Pesticides
Apples	Avocadoes
Bell Peppers	
Kale	
Carrots	Asparagus
Celery	Bananas
Cherries	Blueberries
Grapes	Broccoli
Lettuce	
Nectarines	Kiwi
Peaches	Mangoes
Pears	Onions
Potatoes	
Spinach	Pineapple
Strawberries	Peas

ADOREYOURSELF SUPERFOODS

"The good news is that a large number of cancers can be prevented. It is estimated that as many as two-thirds of all cancer cases are linked to environmental causes. This number may even be higher. Many of these are linked to lifestyle factors that can be modified."
National Institutes of Health[669]

Superfoods can add a super dose of goodness to your health regimen. Please be sure to obtain organically grown superfood products, as any pesticide residues will conflict and nullify the benefits that can otherwise be obtained from these wonderful goodies. Here's a few:

FRUITS, Organic

Acai, Bilberries, Black Cherries, Black Raspberries, Blueberries, Mango, Pineapple, Star fruit, Berries, Bananas, Cherries, Cranberries, Goji Berries, Lemon, Grapefruit, Oranges, Kiwi, Tomato, Peaches, Plums, Apricots, Watermelon, Limes, Nectarines, Apples, Strawberries, Cantelope, Grapes, Pomegranate, Papaya

VEGETABLES and GRAINS, Organic

Bok Choy, Broccoli, Dandelion Greens, Kale, Garlic, Onions, Reishi Mushroom, Beets, Parsley, Rutabaga, Shitake Mushroom, Carrots, Cilanatro, Celery + Root, Endive, Spinach, Leeks, Radish, Scallion, Pumpkin, Turnip, Potato, Parsnip, Amaranth, Brown Rice, Millet, Buckwheat, Quinoa

DAIRY, Organic

Yogurt, Greek Yogurt, Kefir, Cheeses (particularly raw and derived from sheep and goat origin), Whole milk, Cottage Cheese, Goat Milk

OTHER, Organic

Apple Cider Vinegar, Buckwheat, Cocoa raw and dark, Chlorella, Spirulina, Honey (Raw and Manuka varieties), Nutritional Yeast, Seaweed, Kelp, Pumpkin Seeds, Sesame Seeds, Almonds, Walnuts, Pecans, Brazil Nuts, Chia Seeds, Vanilla, Sunflower Seed, Kimchi, Kombucha

HERBS and SPICES, Organic

Alfalfa, Ashwagandha, Burdock Root, Cayenne Pepper, Cilantro, Cinnamon, Mint, Cranesbill, Dandelion Root, Eleuthero, Green Tea, Raspberry Leaf, Red Clover, Lavender Rhodiola, Mint, Rosemary, Oregano, Parsley, Thyme, Turmeric, Pepper, Salt, Basil

NUTRIENTS: You want to make sure you're getting enough of the essential minerals and vitamins into your diet. These are critical to help your body function at its best. Even if we're eating well, supplements can still complement our diet in a big way! Find a high-quality full spectrum mineral and vitamin blend. Opt for one made with real organic ingredients. A good brand will contain all the essential minerals and micronutrients your body needs to thrive including the micronutrients. If you're deficient in any particular minerals you may initially need to take extra amounts to refuel your system, such as extra magnesium or vitamin B12.

ADOREYOURSELF NUTRIENTS

"Thanks to three quarters of a century of "scientific agriculture" with the use of synthetic fertilizers, the soil of our farm lands has been leached of its trace mineral content and our food supply is often times lacking in these essential nutrients, which are not added back to the soil."[670] Hundreds of diseases result from mineral deficiencies. Even if we're eating well, we may not be getting all the nutrients our bodies and minds need to function at their optimum levels. "The basic functions of life cannot be performed without minerals, either as a major part of the function or as a catalytic cofactor (i.e.-RNA, DNA, subcellular and digestive enzymes and the utilization of vitamins). Simply said, minerals are the currency of life."[671]

The 90 Essential Nutrients[672]

60 Minerals, Elements, Metals, Trace Minerals and Rare Earths:

Aluminum, Arsenic, Barium, Beryllium, Boron, Bromine, Calcium, Carbon, Cerium, Chloride, Chromium, Cobalt, Copper, Dysprosium, Erbium, Europium, Gadolinium, Gallium, Germanium, Gold, Hafnium, Holmium, Hydrogen, Iodine, Iron, Lanthanum, Lithium, Lutecium, Magnesium, Manganese, Molybdenum, Neodymium, Nickle, Niobium, Nitrogen, Oxygen, Phosphorous, Potassium, Praseodymium, Rhenium, Rubidium, Samarium, Scandium, Selenium, Silica, Silver, Sodium, Strontium, Sulphur, Tantalum, Terbium, Thulium, Tin, Titanium, Vanadium, Yitterbium, Ytrium, Zinc, Zirconium

16 Vitamins: Vitamin A, Vitamin B1 (Thiamine), Vitamin B2 (Riboflavin), Vitamin B3 (Niacin), Vitamin B5 (Pantothenic Acid), Vitamin B6 (Pyridoxine), Vitamin B12 (Cyanocobalamine), Vitamin C, Vitamin D, Vitamin K, Biotin, Choline, Flavonoids and Bioflavonoids, Folic Acid, Inositol

2-3 Essential Fatty Acids

Omega 3, Omega 6, Omega 9

12 Amino Acids

Valine, Lysine, Threonine, Leucine, Isoleucine, Tryptophan, Phenylalanine, Methionine, Histadine, Arginine, Taurine, Tyrosine

Get your nutrients and protect your health and mind.

Supplementing with good quality minerals, vitamins, omega oils and amino acids can make a major difference in your health and well being.

ADOREYOURSELF KITCHEN

FATS and OILS: Our bodies need fat to help utilize vitamins and minerals efficiently.

Good fats for eating, baking, and cooking include:

- Butter (rBGH free)
- Lard and Tallow (from animals raised ethically)
- Ghee (rBGH free)
- Cold-pressed, unrefined, virgin oils
- Virgin Olive oil
- Unrefined Coconut oil
- Fat from meat raised humanely without steroids, drugs, or rBGH

SALT: People and animals need salt-- sodium chloride is essential for digestion and stomach acid. Heartburn can result from a sodium free diet,[673] without enough our bodies fail at producing enough digestive acids. Common table salt can be contaminated with aluminum and other stuff, though it does have iodine added. Your best bet for health is to switch to Himalayan, Kosher or Sea Salt, then get a good iodine supplement. We really must reduce our plastic pollution, some salts have recently been found contaminated with microplastics.[674]

Good Salt

- Himalayan Salt
- Sea Salt
- Kosher Salt

Unhealthy Salt

Table salt may have fillers, heavy metals

SUGAR "Sugar taken every day produces a continuously overacid condition, and more and more minerals are required from deep in the body in the attempt to rectify the imbalance. Finally, in order to protect the blood, so much calcium is taken from the bones and teeth that decay and general weakening begin. Excess sugar eventually affects every organ in the body." William Dufty, Sugar Blues

Good Sugar

- Raw Honey
- Organic Blackstrap Molasses
- Manuka Honey
- Grade B Maple Syrup, dark amber
- Organic Turbinado sugar
- Organic whole cane sugar
- Organic whole leaf Stevia: only need a pinch,
  1 tsp is equivalent in sweetness to 1 cup of sugar.

Unhealthy Sugar

Refined white sugar
High fructose corn syrup
Fake Sweeteners

SPICES

Source organic spices as well, for many contain pesticides and can be exposed to irradiation.

PREPARE TO RISE LAWS

And so, my fellow Americans:
ask not what your country can do for you —
ask what you can do for your country.
President John Fitzgerald Kennedy
Inaugural Address
January 20, 1961

HOW LAWS ARE MADE

Most laws in the United States begin as bills. A bill begins with an idea. That idea can come from anyone—including you! The idea is sent to Congress, where a Member of the U.S. House of Representatives researches the idea and writes a bill.

Once the bill is written, it is placed in the hopper, and introduced to the rest of the Members of the U.S. House of Representatives. The Members debate the bill, then vote on whether it should become a law or not using the electronic voting system.

After the bill has passed in the House, it is sent to the U.S. Senate. The Members of the Senate debate and vote on the bill. If the bill passes, it is sent to the President of the United States for approval. Once the President signs the bill, it is a law. Now that the bill has become a law, it is a rule that all Americans must follow.

WHAT IS CONGRESS?

The U.S. government is made up of the executive branch, the judicial branch, and the legislative branch. The executive branch, led by the President and the Vice President, enforces our laws. The judicial branch, led by the Supreme Court, interprets our laws. The legislative branch, which makes our laws, is the Congress.

Congress has two parts: the U.S. Senate and the U.S. House of Representatives. Each state has two U.S. Senators and at least one U.S. Representative; the more residents a state has, the more U.S. Representatives it is allowed. There are 100 U.S. Senators and 435 U.S. Representatives.

The laws Congress makes help Americans. There are laws that say kids have to go to school, laws that set standards for vehicle and highway safety, and laws that protect animals and nature. Congress meets in the Capitol in Washington, D.C.

Source: http://kids.clerk.house.gov/young-learners/lesson.html?intID=31

HOW ARE REGULATIONS CREATED?

To better understand our government's regulations as well as the process behind them, the following information details the regulation process and can be found at the EPA's website.[675]

The Basics of the Regulatory Process

"Have you ever wondered how EPA protects the environment? We use a variety of tools and approaches, like partnerships, educational programs, and grants. One of our most significant tools is writing regulations. Regulations are mandatory requirements that can apply to individuals, businesses, state or local governments, non-profit institutions, or others.

Congress passes the laws that govern the United States, but Congress has also authorized EPA and other federal agencies to help put those laws into effect by creating and enforcing regulations. Below, you'll find a basic description of how laws and regulations are developed, what they are, and where to find them, with an emphasis on environmental laws and regulations

Creating a law

Step 1: Congress Writes a Bill

A member of Congress proposes a bill. A bill is a document that, if approved, will become law. To see the text of bills Congress is considering or has considered, go to Congress.gov

Step 2: The President Approves or Vetoes the Bill

If both houses of Congress approve a bill, it goes to the President who has the option to either approve it or veto it. If approved, the new law is called an act or statute.

Step 3: The Act is Codified in the *United States Code*

Once an act is passed, the House of Representatives standardizes the text of the law and publishes it in the *United States Code* (U.S.C.). The U.S.C. is the codification by subject matter of the general and permanent laws of the United States. Since 1926, the U.S.C. has been published every six years. In between editions, annual cumulative supplements are published in order to present the most current information.
United States Code: This database is available from the Government Printing Office (GPO). GPO is the sole agency authorized by the federal government to publish the U.S.C.

Putting the law to work

Once a law is official, here's how it is put into practice: Laws often do not include all the details needed to explain how an individual, business, state or local government, or others might follow the law. The *United States Code* would not tell you, for example, what the speed limit is in front of your house. In order to make the laws work on a day-to-day level, Congress authorizes certain government agencies - including EPA - to create regulations.

LAWS AFFECTING FOOD

THE PURE FOOD & DRUG ACT, June 23, 1906

"The Pure Food and Drug Act was a centerpiece of progressive reforms in the early 20th century. Muckraking journalists had long reported on the appallingly unsanitary conditions of the country's manufacturing plants, especially those in Chicago's meat-packing industry. But it wasn't until the public outcry following the publication of Upton Sinclair's *The Jungle* that Congress moved on legislation that would prevent "the manufacture, sale, or transportation of adulterated or misbranded or poisonous or deleterious foods, drugs or medicines, and liquors."

The version of the bill which became the Pure Food and Drug Act originated in the Senate (S.88), and after being sent to the House it was reported out of the Interstate and Foreign Commerce Committee with amendments on March 7th. It sat unconsidered for three months, causing some to wonder if Speaker Joe Cannon of Illinois was delaying it. On June 21st, with only a few days left to the session, Representative James Mann of Illinois captivated the chamber with a speech about fruit that had been colored with poisonous red dye, and liquor that had been distilled with chemical fillers. The *New York Times* called the debate over the Pure Food bill "one of the wildest times that has been seen this session." After the measure passed, the House and Senate met in conference, settled their differences, and sent the bill back to their respective chambers for final consideration. Following a round of applause, the House approved the conference report on June 29th. President Theodore Roosevelt signed the Pure Food and Drug Act into law the next day. **http://history.house.gov/HistoricalHighlight/Detail/15032393280**

FEDERAL FOOD, DRUG AND COSMETIC ACT OF 1938

This act replaced the original Pure Food and Drugs Act established by President Theodore Roosevelt and Harvey Wiley. Section 408 of the Federal Food, Drug, and Cosmetic Act (FFDCA) authorizes EPA to set tolerances, or maximum residue limits, for pesticide residues on foods. In the absence of a tolerance for a pesticide residue, a food containing such a residue is subject to seizure by the government. Once a tolerance is established, the residue level in the tolerance is the trigger for enforcement actions. That is, if residues are found above that level, the commodity will be subject to seizure.[676]

§342. Adulterated food, Food Additives

A food shall be deemed to be adulterated—

(a) Poisonous, insanitary, etc., ingredients

(1) If it bears or contains any poisonous or deleterious substance which may render it injurious to health; but in case the substance is not an added substance such food shall not be considered adulterated under this clause if the quantity of such substance in such food does not ordinarily render it injurious to health.1 (2)(A) if it bears or contains any added poisonous or added deleterious substance (other than a substance that is a pesticide chemical residue in or on a raw agricultural commodity or processed food, a food additive, a color additive, or a new animal drug) that is unsafe within the meaning of section 346 of this title.677

Unsafe Food Additives678:

(a)Unsafe food additives; exception for conformity with exemption or regulation A food additive shall, with respect to any particular use or intended use of such additives, be deemed to be unsafe for the purposes of the application of clause (2)(C) of section 342(a) of this title, unless—

(1) it and its use or intended use conform to the terms of an exemption which is in effect pursuant to subsection (j) of this section;

(2) there is in effect, and it and its use or intended use are in conformity with, a regulation issued under this section prescribing the conditions under which such additive may be safely used; or

(3) in the case of a food additive as defined in this chapter that is a food contact substance, there is—(A) in effect, and such substance and the use of such substance are in conformity with, a regulation issued under this section prescribing the conditions under which such additive may be safely used; or (B) a notification submitted under subsection (h) of this section that is effective. While such a regulation relating to a food additive, or such a notification under subsection (h)(1) of this section relating to a food additive that is a food contact substance, is in effect, and has not been revoked pursuant to subsection (i) of this section, a food shall not, by reason of bearing or containing such a food additive in accordance with the regulation or notification, be considered adulterated under section 342(a)(1) of this title.

DELANEY AMENDMENT

The Delaney Clause was a part of the 1958 Food Additives Amendment (section 409) to the 1954 Federal Food, Drug and Cosmetic Act (FFDCA). This clause governed regulation of pesticide residues in processed foods. It established that no residues from pesticides found to cause cancer in animals would be allowed as a food additive. This meant that tolerance levels must be based only on the risk of carcinogenicity and that the benefits of the pesticide could not be considered. The Delaney Amendment (Clause) was not renewed by Congress in 1996, but nonetheless we can urge our congresspeople to bring it back or write a new bill reflecting the same principles. "The Delaney Clause, named after Congressman James Delaney of New York and tacked onto the Federal Food, Drugs, and Cosmetic Act of 1958, said, "the Secretary [of the Food and Drug Administration] shall not approve for use in food any chemical additive found to induce cancer in man, or, after tests, found to induce cancer in animals." Not any. Zero."[679]

DSHEA, Dietary Supplement Health and Education Act

In this time of rampant environmental pollution, it would serve us well to protect our access to minerals, vitamins and health supplements. According to health.gov, "The Dietary Supplement Health and Education Act of 1994 (DSHEA, or the Act) was enacted by Congress following public debate concerning the importance of dietary supplements in promoting health, the need for consumers to have access to current and accurate information about supplements, and controversy over the Food and Drug Administration's (FDA) regulatory approach to this product category." [680]

LAWS AFFECTING FOOD

FOOD SAFETY MODERNIZATION ACT, 2011

The Food Safety Modernization Act (FSMA) represents the first major reform to the US Food and Drug Administration (FDA) food safety authority since 1938.

- FSMA requires enhanced regulation of produce from farm to sale and other FDA regulated foods from processing to sale and introduces food defense requirements.
- FSMA alters the role of FDA in food Safety through 5 key changes:

A shift of focus from reaction to prevention including preventing intentional contamination. More authority to inspect and assure compliance with inspection frequencies based on risk. Mandatory recall authority. Authorities to strengthen import safety to assure that US food safety standards are met. Stronger partnerships with other government agencies and private entities. *Summary provided by Food Policy Center University of Minnesota*[681]

SAFE AND ACCURATE FOOD LABELING ACT OF 2015

Otherwise known as the DARK act (Deny Americans Right to Know)

This GMO-backed anti-labeling bill was signed by President Obama in July 2016. Otherwise known as the Big M Protection Act and the DARK act, this law prevents GMO labeling. In a strange meeting in the middle of the night, in conjunction with signing the DARK ACT, the **Roberts-Stabenow Biotech Labeling Act, S. 764** was signed. The RSBLA does require labeling of most GMO derived food, but has limited definition so perhaps not all will fall into the labeled category. Labeling won't be in written but rather in a QR Code that requires us to scan the code with a smart phone and internet access to translate. I guess if we're ever in doubt or have lost our phone we'll just have to resort to good old common sense.

FALCPA Food Allergen Labeling and Consumer Protection

Effective 2006, if a product contains one of the eight top allergens (milk, eggs, soy, wheat, fish, shellfish, peanuts, treenuts) it must be disclosed on the label.

FD&C Section 408: Maximum Residues

Section 408 of the Federal Food, Drug, and Cosmetic Act (FFDCA) authorizes EPA to set tolerances, or maximum residue limits, for pesticide residues on foods. In the absence of a tolerance for a pesticide residue, a food containing such a residue is subject to seizure by the government. Once a tolerance is established, the residue level in the tolerance is the trigger for enforcement actions. That is, if residues are found above that level, the commodity will be subject to seizure.[682]

Federal Meat Inspection Act

The Federal Meat Inspection Act of 1906 (P.L. 59-242) and the Wholesome Meat Act of 1967 (P.L. 90-201) were designed and implemented to provide the public with a safe, wholesome meat supply. Today's consumer relies on the Food Safety and Inspection Service (FSIS) inspectors to ensure this.[28]

LAWS AFFECTING FOOD

FOOD QUALITY PROTECTION ACT OF 1996

Signed into law by President Bill Clinton, this Act effectively ended the protections provided to us through the Delaney Clause. The Delaney Clause was an instrumental part of the 1958 Food Additives Amendment to the 1954 Federal Food, Drug, and Cosmetic Act. Without the protection provided by the Delaney clause, GMOs quietly slipped into the food supply.

GRAS: Generally Recognized as Safe

The Generally Recognized as Safe Clause to the 1958 Food Additives Amendment signed into law by President Eisenhower may have remain unchanged over the years, but the implementation of the law has allowed industry to take advantage.

The FDA does not require all ingredient information from the manufacturer, it is provided on a *voluntary* basis. This law like the Toxic Substance Control Act was designed with the assumption that honest information would be provided. "The agency's (FDA's) attempts to limit these undisclosed GRAS determinations by asking industry to voluntarily inform the FDA about their chemicals are insufficient to ensure the safety of our food in today's global marketplace with a complex food supply. Furthermore, no other developed country in the world has a system like GRAS to provide oversight of food ingredients."[683]

ORGANIC FOODS PRODUCTION ACT OF 1990

Title I: National Standards Governing the Organic Production of Agricultural Products - Directs the Secretary of Agriculture to establish: (1) a national organic production certification program; (2) a label for organically produced and handled agricultural products; (3) a national list of approved and prohibited substances to be included in the organic production standards; and (4) a certifying agent accreditation program. Authorizes State organic certification programs.

USDA National Organic Standards Board (NOSB) definition, April 1995:

1. "Organic agriculture is an ecological production management system that promotes and enhances biodiversity, biological cycles and soil biological activity. It is based on minimal use of off-farm inputs and on management practices that restore, maintain and enhance ecological harmony.

2. "'Organic' is a labeling term that denotes products produced under the authority of the Organic Foods Production Act. The principal guidelines for organic production are to use materials and practices that enhance the ecological balance of natural systems and that integrate the parts of the farming system into an ecological whole.

3. "Organic agriculture practices cannot ensure that products are completely free of residues; however, methods are used to minimize pollution from air, soil and water.

4. "Organic food handlers, processors and retailers adhere to standards that maintain the integrity of organic agricultural products. The primary goal of organic agriculture is to optimize the health and productivity of interdependent communities of soil life, plants, animals and people." USDA[684]

LAWS AFFECTING FOOD

National Organic Standards Board (NOSB)

The National Organic Standards Board (NOSB) is a Federal Advisory Board made up of 15 dedicated public volunteers from across the organic community. Established by the Organic Foods Production Act (OFPA) and governed by the Federal Advisory Committee Act (FACA), the NOSB considers and makes recommendations on a wide range of issues involving the production, handling, and processing of organic products. The NOSB also has special responsibilities related to the National List of Allowed and Prohibited Substances.

The National List of Allowed and Prohibited Substances identifies the synthetic substances that may be used and the nonsynthetic (natural) substances that may not be used in organic crop and livestock production. It also identifies a limited number of non-organic substances that may be used in or on processed organic products.[685]

How Does FDA Evaluate the Safety of GE Plants? During the FDA consultation process, the food developer conducts a safety assessment. This safety assessment identifies the distinguishing attributes of the new traits in the plant and assesses whether any new material in food made from the GE plant is safe when eaten by humans or animals. As part of this assessment, the developer compares the levels of nutrients and other components in the food to those in food from traditionally bred plants or other comparable foods. The developer submits a summary of its safety assessment to FDA for FDA's evaluation. When the safety assessment is received by FDA, our scientists carefully evaluate the data and information. FDA considers the consultation to be complete only when its team of scientists is satisfied that the developer's safety assessment has adequately addressed all safety and other regulatory issues.[686]

PESTICIDES

Decreasing pesticide use will reduce incidences of disease and cancer amongst people & animals.

Federal Insecticide, Fungicide, and Rodenticide Act (FIFRA):

Gives the EPA authority to regulate the sale, use and distribution of pesticides.

Federal Food, Drug, and Cosmetic Act (FFDCA):

Gives the EPA authority to set limits on the amount of pesticide residues allowed on food or animal feed. These limits are called tolerances.

Food Quality Protection Act of 1996 (FQPA):

This act amended FIFRA and FFDCA by increasing the safety standards for new pesticides used on foods. FQPA also required older pesticides and previously established tolerances to be periodically re-assessed using the new, tougher standards.

Pesticide Registration Improvement Act (PRIA):

Establishes the fees and time-lines associated with pesticide registration actions.

Endangered Species Act (ESA): Requires the EPA to assess the risk of pesticides to threatened or endangered species and their habitats.[687]

LAWS AFFECTING FOOD

Federal Insecticide, Fungicide, Rodenticide Act: all pesticides sold or distributed in the United States (including imported pesticides) to be registered by EPA.
Registration is based on evaluation of scientific data and assessment of risks and benefits of a product's use. Label directions control how products are used.

- We can authorize limited use of unregistered pesticides or pesticides registered for other uses to address emergencies and special local needs.
- We can suspend or cancel a product's registration.
http://www.epa.gov/pesticide-registration/about-pesticide-registration

Federal Food, Drug and Cosmetic Act (FFDCA)

Requires us to set pesticide tolerances for all pesticides used in or on food or in a manner that will result in a residue in or on food or animal feed. A tolerance is the maximum permissible level for pesticide residues allowed in or on human food and animal feed.

- Includes strong provisions for protecting infants and children, as well as other sensitive subpopulations.
- Provides for exemption from the requirement for a tolerance.

The Food Quality Protection Act, of 1996

Amended both FIFRA and FFDCA. We must find that a pesticide poses a "reasonable certainty of no harm" before it can be registered for use on food or feed. We must review each pesticide registration at least once every 15 years.

- Several factors must be addressed before a tolerance can be established, including:
- the aggregate, non-occupational exposure from the pesticide (exposure through diet and drinking water and from using pesticides in and around the home);
- the cumulative effects from exposure to pesticides that have a common mechanism of toxicity, that is, two or more pesticide chemicals or other substances that cause a common toxic effect(s) by the same, or essentially the same, sequence of major biochemical events (i.e., interpreted as mode of action);
- whether there is increased susceptibility to infants and children, or other sensitive subpopulations, from exposure to the pesticide; and
- whether the pesticide produces an effect in humans similar to an effect produced by a naturally-occurring estrogen or produces other endocrine-disruption effects.

The Pesticide Registration Improvement Act of 2003 (PRIA) also amended FIFRA and FFDCA. PRIA was reauthorized by the Pesticide Registration Improvement Renewal Act of 2007 and the Pesticide Registration Improvement Extension Act of 2012.
The Endangered Species Act (ESA) requires federal agencies to ensure that any action they authorize, fund, or carry out, will not likely jeopardize the continued existence of any listed species, or destroy or adversely modify any critical habitat for those species.

LAWS AFFECTING FOOD

Inert Ingredients PRN 97-6

Use of term "inert" in Label Ingredients: the phrase "Inert ingredients," may be replaced by the term "Other ingredients. An inert ingredient is simply any ingredient in the product that is not pesticidally active. Unless an inert ingredient is determined to be highly toxic, it is not required to be identified by name or percentage on the label, but the total percentage of such ingredients must be declared. EPA has long known and acknowledged that some inert ingredients are not benign to human health or the environment. The "inert" ingredients in some products may be more toxic or pose greater risks than the active ingredient."[688]

TOXIC SUBSTANCES

TOXIC SUBSTANCES CONTROL ACT

Established in 1976, the TSCA was designed to give the EPA the framework to monitor the thousands of chemicals in use, produced, and imported into the country. While the EPA theoretically has the power to screen and monitor these chemicals, many slip through the cracks and end up in various consumer products. For this and other reasons that favor industry over our own health, safety and well being, many organizations have been trying to reform the TSCA.

FRANK R. LAUTENBERG CHEMICAL SAFETY ACT FOR THE 21ST CENTURY ACT

- Mandates safety reviews for all chemicals in active commerce.
- Requires a safety finding for new chemicals before they can enter the market.
- Replaces TSCA's burdensome cost-benefit safety standard—which prevented EPA from banning asbestos—with a pure, health-based safety standard.
- Explicitly requires protection of vulnerable populations like children and pregnant women.
- Gives EPA enhanced authority to require testing of both new and existing chemicals.
- Sets aggressive, judicially enforceable deadlines for EPA decisions.

Makes more information about chemicals available, by limiting companies' ability to claim information as confidential, and by giving states and health and environmental professionals access to confidential information they need to do their jobs."[689] Became law June 22, 2016.

CERCLA, SUPERFUND

"The Comprehensive Environmental Response, Compensation, and Liability Act -- otherwise known as CERCLA or Superfund -- provides a Federal "Superfund" to clean up uncontrolled or abandoned hazardous-waste sites as well as accidents, spills, and other emergency releases of pollutants and contaminants into the environment. Through CERCLA, EPA was given power to seek out those parties responsible for any release and assure their cooperation in the cleanup."[690]

LAWS AFFECTING FOOD

RCRA, Resource Conservation and Recovery Act [691]

The Resource Conservation and Recovery Act (RCRA) gives EPA the authority to control hazardous waste from the "cradle-to-grave." This includes the generation, transportation, treatment, storage, and disposal of hazardous waste. RCRA also set forth a framework for the management of non-hazardous solid wastes. The 1986 amendments to RCRA enabled EPA to address environmental problems that could result from underground tanks storing petroleum and other hazardous substances.

PROPOSITION 65 (California only)

"Proposition 65 requires California to publish a list of chemicals known to cause cancer, birth defects or other reproductive harm. This list, which must be updated at least once a year, has grown to include approximately 900 chemicals since it was first published in 1987. Proposition 65 became law in November 1986, when California voters approved it by a 63-37 percent margin. The official name of Proposition 65 is the Safe Drinking Water and Toxic Enforcement Act of 1986."[692]

Stockholm Convention on Persistent Organic Pollutants

"The Stockholm Convention on Persistent Organic Pollutants is a global treaty to protect human health and the environment from chemicals that remain intact in the environment for long periods, become widely distributed geographically, accumulate in the fatty tissue of humans and wildlife, and have harmful impacts on human health or on the environment."[409]

WATER

HISTORY OF THE CLEAN WATER ACT[693]

The Federal Water Pollution Control Act of 1948 was the first major U.S. law to address water pollution. Growing public awareness and concern for controlling water pollution led to sweeping amendments in 1972. As amended in 1972, the law became commonly known as the Clean Water Act (CWA).

THE SAFE DRINKING WATER ACT

"The Safe Drinking Water Act (SDWA) was established to protect the quality of drinking water in the U.S. This law focuses on all waters actually or potentially designed for drinking use, whether from above ground or underground sources. The Act authorizes EPA to establish minimum standards to protect tap water and requires all owners or operators of public water systems to comply with these primary (health-related) standards. The 1996 amendments to SDWA require that EPA consider a detailed risk and cost assessment, and best available peer-reviewed science, when developing these standards. State governments, which can be approved to implement these rules for EPA, also encourage attainment of secondary standards (nuisance-related). Under the Act, EPA also establishes minimum standards for state programs to protect underground sources of drinking water from endangerment by underground injection of fluids."[694]

LAWS AFFECTING FOOD

CODEX ALIMENTARIUS & THE WTO

Codex is an international body created after WWII to establish "Food Rules." These rules are slowly being unfolded and incorporated to harmonize global trade. These rules are enforced by the World Trade Organization (WTO). Any member country can have its own laws upended by Codex laws. Our COOL meat labeling, for instance was eliminated because it contradicted Codex, and showed "favoritism" to meat from the USA. If we didn't comply the US could've faced sanctions and fines as determined by the WTO.

In essence what concerns many people is that our own laws can be voided so easily if the WTO comes calling. Already in our country Big Ag and the pesticide makers have incredible control over food laws, food safety and labeling. Most of the pesticide makers also dominate pharmaceuticals, so perhaps they're not so interested in whether we're healthy or not. In any case let us take heed and protect ourselves and protect our country from unlawful law making that could affect our health.

Back in 2005 Representative Ron Paul shared his concerns about Codex[695]:

"Make no mistake about it: those international standards are moving steadily toward the Codex regime and its draconian restrictions on health freedom. Pharmaceutical companies have spent billions of dollars trying to get Washington to regulate your dietary supplements. So far, that effort has failed, in part because of a 1994 law called the Dietary Supplement Health and Education Act. Big Pharma and the medical establishment hate this Act because it allows consumers some measure of freedom to buy the supplements they want.

The largely government-run "healthcare" establishment, including the nominally private pharmaceutical companies, want government to control the dietary-supplement industry so that only they can manufacture and distribute supplements providing any real benefit. If this takes place, as it has in Europe, the high-potency, beneficial supplements that you can now buy over the counter will be available, if at all, only by prescription and at a much higher cost. This alone is sufficient reason for Congress to oppose the unconstitutional, freedom-destroying CAFTA bill. FDA and Congress are also working (FDA quite openly, Congress more covertly) toward the goal of harmonizing our health laws with Codex Alimentarius standards and guidelines."

FOOD RECALLS

From the USDA here's a breakdown of reasons for recall.[696]

Bacteria	Associated Foods	Symptoms and Potential Impact	Prevention
Campylobacter jejuni	Contaminated water, raw or unpasteurized milk, and raw or undercooked meat, poultry, or shellfish.	Diarrhea (sometimes bloody), cramping, abdominal pain, and fever that appear 2 to 5 days after eating; may last 7 days. May spread to bloodstream and cause a life- threatening infection.	Cook meat and poultry to a safe minimum internal temperature; do not drink or consume unpasteurized milk or milk products; wash your hands after coming in contact with feces.
Clostridium botulinum	Improperly canned foods, garlic in oil, vacuum-packed and tightly wrapped food.	Bacteria produce a nerve toxin that causes illness, affecting the nervous system. Toxin affects the nervous system. Symptoms usually appear 18 to 36 hours, but can sometimes appear as few as 6 hours or as many as 10 days after eating; double vision, blurred vision, drooping eyelids, slurred speech, difficulty swallowing, dry mouth, and muscle weakness. If untreated, these symptoms may progress causing muscle paralysis and even death.	Do not use damaged canned foods or canned foods showing signs of swelling, leakage, punctures, holes, fractures, extensive deep rusting, or crushing/denting severe enough to prevent normal stacking. Follow safety guidelines when home canning food. Boil home canned foods for 10 minutes before eating to ensure safety. (Note: Safe home canning guidelines may be obtained from State University or County Extension Office).
Clostridium perfringens	Meats, meat products and gravy Called "the cafeteria germ" because many outbreaks result from food left for long periods in steam tables or at room temperature.	Intense abdominal cramps nausea, and diarrhea may appear 6 to 24 hours after eating; usually last about 1 day, but for immune comprised individuals, symptoms may last 1 to 2 weeks. Complications and/or death can occur only very rarely.	Keep hot foods hot and cold foods cold! Once food is cooked, it should be held hot, at an internal temperature of 140 °F or above. Use a food thermometer to make sure. Discard all perishable foods left at room temperature longer than 2 hours; 1 hour in temperatures above 90 °F.

Cryptosporidium	Soil, food, water, contaminated surfaces. Swallowing contaminated water, including that from recreational sources, (e.g., a swimming pool or lake); eating uncooked or contaminated food; placing a contaminated object in the mouth.	Dehydration, weight loss, stomach cramps or pain, fever, nausea, and vomiting; respiratory symptoms may also be present. Symptoms begin 2 to 10 days after becoming infected, and may last 1 to 2 weeks. Immune-comprised individuals may experience a more serious illness.	Wash your hands before and after handling raw meat products, and after changing diapers, going to the bathroom, or touching animals. Avoid water that might be contaminated. (Do not drink untreated water from shallow wells, lakes, rivers, springs, ponds, and streams.)
*Escherichia coli*O157:H7	Uncooked beef (especially ground beef), unpasteurized milk and juices (e.g., "fresh" apple cider); contaminated raw fruits and vegetables, or water. Person to person contamination can also occur.	Severe diarrhea (often bloody diarrhea), abdominal cramps, and vomiting. Usually little or no fever. Can begin 2 to 8 days, but usually 3-4 days after consumption of contaminated food or water and last about 5 to 7 days depending on severity. Children under 5 are at greater risk of developing hemolytic uremic syndrome (HUS), which causes acute kidney failure.	Cook hamburgers and ground beef to a safe minimum internal temperature of 160°F. Drink only pasteurized milk, juice, or cider. Rinse fruits and vegetables under running tap water, especially those that will not be cooked. Wash your hands with warm water and soap after changing diapers, using the bathroom, handling pets or having any contact with feces.
Listeria monocytogenes	Ready-to-eat foods such as hot dogs, luncheon meats, cold cuts, fermented or dry sausage, and other deli-style meat and poultry. Also, soft cheeses made with unpasteurized milk. Smoked seafood and salads made in the store such as ham salad, chicken salad, or seafood salad.	Fever, muscle aches, and sometimes gastrointestinal symptoms such as nausea or diarrhea. If infection spreads to the nervous system, symptoms such as headache, stiff neck, confusion, loss of balance, or convulsions can occur .Those at risk (including pregnant women and newborns, older adults, and people with weakened immune systems) may later develop more serious illness; death can result from Listeria. Can cause severe problems with pregnancy, including miscarriage or death in newborns.	Cook raw meat, poultry and seafood to a safe minimum internal temperature; prevent cross contamination, separating ready to eat foods from raw eggs, and raw meat, poultry, seafood, and their juices; wash your hands before and after handling raw meat ,poultry, seafood and egg products. Those with a weakened immune system should avoid eating hot dogs, and deli meats, unless they are reheated to 165 ºF or

			steaming hot. Do not drink raw (unpasteurized) milk or foods that have unpasteurized milk in them, (e.g. soft cheeses). Do not eat deli salads made in store, such as ham, egg, tuna or seafood salad.
Salmonella (over 2300 types)	Raw or undercooked eggs, poultry, and meat; unpasteurized milk and juice; cheese and seafood; and contaminated fresh fruits and vegetables.	Diarrhea, fever, and abdominal cramps usually appear 12 to 72 hours after eating; may last 4 to 7 days. In people with weakened immune system, the infection may be more severe and lead to serious complications, including death.	Cook raw meat, poultry, and egg products to a safe temperature. Do not eat raw or undercooked eggs. Avoid consuming raw or unpasteurized milk or other dairy products. Produce should be thoroughly washed before consuming.
Shigella (over 30 types)	Person-to-person by fecal-oral route; fecal contamination of food and water. Most outbreaks result from food, especially salads, prepared and handled by workers using poor personal hygiene.	Disease referred to as "shigellosis" or bacillary dysentery. Diarrhea (watery or bloody) , fever, abdominal cramps; 1 to 2 days from ingestion of bacteria and usually resolves in 5 to 7 days	Hand washing is a very important step to prevent shigellosis. Always wash your hands with warm water and soap before handling food and after using the bathroom, changing diapers or having contact with an infected person.
Staphylococcus aureus	Commonly found on the skin and in the noses of up to 25% of healthy people and animals. Person-to-person through food from improper food handling. Multiply rapidly at room temperature to produce a toxin that causes illness. Contaminated milk, cheese.	Severe nausea, abdominal cramps, vomiting, and diarrhea occur 30 minutes to 6 hours after eating; recovery from 1 to 3 days — longer if severe dehydration occurs.	Because the toxins produced by this bacterium are resistant to heat and cannot be destroyed by cooking, preventing the contamination of food before the toxin can be produced is important. Keep hot foods hot (over 140°F) and cold foods cold (40°F or under); wash your hands with

			warm water and soap and wash kitchen counters with hot water and soap before and after preparing food.
Vibrio vulnificus	Uncooked or raw seafood (fish or shellfish); oysters	In healthy persons symptom include diarrhea, stomach pain, and vomiting May result in a blood infection and death for those with a weakened immune systems particularly with underlying liver disease.	Do not eat raw oysters or other raw shellfish; cook shellfish (oysters, clams, mussels) thoroughly. Prevent cross-contamination by separating cooked seafood and other foods from raw seafood and its juices. Refrigerate cooked shellfish within two hours after cooking.

ENDNOTES

PESTICIDES

[1] Neurodevelopment and Endocrine Disruption, Theo Colburn, Environmental Health Perspectives, June 2004; 112, p. 944-949, https://www.ncbi.nlm.nih.gov/pmc/articles/PMC1247186/#b47-ehp0112-000944.
Pesticide use in the U.S. and policy implications: a focus on herbicides.
Short P[1], Colborn T. https://www.ncbi.nlm.nih.gov/pubmed/10188206

[2] National Institute of Environmental Health Sciences, https://www.niehs.nih.gov/health/topics/agents/pesticides/

[3] http://www.ncbi.nlm.nih.gov/pmc/articles/PMC2946087/, Alavanja MCR. Pesticides Use and Exposure Extensive Worldwide. *Reviews on environmental health*. 2009;24(4):303-309. Donaldson D, Kiely T, Grube A. Pesticide's industry sales and usage 1998-1999 market estimates. US Environmental Protection Agency; Washington (DC): Report No. EPA-733-R-02-OOI. Available from: http://www.epa.gov/oppbead/ pesticides/99 pestsales/market-estimates.pdf

[4] 2.4_D Herbicide $ GMO Crops: Pets, Wildlife and 2,4-D, June 22, 2014, Environmental Working Group, http://www.ewg.org/research/24D/pets-wildlife-24D

[5] Trump Admin Appeals Ruling Ordering EPA to Ban Pesticide, 9/24/18, https://thehill.com/policy/energy-environment/408173-trump-admin-appeals-ruling-ordering-epa-to-ban-pesticide

[6] EPA Fact Sheet, Chlorpyrifos, https://www.epa.gov/ingredients-used-pesticide-products/chlorpyrifos

[7] National Pesticide Information Center, Chlorpyrifos fact sheet, http://npic.orst.edu/factsheets/chlorpgen.html

[8] Herbicide Paraquat Again Linked to Parkinson's Symptoms in the Brain, Beyond Pesticides, https://beyondpesticides.org/dailynewsblog/2018/02/herbicide-paraquat-linked-parkinsons-symptoms-brain/

[9] Swedes to Sue Commission over Paraquat, Roger Falk, Politico, European Voice, 2/11/04, https://www.politico.eu/article/swedes-to-sue-commission-over-paraquat/

[10] Chemicals Implicated, Beyond Pesticides, https://beyondpesticides.org/programs/bee-protective-pollinators-and-pesticides/chemicals-implicated

[11] EU Member States Support Near-Total Neonicotinoids Ban, Matt McGrath, BBC, April 27, 2018, https://www.bbc.com/news/science-environment-43910536

[12] Certain Fungicides May Play a Role in Autism, Neurodegenerative Diseases, National Institute of Environmental Health Sciences, Pearson BL, Simon JM, McCoy ES, Salazar G, Fragola G, Zylka MJ. 2016. Identification of chemicals that mimic transcriptional changes associated with autism, brain aging and neurodegeneration. Nat Commun (7):11173.

[13] Combined Toxicity of Insecticides and Fungicides Applied to California Almond Orchards to Honey Bee Larvae and Adults Andrea Wade, Chia-Hua Lin, Colin Kurkul, Erzsébet Ravasz Regan, and Reed M. Johnson, College of Wooster, Ohio State University, January 8, 2019, http://www.mdpi.com/2075-4450/10/1/20/pdf

[14] Dicamba Fact Sheet, Caroline Cox, Journal of Pesticide Reform, Spring 1994, https://www.panna.org/sites/default/files/dicamba-NCAP.pdf

[15] The EPA Says Farmers Can Keep Using Weedkiller Blamed for Vast Crop Damage, Dan Charles, November 1, 2018, National Public Radio, https://www.npr.org/sections/thesalt/2018/11/01/662918255/the-epa-says-farmers-can-keep-using-weedkiller-blamed-for-vast-crop-damage

[16] Pesticide use in the U.S. and Policy Implications: A Focus on Herbicides, Short, P., Colborn, T. Toxicology and Industrial Health, March Jan-March; 15 (1-2): 240-75. https://www.ncbi.nlm.nih.gov/pubmed/10188206

[17] 2,4-D: The Most Dangerous Pesticide You've Never Heard Of, Danielle Sedbrook, NRDC, March 15, 2016, https://www.nrdc.org/stories/24-d-most-dangerous-pesticide-youve-never-heard

[18] Enlist Duo is Back Again, So We're Back in Court, Peter Lehner, March 24, 2017, Earth Justice, https://earthjustice.org/blog/2017-march/enlist-duo-is-back-again-so-we-re-back-in-court

[19] Cancer Causing Pesticide 'Garbage' Taints Tap Water for Millions in California, Bill Walker, Emily Wathen, Dve Andrews, Environmental Working Group, April 11, 2017, https://www.ewg.org/research/cancer-causing-pesticide-garbage-taints-tap-water-millions-california

[20] California Strawberry Industry is Hooked on Dangerous Pesticide, Bernice Yeung, Kendall Taggart, Andrew Donohue, The Center for Investigative Reporting, Nov 10, 2014, The Guardian, https://www.theguardian.com/us-news/2014/nov/10/-sp-california-strawberry-industry-pesticides

[21] Carbaryl, EPA fact sheet, https://www.epa.gov/sites/production/files/2016-09/documents/carbaryl.pdf

[22] Carbaryl, Extoxnet, http://pmep.cce.cornell.edu/profiles/extoxnet/carbaryl-dicrotophos/carbaryl-ext.html

[23] Atrazine in Water Tied to Hormonal Irregularities, Lindsey Konkel, Environmental Health News, Nov 28, 2011, Scientific American Magazine, https://www.scientificamerican.com/article/atrazine-water-tied-hormonal-irregularities/

[24] Toxic Substance Portal- Atrazine, Agency for Toxic Substances, September 2003, https://www.atsdr.cdc.gov/phs/phs.asp?id=336&tid=59

[25] Glyphosate, Pathways to Modern Diseases III: Manganese, Neuorological Diseases and Associated Pathologies, Anthony Samsel, Stephanie Seneff, March 24, 2015, Surgical Neurology International, https://www.ncbi.nlm.nih.gov/pmc/articles/PMC4392553/

[26] https://www.baumhedlundlaw.com/toxic-tort-law/monsanto-roundup-lawsuit/where-is-glyphosate-banned/

[27] Trends in Glyphosate Herbicide Use in the United States and Globablly, Charles M. Benbrook, Environmental Sciences Europe, 2016 28:3, https://enveurope.springeropen.com/track/pdf/10.1186/s12302-016-0070-0?site=enveurope.springeropen.com

[28] Weedkiller found in Granola and Crackers, Internal FDA Emails Show, Carey Gillam, Apr 30, 2018, The Guardian, https://www.theguardian.com/us-news/2018/apr/30/fda-weedkiller-glyphosate-in-food-internal-emails

[29] Weed-Whacking Herbicide Proves Deadly to Human Cells, Crystal Gammon, Scientific American, June 23, 2009, https://www.scientificamerican.com/article/weed-whacking-herbicide-p/

[30] Behavioral and Immunohistochemical Study of the Effects of Subchronic and Chronic Exposure to Glyphosate in Mice, Yassine Ait Bali, Saadia Ba-Mhamed, Mohamed Bennis, Frontiers in Behavioral Neuroscience, Aug 8, 2017, https://www.ncbi.nlm.nih.gov/pmc/articles/PMC5550406/

[31] Misgivings About How a Weedkiller Affects the Soil, Stephanie Strom, New York Times, Sept 19, 2013, https://www.nytimes.com/2013/09/20/business/misgivings-about-how-a-weed-killer-affects-the-soil.html

[32] Atrazine Exposure and Reproductive Dysfunction through the Hypothalamus-Pituitary-Gonadal Axis, Sara E. Wirbisky, Jennifer L. Freeman, School of Health Sciences, Purdue University, August 6, 2015, https://www.mdpi.com/2305-6304/3/4/414/pdf

[33] 2,4-D Hazardous Substance Fact Sheet, New Jersey Department of Health Right to Know, April 2017, https://nj.gov/health/eoh/rtkweb/documents/fs/0593.pdf

[34] Congress Questions EPA about Dow's Enlist Duo Pesticide Risks, Patricia Callahan, Chicago Tribune, Feb 15, 2016, http://www.chicagotribune.com/news/watchdog/ct-epa-pesticides-dow-met-20160214-story.html

[35] Paraquat Information Center, https://paraquat.com/en/use/crops

[36] Study Uncovers Cause of Pesticide Exposure, Parkinson's Link, Professor Scott Ryan, University of Guelph, May 23, 2018, https://www.sciencedaily.com/releases/2018/05/180523133158.htm

[37] Neonicotinoids, Highly Hazardous Pesticides, Pesticide Action Network Asia and Pacific, November 2011, http://www.panna.org/sites/default/files/PAN%20AP%20pesticides-factsheet-hhps-neonicotinoids.pdf

[38] Agricultural Fungicides Are 'Bad News for Neurons', study suggests, Ian Sample, The Guardian, March 31, 2016, https://www.theguardian.com/science/2016/mar/31/agricultural-fungicides-are-bad-news-for-neurons-study-suggests

[39] In Bee Decline, Fungicides Emerge as Improbable Villain, Cornell University, Nov 14, 2017, https://phys.org/news/2017-11-bee-decline-fungicides-emerge-improbable.html

[40] What's on My Food, Foods with Chlorpyrifos Residue, Pesticide Action Network, http://www.whatsonmyfood.org/pesticide.jsp?pesticide=160

[41] The Most Widely Used Pesticide, One Year Later, Xindi Hu, Harvard University, April 17, 2018, http://sitn.hms.harvard.edu/flash/2018/widely-used-pesticide-one-year-later/

[42] Glufosinate Market Worth 2.34 Billon USD by 2022, Markets and Markets, Feb 2017, https://www.marketsandmarkets.com/Market-Reports/glufosinate-market-191789620.html

[43] Safety Assessment including Current and Emerging Issues in Toxicologic Pathology, Ramesh C. Gupta, James W. Crissman, Haschedk and Rousseaux's Handbook of Toxicologic Pathology (Third Edition) 2013, Ch. 42 Agricultural Chemicals,https://www.sciencedirect.com/science/article/pii/B978012415759000042X, https://www.sciencedirect.com/topics/agricultural-and-biological-sciences/glufosinate

[44] Glufosinate, A Herbicide Used with Genetically Modified Crops: Ignored Side Effects, Prof. Joe Cummins, Feb 12, 2002, Institute for Agriculture and Trade Policy,

https://www.iatp.org/news/glufosinate-a-herbicide-used-with-genetically-modified-crops-ignored-side-effects

[45] Cholinesterase Inhibitors: Agency for Toxic Substances and Disease Registry, https://www.atsdr.cdc.gov/csem/csem.asp?csem=11&po=5

[46] Endocrine Disruptors, National Institute of Environmental Health Sciences, https://www.niehs.nih.gov/health/topics/agents/endocrine/index.cfm

[47] President's Cancer Panel Report: https://deainfo.nci.nih.gov/advisory/pcp/annualreports/pcp08-09rpt/pcp_report_08-09_508.pdf

[48] Roundup Lawsuit Public Documents, Baum Hedlund Aristei Goldman, Los Angeles, California, https://www.baumhedlundlaw.com/toxic-tort-law/monsanto-roundup-lawsuit/monsanto-secret-documents-page-five/

[49] Monsanto Ordered to Pay $289m as jury rules weedkiller caused man's cancer, Sam Levin, Patrick Greenfield, Aug 11, 2018, the Guardian, https://www.theguardian.com/business/2018/aug/10/monsanto-trial-cancer-dewayne-johnson-ruling

[50] Monsanto No More: Agri-Chemical Giant's Name Dropped in Bayer Acquisition, Camila Domonoske, June 4, 2018, National Public Radio, https://www.npr.org/sections/thetwo-way/2018/06/04/616772911/monsanto-no-more-agri-chemical-giants-name-dropped-in-bayer-acquisition

[51] Lawsuit documents Reveal Monsanto's Counterfeit Science Campaign, 2018, Union of Concerned Scientists, https://www.ucsusa.org/publications/got-science/2017/got-science-april-2017

[52] EPA Toxicologist Letter on Glyphosate, March 24, 2013, https://www.baumhedlundlaw.com/epa-official-helped-monsanto-kill-study/

[53] Unidentified Inert Ingredients in Pesticides: Implications for Human and Environmental Health, Caroline Cox, Michael Surgan, December 2006, Environmental Health Perspectives, p 1803-1806, https://www.ncbi.nlm.nih.gov/pmc/articles/PMC1764160/

[54] President's Cancer Panel Report, 2008-2009, Reducing Environmental Cancer Risk, p.45 https://deainfo.nci.nih.gov/advisory/pcp/annualreports/pcp08-09rpt/pcp_report_08-09_508.pdf

[55] Weed Whacking Herbicide Proves Deadly to Human Cells, Crystal Gammon, June 23, 2009, Scientific American, https://www.scientificamerican.com/article/weed-whacking-herbicide-p/

[56] Major Pesticides are More Toxic to Human Cells Than Their Declared Active Principles, Robin Mesnage, Nicolas Defarge, Joel Spiroux de Vendomois, Gilles-Eric Seralini, Biomed Research International, Feb 26, 2014, https://www.ncbi.nlm.nih.gov/pmc/articles/PMC3955666/

[57] Serious Birth Defect on the Rise, CDC Researchers Say, Jen Christensen, Jan 22, 2016, https://www.cnn.com/2016/01/22/health/birth-defect-gastroschisis-increase/index.html

[58] Expected New Cancer Cases and Deaths in 2020, U.S. Centers for Disease Control, https://www.cdc.gov/cancer/dcpc/research/articles/cancer_2020.htm

[59] The Growing Crisis of Chronic Disease in the United States, Partnership to Fight Chronic Disease, https://www.fightchronicdisease.org/sites/default/files/docs/GrowingCrisisofChronicDiseaseintheUSfactsheet_81009.pdf

[60] Brain Cancer Mortality in the United States, 1986 to 1995: A Geographic Analysis, Zixing Fang, Martin Kulldorff, David I Gregorio, Neuro-Oncology July 6, 2004, p 179-187, https://www.ncbi.nlm.nih.gov/pmc/articles/PMC1872002/

[61] Pesticide Industry Propaganda: The Real Story: Myth 3: Cancer Rates are Decreasing, Environmental Working Group, May 1, 1995, https://www.ewg.org/research/industrys-myths/myth-3-cancer-rates-are-decreasing

[62] EPA Pesticides Industry Sales and Usage, 2006 and 2007 Market Estimates, http://www.epa.gov/sites/production/files/2015-10/documents/market_estimates2007.pdf
[63] Pesticide Use and Exposure Extensive Worldwide, Michael C.R. Alavanja, Dr. P.H., Rev Environmental Health, PMCID: PMC2946087, Sept 27, 2010, https://www.ncbi.nlm.nih.gov/pmc/articles/PMC2946087/
[64] Organic Pesticides: Not an Oxymoron, NPR, Maureen Langlois, June 17, 2011, https://www.npr.org/sections/health-shots/2011/06/18/137249264/organic-pesticides-not-an-oxymoron
[65] Chemical Trespass, Pesticide Action Network, May 2004, https://www.panna.org/sites/default/files/ChemTres2004Eng.pdf
Third National Report on Human Exposure to Environmental Chemicals, July 2005, Centers for Disease Control, NCEH Pub. No. 05-0570, https://clu-in.org/download/contaminantfocus/pcb/third-report.pdf
[66] North America to Drive Global Fungicides Market: Lucintel Estimates Fungicides Market to Reach US $21.42 Billion in 2017,Oct 4, 2012,Cision PR Web, http://www.prweb.com/releases/2012/10/prweb9945474.htm
[67] Fungicide Use Surges, Largely Unmonitored, Brett Israel, Environmental Health News Feb 22, 2013, Scientific American, https://www.scientificamerican.com/article/fungicide-use-surges-largely-unmonitored/
[68] Chronic exposures to fungicide pyrimethanil: multi-organ effects on Italian tree frog (*Hyla intermedia*) Ilaria Bernabò,Antonello Guardia, Rachele Macirella, Sandro Tripep, Elvira BrunellSi, Scientific Reports, July 31, 20, https://www.nature.com/articles/s41598-017-07367-6
[69] Research Shows Fungicide Affects Honey Bee Health, Entomology Today, July 25, 2013, https://entomologytoday.org/2013/07/25/research-shows-fungicide-affects-honey-bee-health/
[70] New Study Links Pesticide Use to Thryoid Disease in Women, https://beyondpesticides.org/dailynewsblog/2010/02/new-study-links-pesticide-use-to-thyroid-disease-in-women/
[71] Children's Health and the Environment, World Health Organization Training for the Health Sector, July 2008, slide p. 8, https://www.who.int/ceh/capacity/Pesticides.pdf
[72] The Same Pesticides Linked to Bee Declines Might Also Threaten Birds, Elizabeth Royte, Spring 2017, https://www.audubon.org/magazine/spring-2017/the-same-pesticides-linked-bee-declines-might
[73] State of the World's Birds, Birdlife International,2018, https://www.birdlife.org/sites/default/files/attachments/BL_ReportENG_V11_spreads.pdf
[74] Higher Levels of Herbicide Found in Drinking Water May Pose Health Risk, Kari Lydersen, Aug 25, 2009, http://www.washingtonpost.com/wp-dyn/content/article/2009/08/24/AR2009082403051.html
[75] New Aspects on Atrazine Biodegradation, Luciane Sene[I, *]; Attilio Converti[II]; Geslaine Aparecida Ribeiro Secchi[I]; Rita de Cássia Garcia Simão[I] Brazilian Archives of Biology and Technology, vol.53 no.2 Curitiba Mar./Apr. 2010, http://www.scielo.br/scielo.php?pid=S1516-89132010000200030&script=sci_arttext&tlng=es
[76] Atrazine, Pesticide Action Network, http://www.panna.org/resources/atrazine
[77] Concentrations of Glyphosate and Atrazine Compounds in 100 Midwest United States Streams 2013, USGS, https://www.sciencebase.gov/catalog/item/57bb51ece4b03fd6b7dd04de

[78] Dichlorodiphenyltrichloroethane (DDT): ubiquity, persistence, and risks. *Turusov V, Rakitsky V, Tomatis L*, Environmental Health Perspectives. 2002 Feb; 110(2):125-8., https://www.ncbi.nlm.nih.gov/pmc/articles/PMC4947579/, Chemical Pesticides and Human Health: The Urgent Need for a New Concept in Agriculture Polyxeni Nicolopoulou-Stamati,[1,*] Sotirios Maipas,[1] Chrysanthi Kotampasi,[1] Panagiotis Stamatis,[1] and Luc Hens[2]

[79] Lee DH, Lee IK, Song K, Steffes M, Toscano W, Baker BA, and Jacobs DR Jr, 2006, *A Strong Dose-Response Relation Between Serum Concentrations of Persistent Organic Pollutants and Diabetes*, Diabetes Care, 29:1638-1644, http://care.diabetesjournals.org/content/29/7/1638.full

[80] Persistent Organic Pollutants: A Global Issue, A Global Response, https://www.epa.gov/international-cooperation/persistent-organic-pollutants-global-issue-global-response

[81] Persistent Organic Pollutants and Pesticides, UN Environment, http://www.cep.unep.org/publications-and-resources/marine-and-coastal-issues-links/persistent-organic-pollutants-pops-and-pesticides

[82] Organophosphates: A Common But Deadly Pesticide, Ker Than, July 18, 2013, National Geographic, https://news.nationalgeographic.com/news/2013/07/130718-organophosphates-pesticides-indian-food-poisoning/

[83] Cover Up, Bob Woffinden, Aug 24, 2001, The Guardian US Edition, https://www.theguardian.com/education/2001/aug/25/research.highereducation

[84] Organophosphates, Illinois Department of Public Health Emergency Preparedness, http://www.idph.state.il.us/Bioterrorism/factsheets/organophosphate.htm

[85] EPA: Data Requirements for Pesticide Registration, https://www.epa.gov/pesticide-registration/data-requirements-pesticide-registration

[86] Prevention and Disposal of Obsolete Pesticides, Food and Agricultural Organization of the United Nations, http://www.fao.org/agriculture/crops/obsolete-pesticides/why-problem/pesticide-bans/en/

[87] Special Report: Why Brazil Has A Big Appetite For Banned Pesticides, Paola Prada, Reuters, April 2, 2015,https://www.reuters.com/article/us-brazil-pesticide-specialreport/special-report-why-brazil-has-a-big-appetite-for-banned-pesticides-idUSKBN0MT1Q820150402

[88] Setting Tolerances for Pesticide Residues in Foods, EPA, https://www.epa.gov/pesticide-tolerances/setting-tolerances-pesticide-residues-foods

[89] Gut Wrenching: New Studies Reveal the Insiduous Effects of Glyphosate, Dr. Pamela Coleman, March 26, 2014, Cornucopia Institute, https://www.cornucopia.org/2014/03/gut-wrenching-new-studies-reveal-insidious-effects-glyphosate/

[90] Tryptophan Metabolism and White Matter Integrity in Schizophrenia, Joshua Chiappelli,[1,*] Teodor T Postolache,[2,3,4] Peter Kochunov,[1] Laura M Rowland,[1] S Andrea Wijtenburg,[1]Dinesh K Shukla,[1] Malle Tagamets,[1] Xiaoming Du,[1] Anya Savransky,[1] Christopher A Lowry,[5] Adem Can,[2]Dietmar Fuchs,[6] and L Elliot Hong[1], Neuropsychopharmacology. 2016 Sep; 41(10): 2587–2595., https://www.ncbi.nlm.nih.gov/pmc/articles/PMC4987857/

[91] Organic Imports Continue to Rise Alongside Organic Demand, Research Shows, Colin O'Neil, Ag Mag, Environmental Working Group, Oct 25, 2017, https://www.ewg.org/agmag/2017/10/organic-imports-continue-rise-alongside-organic-demand-research-shows

[92] What's On My Food, Grapes, Pesticide Action Network, http://www.whatsinmyfood.org/food.jsp?food=GRG

[93] Exposure to Common Pesticides May Affect Human Brain; Effects Similar to Autism and Alzheimer's, Susan Scutti, April 1, 2016, https://www.medicaldaily.com/fungicides-human-brain-autism-spectrum-disorder-alzheimers-disease-380352

[94] NRDC to EPA: Red Flags on Imidacloprid Health Risks, Jennifer Sass, Nov 29, 2017, https://www.nrdc.org/experts/jennifer-sass/nrdc-epa-red-flags-imidacloprid-health-risks

[95] Boscalid, Federal Register, https://www.federalregister.gov/documents/2015/03/18/2015-06141/boscalid-pesticide-tolerances

[96] Disturbing New Evidence About What Common Pesticides Can Do to Brains, Tom Philpott, April 13, 2016, Mother Jones, https://www.motherjones.com/food/2016/04/what-are-these-widely-used-fungicides-doing-us/

[97] Fungicide Contamination Reduces Beneficial Fungi in Bee Bread Based on An Area-Wide Field Study in Honey Bee, Apis mellifera, Colonies, Jay A. Yoder, Andrew J. Jajack, Andrew E. Rosselot, Terrance J. Smith, Mary Clare Yerke, Diana Sammataro, Journal of Toxicology and Environmental Helath, Part A, 76:597-600, 2013, Taylor and Francis, LLC, https://naldc.nal.usda.gov/download/57094/PDF

[98] Thyroid Disrupting Chemicals and Brain Development: An Update, Bilal B Mughal, Jean-Baptiste Fini, Barbara A Demeneix, Endocrine Connections, April, 2018, https://www.ncbi.nlm.nih.gov/pmc/articles/PMC5890081/

[99] Toxicity of Pesticides to Pollinators and Beneficials, University of Massachussetts Amherst, Center for Agriculture, Food and the Environment, https://ag.umass.edu/fruit/ne-small-fruit-management-guide/appendices-resource-material-listings-conversion-tables-0

[100] The Role of Fenhexamid on the Proliferation of Ovarian Cancer BG-1 Cells, Anxing Fei1, Handong Fu3, Hong Jiang, Liping Wei1, Hongxia Zhang, Anqiong Fei, Yan Zhang, Tiantian Zou, Shuzhen Gao, Lin Li, Hong Jiang, Min Zhou, Hui Xing, Yanli Huang, International Journal Clinical and Experimental Pathology, April 15, 2018; 11(4);2025-2031, http://www.ijcep.com/files/ijcep0059707.pdf

[101] What's on my Food, Apples, Pesticide Action Network, http://www.whatsinmyfood.org/food.jsp?food=AP

[102] Chemical Banned in Europe is Probably On Your Apple, John Upton, Grist Magazine, April 25, 2014, https://grist.org/food/chemical-banned-in-europe-is-probably-on-your-apple/

[103] Diphenylamine Safety Data Sheet according to the Federal Register, Lab Chem, Jan 7, 2015, http://www.labchem.com/tools/msds/msds/LC13610.pdf

[104] Acetamiprid, Pesticide Properties Database, University of Hertfordshire, https://sitem.herts.ac.uk/aeru/ppdb/en/Reports/11.htm

[105] NRDC to EPA: Red Flags on Imidacloprid Health Risks, Jennifer Sass, Natural Resources Defense Council, November 29, 2017, https://www.nrdc.org/experts/jennifer-sass/nrdc-epa-red-flags-imidacloprid-health-risks

[106] What's On My Food, Sweet Bell Peppers, Pesticide Action Network, http://www.whatsinmyfood.org/food.jsp?food=PP

[107] Gateway on Pesticide Hazards and Safe Pest Management, Thiamethoxam, Beyond Pesticides, https://www.beyondpesticides.org/resources/pesticide-gateway?pesticideid=289

[108] Chlorpyrifos Fact Sheet, National Pesticide Information Center, npic.orst.edu/factsheets/chlorpgen.html
[109] What's On My Food, Strawberries, Pesticide Action Network, http://www.whatsinmyfood.org/food.jsp?food=ST
[110] Captan, Extoxnet, Cornell University, http://pmep.cce.cornell.edu/profiles/extoxnet/24d-captan/captan-ext.html
[111] What's On My Food, Corn, Pesticide Action Network, http://www.whatsinmyfood.org/food.jsp?food=CO
[112] Malathion 'Probably Carcinogenic to Humans' WHO Agency Concludes, CBC News, March 20, 2015, https://www.cbc.ca/news/canada/manitoba/malathion-probably-carcinogenic-to-humans-who-agency-concludes-1.3004084
[113] What's On My Food, Potatoes, Pesticide Action Network, http://www.whatsinmyfood.org/food.jsp?food=PO
[114] What's On My Food, Wheat, Pesticide Action Network, http://www.whatsinmyfood.org/food.jsp?food=WF
[115] Actions of the Endocrine Disruptor Methoxychlor and its Estrogenic Metabolite on in Vitro Embryonic Rat Seminiferous Cord Formation and Perinatal Testis Growth, Cupp AS, Skinner MK, Reproductive Toxicology, May-June 2015, https://www.ncbi.nlm.nih.gov/pubmed/11390175
[116] What's On my Food, Peaches, Pesticide Action Network, http://www.whatsinmyfood.org/food.jsp?food=PC
[117] Chlorpyrifos, The Toxic Pesticide Harming Our Children and Environment, Earth Justice, https://earthjustice.org/features/what-you-need-to-know-about-chlorpyrifos
[118] What's On My Food, Kale, Pesticide Action Network, http://www.whatsinmyfood.org/food.jsp?food=GK
[119] What's On My Food, Cilantro, Pesticide Action Network, http://www.whatsinmyfood.org/food.jsp?food=CL
[120] Pesticides in Marijuana Pose a Growing Problem for Cannabis Consumers, Alicia Lozano, Oct 27, 2016, LA Weekly, https://www.laweekly.com/news/pesticides-in-marijuana-pose-a-growing-problem-for-cannabis-consumers-7526808
[121] EPA: This Pesticide is Killing Bees. (Pssst, it's Also In Some of Your Weed), Ricardo Baca, The Cannabist Denver Post Jan 8, 2016, https://www.thecannabist.co/2016/01/08/imidacloprid-pesticide-chemical-bees-marijuana-pot/46262/
[122] https://ehp.niehs.nih.gov/EHP515/ *Effects of Neonicotinoid Exposure on Human Health, A Systematic Review* Cimino AM, Boyles AL, Thayer KA, Perry MJ, 2017. Environmental Health Perspectives 125: 155-162
[123] 14th Report on Carcinogens 2016, National Institute of Health, National Toxicology Program, https://ntp.niehs.nih.gov/ntp/roc/content/introduction_508.pdf
[124] Neurotoxicity of Pesticides; A brief review, Lucio G Costa, Marina Guizzetti, Annabella Vitalone, Frontiers in Bioscience, A Journal and Virtual Library, 2008, https://ohsu.pure.elsevier.com/en/publications/neurotoxicity-of-pesticides-a-brief-review
[125] Effect of Endocrine Disrupting Pesticides: A Review, Wissem Mnif, Aziza Ibn Hadj Hassine, Aicha Bouaziz, Aghleb Bartegi, Olivier Thomas, Benoit Roig, International Jounal of Environmental Research and Public Health, 2011 Jun; 8(6):2265-2303, https://www.ncbi.nlm.nih.gov/pmc/articles/PMC3138025/#b65-ijerph-08-02265

[126] CDC: Reproductive Health and the Workplace: Pesticides, National Institute for Occupational Safety and Health, Centers for Disease Control, https://www.cdc.gov/niosh/topics/repro/pesticides.html

[127] New Scientific Paper: Broad Class of Pesticides Puts Children At Risk For Reduced IQ, Learning Disabilities, Natural Resources Defense Council, https://www.nrdc.org/media/2018/181024-0. And Berkely University School of Public Health, Oct 24, 2018, https://sph.berkeley.edu/new-scientific-paper-broad-class-pesticides-puts-children-risk-reduced-iq-learning-disabilities

[128] Pesticide-Induced Diseases: Learning/Development Disorders, Beyond Pesticides, https://www.beyondpesticides.org/resources/pesticide-induced-diseases-database/learningdevelopmental

[129] The Toxins That Threaten Our Brains, James Hamblin, Mar 18, 2014, The Atlantic, https://www.theatlantic.com/health/archive/2014/03/the-toxins-that-threaten-our-brains/284466/

[130] Cancer Health Effects of Pesticides, Systemic Review, K.L. Bassil, C. Vakil, M. Sanborn, D.C. Cole, J.S. Kaur, K.J. Kerr, Canada Family Physicians, Oct 2007, Official Publication of the College of Family Physicians of Canada, https://www.ncbi.nlm.nih.gov/pmc/articles/PMC2231435/

[131] Respiratory Disease and pesticide Exposure: A Case-Control Study in Lebanon, Pascale Salameh, Mirna Waked, Isabelle Baldi, Patrick Brochard, Bernadette Abi Saleh, Journal of Epidemiology and Community Health, Mar 2006 60(3): 256-261, https://www.ncbi.nlm.nih.gov/pmc/articles/PMC2465555/

[132] New Study Suggests Kidney Disease May Be Linked to Pesticide Exposure, Bhavya Khullar, Sept 8, 2017, Down to Earth, https://www.downtoearth.org.in/news/health/new-study-suggests-kidney-disease-may-be-linked-to-pesticide-exposure-58632

[133] Parkinson's Disease and Pesticides, What's the Connection, Brad Stetka, Scientific American, April 8, 2014, https://www.scientificamerican.com/article/parkinsons-disease-and-pesticides-whats-the-connection/

[134] Environmentally-Caused Disease Crisis? Pesticide Damage to DNA Found "Programmed" Into Future Generations, Ken Roseboro, Aug 16, 2018, Ecowatch, https://www.ecowatch.com/generational-harm-of-pesticides-2596453994.html

[135] Pesticide Exposure and Risk of Alzheimer's Disease: A Systematic Review and Meta-Analysis, Dandan Yan, Yunjian Zhang, Liegang Liu, Hong Yan, Scientific Reports, Sept 1, 2016, https://www.ncbi.nlm.nih.gov/pmc/articles/PMC5007474/

[136] Bees on the Brink: Study Shows Pesticide Exposure Can Dramatically Affect Their Social Behavior, Peter Reuell, Harvard University Gazette, Nov 16, 2018, https://news.harvard.edu/gazette/story/2018/11/pesticide-exposure-can-dramatically-impact-bees-social-behaviors/

[137]High Pesticide Exposure Events and Olfactory Impairment among U.S. Farmers
Srishti Shrestha, Freya Kamel, David M. Umbach, Laura E. Beane Freeman,Stella Koutros,Michael Alavanja,Aaron Blair,Dale P. Sandler,Honglei Chen, 16 January 2019
Michigan State University, National Institute of Health and National Cancer Institute Study, https://beyondpesticides.org/dailynewsblog/2019/01/acute-pesticide-incidents-may-lead-to-loss-of-smell/

[138] Study Links Exposure to Common Pesticide with ADHA in Boys, Cinncinnati Children's Hospital, June 1, 2015, https://www.cincinnatichildrens.org/news/release/2015/study-links-pesticide-ADHD-in-boys-06-01-2015
[139] Study Links Mother's Pesticide Levels with Autism in Children, American Psychiatric Association, Aug 16, 2018, https://www.psychiatry.org/newsroom/news-releases/study-links-mothers-pesticide-levels-with-autism-in-children
[140] Food Allergies? Pesticides in Tap Water May Be To Blame, American College of Allergy, Asthma and Immunology, Dec 3, 2012, https://acaai.org/news/food-allergies-pesticides-tap-water-might-be-blame
[141] Pesticides: Health Effects in Drinking Water, Nancy M. Trautman, Keith S. Porter, Robert J. Wagenet, Pesticide Safety Education Program, Cornell Universtiy Cooperative Extension, http://psep.cce.cornell.edu/facts-slides-self/facts/pes-heef-grw85.aspx
[142] Pesticides and the Loss of Biodiversity, Richard Isenring, PAN Europe, March 2010, https://www.pan-europe.info/old/Resources/Briefings/Pesticides_and_the_loss_of_biodiversity.pdf
[143] Pesticide Exposure in Children, American Academy of Pediatrics, May 1, 2013, Council on Environmental Health, http://pediatrics.aappublications.org/content/130/6/e1757
[144] Lu C, Toepel K, Irish R, Fenske RA, Barr DB, Bravo R. *Organic Diets Significantly Lower Children's Dietary Exposure to Organophosphorus Pesticides.* Environmental Health Perspectives, 2006;114(2):260–263pmid:16451864, https://www.ncbi.nlm.nih.gov/pmc/articles/PMC1367841/
[145] Report: Pesticide Exposure Linked with Childhood Cancer and Lower IQ, Carina Storrs, Sept 14, 2015, CNN, https://www.cnn.com/2015/09/14/health/pesticide-exposure-childhood-cancer/index.html
[146] Atrazine At A Glance, Breast Cancer Prevention Partners, https://www.bcpp.org/resource/atrazine/
[147] Neurodevelopment and Endocrine Disruption, Theo Colburn, Environmental Health Perspectives June 2004, 112(9):944-949, https://www.ncbi.nlm.nih.gov/pmc/articles/PMC1247186/#b47-ehp0112-000944
[148] A Silent Pandemic: Industrial Chemicals Are Impairing the Brain Development of Children Worldwide, Harvard School of Public Health, Nov 7, 2006, http://archive.sph.harvard.edu/press-releases/2006-releases/press11072006.html
[149] Cover-Up, The Spanish Cooking Oil Scandal, Bob Woffinden, Aug 24, 2001, The Guardian, https://www.theguardian.com/education/2001/aug/25/research.highereducation
[150] Contaminated School Meal Kills 25 Indian Children, Reuters, July 17, 2013, https://www.reuters.com/article/us-india-chidren-poison/contaminated-school-meal-kills-25-indian-children-idUSBRE96G0AY20130717
[151] Organophosphates: A Common but Deadly Pesticide, Ker Than, National Geographic, July 18, 2013, https://news.nationalgeographic.com/news/2013/07/130718-organophosphates-pesticides-indian-food-poisoning/
[152] Cholinesterase Inhibition, Extoxnet, Cornell University, Sept 1993, http://pmep.cce.cornell.edu/profiles/extoxnet/TIB/cholinesterase.html

[153] Carbaryl, National Pesticide Information Center, http://npic.orst.edu/factsheets/carbarylgen.html

[154] Shukla, Yogeshwer & Antony, Mary & Kumar, Sushil & Mehrotra, N.K. (1988). Tumour-promoting ability of mancozeb, a carbamate fungicide, on mouse skin. Carcinogenesis. 9. 1511-2. 10.1093/carcin/9.8.1511, https://www.researchgate.net/publication/20020246_Tumour-promoting_ability_of_mancozeb_a_carbamate_fungicide_on_mouse_skin

[155] Carbaryl exposure and incident cancer in the Agricultural Health Study Rajeev Mahajan, Aaron Blair, Joseph Coble, Charles F. Lynch, Jane A. Hoppin, Dale P. Sandler and Michael C.R. Alavanja, International Journal of Cancer, 121, 1799-1805, 2007, https://onlinelibrary.wiley.com/doi/pdf/10.1002/ijc.22836

[156] Roundup Class Action Lawsuit, Prosecutor's Website, https://www.baumhedlundlaw.com/toxic-tort-law/monsanto-roundup-lawsuit/roundup-class-action-lawsuit/

[157] Glyphosate, a Chelating Agent—Relevant for Ecological Risk Assessment? Martha Mertens, Sebastian Hoss, Gunter Heumann, Joshua Afzal, Wolfram Reichenbecher, Environmental Science and Pollution Research International, Jan 2, 2018, https://www.ncbi.nlm.nih.gov/pmc/articles/PMC5823954/

[158] Glyphosate Perturbs the Gut Microbiota of HoneyBees, Erick V.S. Motta, Kasie Raymann, Nancy A. Moran, Proceedings of the National Academy of Sciences of the United States of America, Oct 9, 2018, https://www.pnas.org/content/115/41/10305

[159] Monsanto Documents, Results Lifetime Carcinogenicity Study in Mice, December 26, 1984, https://www.baumhedlundlaw.com/pdf/monsanto-documents/Monsanto-Study-Lifetime-Carcinogenicit-Study-in-Mice.pdf

[160] Monsanto Documents, Evaluation of the Potential Genotoxicy of Glyphosate, Glyphosate Mixtures and Component Surfactants, James M. Parry, https://www.baumhedlundlaw.com/pdf/monsanto-documents/Dr-James-Parry-Glyphosate-Review-Evaluation-of-the-potential-genotoxicity-of-Glyphosate-Glyphosate-mixtures-and-component-surfactants-1999.pdf

[161] Dietary Magnesium Intake and Risk of Stroke: A Meta-Analysis of Prospective Studies, Susanna C Larrson, Nicola Orsini, Alicja Wolk, American Journal of Clinical Nutrition, Dec 28, 2011, https://academic.oup.com/ajcn/article/95/2/362/4576752

[162] Maternal Residential Exposure to Agricultural Pesticides and Birth Defects in a 2003-2005 North Carolina Birth Cohort, Kristen M. Rappazzo, Joshua L. Warren, Robert E. Meyer, Amy H. Herring, Alison P. Sanders, Naomi C. Brownstein, Thomas J. Luben, Birth Defects Research, A Clin Mol Teratology, April 1, 2017, https://www.ncbi.nlm.nih.gov/pmc/articles/PMC4833532/

[163] Pesticides in Paradise: Hawaii's Spike in Birth Defects Puts Focus on GM Crops, Christopher Pala, Aug 23, 2015, The Guardian, http://www.theguardian.com/us-news/2015/aug/23/hawaii-birth-defects-pesticides-gmo

[164] Pesticides in Paradise: Hawaii's Health & Environment At Risk, Center for Food Safety, May 6, 2015, https://www.centerforfoodsafety.org/reports/3901/pesticides-in-paradise-hawaiis-health-and-environment-at-risk

[165] Birth Defects in Wildlife: The Role of Environmental Contaminants as Inducers of Reproductive and Development Dysfunction, Hamlin HJ, Guilletter LF Jr, April 2010, Systems

Biology in Reproductive Medicine, Vol 56, 2010 Issue 2, http://www.ncbi.nlm.nih.gov/pubmed/20377310

[166] Life Threatening Super Fungus Spreading Across the United States, CDC Warns, Bobby Cherry, April 9, 2019, WMUR ABC News, https://www.wmur.com/article/life-threatening-super-fungus-spreading-across-the-united-states-cdc-warns/27089336

[167] US Department of State, Montreal Protocolon Substances that Deplete the Ozone Layer, https://www.state.gov/e/oes/eqt/chemicalpollution/83007.htm

[168] Sulfuryl Fluoride Face Sheet, National Pesticide Information Center, http://npic.orst.edu/factsheets/sfgen.pdf

[169] New Greenhouse Gas Identified, David Chandler, MIT News, March 11, 2009, http://news.mit.edu/2009/prinn-greenhouse-tt0311

[170] California Department of Pesticide Regulation, March 3, 2017, https://www.cdpr.ca.gov/docs/risk/rcd/establishing_sulfuryl_fluoride.pdf; National Institutes of Health, U.S. National Library of Medicine,Toxnet, Sulfuryl Fluoride, https://toxnet.nlm.nih.gov/cgi-bin/sis/search/a?dbs+hsdb:@term+@DOCNO+828; United States EPA Risk Assessment, Human Health Risk Assessment for Sulfuryl Fluoride and Fluoride Anion Addressing the Section 3 Registration of Sulfuryl Fluoride as a Fumigant for Foods and Food Processing Facilities, Jan 18, 2006, http://www.fluoridealert.org/wp-content/pesticides/sf.hra-jan18.2006.pdf;

[171] "Prostate cancer and toxicity from critical use exemptions of methyl bromide: Environmental protection helps protect against human health risks" Lygia T Budnik, Stefan Kloth, Marcial Velasco-Garrido, and Xaver Bau, Environ Health. 2012; 11: 5., https://www.ncbi.nlm.nih.gov/pmc/articles/PMC3807750/

[172] Methyl Bromide Pesticide in Paradise Poisoning Case Still Used in U.S. Crops, Should You Worry About Pesticides on Fruit, Bill Briggs, NBC News, May 15, 2014, https://www.nbcnews.com/health/health-news/pesticide-vacation-n336576

[173] Prostate Cancer and Toxicity from Critical Use Exemptions of Methyl Bromide: Environmental Protection Helps Protect Against Human Health Risks, Lygia T Budnik, Stefan Kloth, Marcial Velasco-Garrido, Xaver Baur, Environmental Health, Jan 27, 2012, https://www.ncbi.nlm.nih.gov/pmc/articles/PMC3807750/

[174] Chloropicrin, EPA RED Fact Sheet, July 10, 2008, https://www3.epa.gov/pesticides/chem_search/reg_actions/reregistration/fs_PC-081501_10-Jul-08.pdf

[175] Stimulation of Nitrous Oxide Production Resulted from Soil Fumigation with Chloropicrin, Atmospheric Environment, K. Spokas, D. Wang, May 16, 2003, https://www.ars.usda.gov/ARSUserFiles/41695/reprints/ae2003.pdf

[176] EPA: Overview of Greenhouse Gases, Nitrous Oxide, https://www.epa.gov/ghgemissions/overview-greenhouse-gases

[177] Should Citrus Farmers Use Antibiotics To Combat Greening Disease, Maryn McKenna,March 1, 2016, National Geographic, https://www.nationalgeographic.com/people-and-culture/food/the-plate/2016/03/01/should-citrus-farmers-use-antibiotics-to-combat-greening-disease/

[178] Fungicide: Mode of Action and Possible Impact on Nontarget Organisms, Chao Yang, Chantal Hamel, Vladimir Vujanovic, Yantai Gan, International Scholary Research Notices Ecology, Volume 2011, Sept 5, 2011, Article ID 130289, https://www.hindawi.com/journals/isrn/2011/130289/

[179] PRN 97-6: Use of Term "Inert"in the Label Ingredients Statement, EPA, Pesticide Registration, https://www.epa.gov/pesticide-registration/prn-97-6-use-term-inert-label-ingredients-statement

[180] Chlorodifluoromethane (Freon 22) CAS NO. 75-45-6, Fluroide Action Network, http://www.fluoridealert.org/wp-content/pesticides/chlorodifluoromethane-page.htm, US EPA, Inert Ingredients of Pesticide Products, https://www.epa.gov/sites/production/files/2015-10/documents/fr52.pdf

[181] An Update of the Worldwide Integrated Assessment (WIA) on Systemic Insecticides, Part 3: Alternatives to Systemic Insecticides, Lorenzo Furlan, Alberto Pozzebon,Carlo Duso,Noa Simon-Delso,Francisco Sánchez-Bayo,Patrice A. Marchand,Filippo Codato,Maarten Bijleveld van Lexmond,Jean-Marc Bonmatin, Environmental Science and Pollution Research, Feb 25, 2018, https://link.springer.com/article/10.1007%2Fs11356-017-1052-5

[182] Fertilizer Use Responsible for Increase in Nitrous Oxide in Atmosphere, Robert Sanders, University of California Berkeley, Berkeley News, April 2, 2012, https://news.berkeley.edu/2012/04/02/fertilizer-use-responsible-for-increase-in-nitrous-oxide-in-atmosphere/

[183] GMOs and Toxic Pesticides, Greenpeace, https://www.greenpeace.org/usa/sustainable-agriculture/issues/gmos/

[184] Multiple Herbicide Resistant Weeds and The Challenges Ahead, University of Nebraska, Lincoln, Institute of Agriculture and Natural Resources, https://cropwatch.unl.edu/multiple-herbicide-resistant-weeds-and-challenges-ahead

[185] Deadly Fungal 'Superbug' Spreads Worldwide, Alarming Scientists, Stephanie Pappas, Live Science, April 8, 2019, https://www.livescience.com/65181-candida-auris-spreading.html

[186] Ignoring Adjuvant Toxicity Falsifies the Safety Profile of Commercial Pesticides, Robin Mesnage, Micahel N. Antoniou, Frontiers in Public Health, Jan 22, 2018, https://www.ncbi.nlm.nih.gov/pmc/articles/PMC5786549/

[187] "Pesticide Mixtures May Increase Health Risks But Are Still Unregulated by California, UCLA Report Says," Carla Denly, Assistant Dean for Communications, UCLA Fielding School of Public Health, Feb 17, 2016, https://ph.ucla.edu/news/press-release/2016/feb/pesticide-mixtures-may-increase-health-risks-are-still-unregulated

[188] EPA Unlawfully Approved Pesticide Enlist Duo, Says NRDC, Natural Resources Defense Council, March 21, 2017, https://www.nrdc.org/media/2017/170321-1

[189] Pesticides in Paradise: Hawaii's Spike in Birth Defects Puts Focus on GM Crops, Christopher Pala in Waimea, The Guardian, Aug 23, 2015, https://www.theguardian.com/us-news/2015/aug/23/hawaii-birth-defects-pesticides-gmo,

[190] Environmental Impacts of Pesticides, Pesticide Action Network North America, PANNA, http://www.panna.org/resources/environmental-impacts

[191] Reducing Environmental Cancer Risk, What We Can Do Now, 2008-2009 Annual Report, Presiden't Cancer Panel, https://deainfo.nci.nih.gov/advisory/pcp/annualreports/pcp08-09rpt/pcp_report_08-09_508.pdf
[192] The Truth about Cats and Dogs and Lawn Chemicals, Paul Schramski, Sanford Lewis, 2008, Pesticide Watch, https://pesticidewatch.org/sites/default/files/pets_guide_draft_final.pdf
[193] Refuse to Use Chemlawn, Be Truly Green, Matthew Wilson, Jay Rasku, 2005, Toxics Action Center, https://toxicsaction.org/wp-content/uploads/refuse-to-use-chemlawn.pdf
[194] Tips for A Lush Organic Lawn, Break Your Lawn's Addiction to Synthetic Fertilizers, Pesticides and Herbicides, Keith Pandolfi, This Old House Magazine, https://www.thisoldhouse.com/ideas/tips-lush-organic-lawn
[195] The Facts About Lawn Chemicals, EPA and Mid America Regional Council, Kansas City, MO, https://cfpub.epa.gov/npstbx/files/marc_lawnchemicals.pdf

GMOS

[196] Transgenic Crops' Built In Pesticide Found To Be Contaminating Waterways, Tom Laskawy, Grist Magazine, Sept 30, 2010, https://grist.org/article/food-2010-09-29-transgenic-crops-found-to-be-contaminating-waterways/
[197] "GMO Crops Mean More Herbicide, Not Less," Beth Hoffman, Forbes Magazine, July 2, 2013, https://www.forbes.com/sites/bethhoffman/2013/07/02/gmo-crops-mean-more-herbicide-not-less/#66e15afa3cd5
[198] Are You Ready for the New Wave of Genetically Engineered Foods?, Stacy Malkan, US Right to Know (USRTK) March 16, 2018, (Common Ground Magazine, March 2018), https://usrtk.org/gmo/newgmos/
[199] Genetically Modified Plants and Human Health, Suzie Key, Julian K-C Ma, Pascal MW Drake, Journal of the Royal Society of Medicine, June 1, 2008, https://www.ncbi.nlm.nih.gov/pmc/articles/PMC2408621/
[200] Immune Reponse, U.S. National Library of Medicine, https://medlineplus.gov/ency/article/000821.htm
[201] Current GMO Crops, GMO Answers, https://gmoanswers.com/current-gmo-crops
[202] "GM Golden Rice Gets Approval From Food Regulators in the US", Andy Coghlan, New Scientist, May 30, 2018, https://www.newscientist.com/article/mg23831802-500-gm-golden-rice-gets-approval-from-food-regulators-in-the-us/
[203] What's in Your Milk, An Expose on the Dangers of Genetically Engineered Milk, Dr. Samuel Epstein, Organic Consumers Association, Jan 3, 2007, https://www.organicconsumers.org/news/whats-your-milk-expose-dangers-genetically-engineered-milk
[204] "FDA Paves Way For GMO Salmon to Hit the Market", Helena Bottemiller Evich, Liz Crampton, Politico, March 8, 2019, https://www.politico.com/story/2019/03/08/fda-salmon-1253697
[205] "Why is Glyphosate Sprayed on Crops Right Before Harvest?", Ken Roseboro, EcoWatch, March 5, 2016, https://www.ecowatch.com/roundup-cancer-1882187755.html
[206] Objecting to Glyphosate Desiccation, Safe Food Matters, Oct 30, 2017, https://safefoodmatters.org/2017/10/30/objecting-to-glyphosate-desiccation/
[207] Not in Our Bread, Glyphosate-the Active Ingredient in Monsanto's Roundup- is the Most Widely Sold Weedkiller in the World, Soil Association of Scotland, https://www.soilassociation.org/our-campaigns/not-in-our-bread/

[208] What is Glyphosate? Soil Assocation of Scotland, https://www.soilassociation.org/our-campaigns/not-in-our-bread/what-is-glyphosate/

[209] See 205, https://www.ecowatch.com/why-is-glyphosate-sprayed-on-crops-right-before-harvest-1882187755.html

[210] Organic Diet Intervention Significantly Reduces Urinary Pesticide Levels in U.S. Children and Adults, Carly Hyland, Asa Bradman, Roy Gerona, Sharyle Patton, Igor Zakharevich, Robert B. Gunier, Kendra Klein, Environmentla Research, Volume 171, April 2019, Pages 568-575, https://www.sciencedirect.com/science/article/pii/S0013935119300246

[211] How "Extreme Levels" of Roundup in Food Became the Industry Norm, Thomas Bohn, Marek Cuhra, Independent Science News, March 24, 2014, https://www.independentsciencenews.org/news/how-extreme-levels-of-roundup-in-food-became-the-industry-norm/

[212] See 211

[213] Statement of Michael M. Landa, J.D. Director, Center for Food Safety and Applied Nutrition, FDA Food and Drug Administration, Department of Health and Human Services, December 10, 2014, https://docs.house.gov/meetings/IF/IF14/20141210/102797/HHRG-113-IF14-Wstate-LandaM-20141210.pdf

[214] The FDA Does Not Test Whether GMOs Are Safe, USRTK, US Right to Know, https://usrtk.org/the-fda-does-not-test-whether-gmos-are-safe/

[215] Roundup Class Action Lawsuit, https://www.baumhedlundlaw.com/toxic-tort-law/monsanto-roundup-lawsuit/roundup-class-action-lawsuit/, United States District Court, District of California, Roundup Products Liability Litigation, http://www.cand.uscourts.gov/VC/roundupmdl

[216] Weed-Whacking Herbicide Proves Deadly to Human Cells, Crystal Gammon, June 23, 2009, http://www.scientificamerican.com/article/weed-whacking-herbicide-p/

[217] American Academy of Environmental Medicine, Genetically Modified Foods, http://www.aaemonline.org/gmo.php

[218] Republished Study: Long-Term Toxicity of a Roundup Herbicide and a Roundup-Tolerant Genetically Modified Maize, Gilles-Eric Seralini, Emilie Clair, Robin Mesnage Steeve Gress, Nicolas Defarge, Manuela Malatesta, Dider Hennequin, Joel SPiroux de Vendomois, Environmental Sciences Europe, 2014, https://enveurope.springeropen.com/track/pdf/10.1186/s12302-014-0014-5?site=enveurope.springeropen.com

[219] Agricultural Health Study, National Institutes of Health, https://aghealth.nih.gov/news/2017.html

[220] Glyphosate, Hard Water and Nephrotoxic Metals: Are They the Culprits Behind the Epidemic of Chronic Kidney Disease of Unknown Etiology in Sri Lanka? Channa Jayasumana,[1,2,*] Sarath Gunatilake,[2,†] and Priyantha Senanayake, Feb 11, 2014, International Journal of Environmental Research and Public Health, https://www.ncbi.nlm.nih.gov/pmc/articles/PMC3945589/

[221] Glyphosate, Pathways to Modern Diseases II, Celiac Sprue and Gluten Intolerance, Anthony Samsel, Stephanie Seneff, Dec 2013, https://www.ncbi.nlm.nih.gov/pmc/articles/PMC3945755/

[222] Glyphosate, a chelating agent—relevant for ecological risk assessment? Martha Mertens,[1] Sebastian Höss,[1] Günter Neumann,[2] Joshua Afzal,[2] and Wolfram Reichenbecher, Environmental Science and Pollution Research International, 2018; 25(6): 5398-5317, https://www.ncbi.nlm.nih.gov/pmc/articles/PMC5823954/#CR172

[223] Weedkiller Found in Granola and Crackers, Internal FDA Emails Show, Carey Gillam, The Guardian, April 30, 2018, https://www.theguardian.com/us-news/2018/apr/30/fda-weedkiller-glyphosate-in-food-internal-emails,

Pesticide Linked to Cancer is in Nearly Every US Food: Report, Lia Eustachewich, New York Post, April 30, 2018, https://nypost.com/2018/04/30/pesticide-linked-to-cancer-is-in-nearly-every-us-food-report/

[224] Glyphosate based- herbicide exposure affects gut microbiota, anxiety and depression-like behaviors in mice, Yassine Aitbali, Saadia Ba-M'hamed, Najoua Elhidar, Ahmed Nafis, Nabila Soraa, Mohammed Bennis, Neurotoxicology and Teratology, 2018 May-Jun; 67:44-49, https://www.ncbi.nlm.nih.gov/pubmed/29635013.

[225] Glyphosate-based herbicides are toxic and endocrine disruptors in human cell lines, Ganier C, Dumont C, Benachour N, Clair E, Chagnon MC, Seralini GE, Toxicology, August 21, 2009, https://www.ncbi.nlm.nih.gov/pubmed/19539684

[226] Perinatal exposure to glyphosate-based herbicide alters the thyrotrophic axis and causes thyroid hormone homeostasis imbalance in male rats, Janaina Sena de Souza, Marina Malta Letro Kizys, Rodrigo Rodrigues da Conceicao, Gabriel Glebocki, Renata Marino Romano, Tania Maria Ortiga-Carvalho, Gisele Giannocco, Ismael Dale Cotrium Guerreiro da Silva, Magnus Regios Dias da Silva,Marco Aurelio Romano, Maria Izabel Chiamolera, Toxicology, Vol 377, Feb 15, 2017, pgs 25-37, https://www.sciencedirect.com/science/article/pii/S0300483X16302645

[227] https://www.ncbi.nlm.nih.gov/pmc/articles/PMC4392553/ Glyphosate, Pathways to Modern Diseases III: Manganese, Neurological Diseases, and Associated Pathologies, Anthony Samsel, Stephanie Seneff, Surgery Neurology International, March 24, 2015,

[228] High Rates of Suicide, Depression Linked to Farmers' Use of Pesticides, Brian Bienkowski, Scientific American, Environmental Health News, Oct 6, 2014, https://www.scientificamerican.com/article/high-rates-of-suicide-depression-linked-to-farmers-use-of-pesticides/?redirect=1

[229] "By the Numbers, Antidepressant Use on the Rise," Lea Winerman, November 2017, Vol 48, No 10, American Psychological Association, https://www.apa.org/monitor/2017/11/numbers.aspx

[230] Prescription Sleep Aid Use Among Adults: United States, 2005–2010 Yinong Chong, Ph.D.; Cheryl D. Fryar, M.S.P.H.; and Qiuping Gu, M.D., Ph.D, August 2013, https://www.cdc.gov/nchs/data/databriefs/db127.pdf

[231] Thyroid Cancer Rates Triple, and Scientists Look for Cause, Amanda Onion, March 31, 2017, Live Science, https://www.livescience.com/58489-thyroid-cancer-rates-tripled.html

[232] Monsanto Papers, Baum Hedlund Aristei Goldman, https://www.baumhedlundlaw.com/toxic-tort-law/monsanto-roundup-lawsuit/monsanto-secret-documents/

[233] Monsanto Papers Secret Documents, https://www.baumhedlundlaw.com/toxic-tort-law/monsanto-roundup-lawsuit/monsanto-secret-documents-page-five/
Roundup Ready Crops, Source Watch,
http://www.sourcewatch.org/index.php/Roundup_Ready_Crops

[234] Mystery Science: More Details on Strange Organism That Could Destroy Monsanto, Melanie Warner, CBS News, May 5, 2011, https://www.cbsnews.com/news/mystery-science-more-details-on-the-strange-organism-that-could-destroy-monsanto/

[235] Potentially Dangerous Virus Gene Hidden in Commercial GM Crops, Dr. Jonathan Latham, Dr. Allison Wilson, Science in Society, Jan 28, 2013, http://www.i-sis.org.uk/Potentially_Dangerous_Virus_Gene_in_GM_Crops.php

[236] What's a GMO? Institute for Responsible Technology,
https://responsibletechnology.org/gmo-education/faqs/

[237] Growing Doubt: A Scientist's Experience of GMOs, Jonathan Latham, PhD, Independent Science News, Aug 31, 2015, https://www.independentsciencenews.org/health/growing-doubt-a-scientists-experience-of-gmos/

[238] Bean Accounting: Are Soy-Based Food Products Safe and Healthy as Advertised? Scientific American, Earth Talk, Roddy Scheer, Doug Moss,
https://www.scientificamerican.com/article/how-safe-is-soy/

[239] Recent Trends in GE Adoption, USDA, https://www.ers.usda.gov/data-products/adoption-of-genetically-engineered-crops-in-the-us/recent-trends-in-ge-adoption.aspx

[240] These Charts Show Every Genetically Modified Food People Already Eat in the U.S., David Johnson, Siobhan O'Connor, April 30, 2015, Time Magazine, http://time.com/3840073/gmo-food-charts/

[241] Corn, NonGMO Project, https://www.nongmoproject.org/high-risk/corn/

[242] Are Bt Crops Safe, Mike Mendelsohn, John Kough, Zigfridais Vaituzis, Keith Matthews, Nature Biotechnology, Vol 21, Number 9, September 2003,
https://www.epa.gov/sites/production/files/2015-08/documents/are_bt_crops_safe.pdf

[243] Monsanto Faces Blowback Over Cancer Cover-Up, Philip Bethge, Spiegel International, Oct 24, 2017, http://www.spiegel.de/international/world/monsanto-papers-reveal-company-covered-up-cancer-concerns-a-1174233.html

[244] Gene Design 2- Gene Constructs, Bt Expression, Plant and Soil Sciences E Library, USDA National Insutitute of Food and Agriculture,
http://passel.unl.edu/pages/informationmodule.php?idinformationmodule=959031259&topicorder=4&maxto=9

[245] **Maternal and fetal exposure to pesticides associated to genetically modified foods in Eastern Townships of Quebec, Canada**, Aziz Aris, Samuel Leblanc, Reproductive Toxicology, Vol 31, Issue 4, May 2011, Pages 528-533,
https://www.sciencedirect.com/science/article/pii/S0890623811000566?via%3Dihub

[246] The Good, The Bad and the Ugly Side of GMOs And Their Link to IBD, Digestive Medical Solutions, http://digestivemedicalsolutions.com/the-good-the-bad-and-the-ugly-side-of-gmos-and-their-link-to-ibd

[247] GMO Corn Causes Liver, Kidney Problems in Rats: Study, Reuters, March 13, 2007, https://www.reuters.com/article/us-monsanto-greenpeace/gmo-corn-causes-liver-kidney-problems-in-rats-study-idUSL1346840020070313

[248] Toxic Pollen from Widely Planted, Genetically Modified Corn Can Kill Monarch Butterflies, Cornell Study Shows, Blaine Friedlander, Cornell University Chronicle, April 19, 1999, http://news.cornell.edu/stories/1999/04/toxic-pollen-bt-corn-can-kill-monarch-butterflies

[249] Developmental exposure to glyphosate-based herbicide and depressive-like behavior in adult offspring: Implication of glutamate excitotoxicity and oxidative stress, DaianeCattani[ab]Patrícia AcordiCesconetto[ab]Mauren KrugerTavares[a]Eduardo BenedettiParisotto[ab]Paulo AlexandreDe Oliveira[c]Carla Elise HeinzRieg[ab]Marina ConcliLeite[d]Rui Daniel SchröderPrediger[c]Nestor CubasWendt[a]GuilhermeRazzera[a]Danilo WilhelmFilho[b]ArianeZamon, Toxicology, Volume 387, July 15, 2017, Pages 67-80, https://www.sciencedirect.com/science/article/pii/S0300483X17301683

[250] Compositional differences in soybeans on the market: Glyphosate accumulates in Roundup Ready GM soybeans, T.Bøhn[ab]M.Cuhra[ab]T.Traavik[ab]M.Sanden[c]J.Fagan[d]R.Primicerio[b], Food Chemistry, Vol 153, June 15, 2014, Pgs 207-215, https://www.sciencedirect.com/science/article/pii/S0308814613019201

[251] The Whole Soy Story, Nutrition Digest, Kaayla T. Daniel, PhD, CCN, Fall 2005, American Nutrition Association, Vol 38, No. 2, http://americannutritionassociation.org/newsletter/whole-soy-story

[252] Childhood food allergies, An evolutionary mismatch hypothesis, Paul W Turke, Evolution, Medicine and Public Health,Octobe 4, 2017, https://www.ncbi.nlm.nih.gov/pmc/articles/PMC5861434/; Evolution of Guidelines on Peanut Allergy and Peanut Introduction in Infants: A Review., Anvari S[1], Chokshi NY[2], Kamili QU[3], Davis CM[1], JAMA Pediatrics Jan 1, 2017, https://www.ncbi.nlm.nih.gov/pubmed/27820622

[253] (see also 224) Glyphosate based- herbicide exposure affects gut microbiota, anxiety and depression-like behaviors in mice, Aitbali Y[1], Ba-M'hamed S[1], Elhidar N[2], Nafis A[2], Soraa N[3], Bennis M[4]. Neurotoxicology and Teratology, May 2018, https://www.ncbi.nlm.nih.gov/pubmed/29635013

[254] CDC Data and Statistics, Inflammatory Bowel Disease Prevalence (IBD) in the United States, https://www.cdc.gov/ibd/data-statistics.htm

[255] Acid Reflux 50% More Common Than Ten Years Ago, Catharine Paddock PhD, Medical News Today, Dec 25, 2011, https://www.medicalnewstoday.com/articles/239665.php

[256] Industrial Food Production, Union of Concerned Scientists, https://www.ucsusa.org/our-work/food-agriculture/our-failing-food-system/industrial-agriculture
Monocultures in America: A System that Needs More Diversity, University of Massachusetts Amherst, College of Natural Sciences, Julia Anderson, Emily Hespeler, Steven Swiren, Dec 5, 2017, https://blogs.umass.edu/natsci397a-eross/monocultures-in-america-a-system-that-needs-more-diversity/

[257] Battle Over Phosphate Mining Roils Small Florida Town, PBS News Hour, Oct 31, 2018, https://www.pbs.org/newshour/show/battle-over-phosphate-mining-roils-small-fla-town

[258] "Fertilizer Use Responsible for Increase in Nitrous Oxide in Atmosphere", Robert Sanders, UC Berkeley University, April 2, 2012, https://news.berkeley.edu/2012/04/02/fertilizer-use-responsible-for-increase-in-nitrous-oxide-in-atmosphere/

[259] Failure to Yield, Evaluating the Performance of Genetically Engineered Crops (2009), Union of Concerned Scientists, http://www.ucsusa.org/food_and_agriculture/our-failing-food-system/genetic-engineering/failure-to-yield.html#.Wgs3KhNSx3k

[260]http://www.ucsusa.org/sites/default/files/legacy/assets/documents/food_and_agriculture/failure-to-yield.pdf (see 258)

[261] Monsanto Loses Millions of Dollars After Indian Farmers Switch to Indigenous Seeds, March 20, 2017, https://www.fooddemocracynow.org/blog/2017/mar/20-2

[262] Recombinant Bovine Growth Hormone, American Cancer Society, https://www.cancer.org/cancer/cancer-causes/recombinant-bovine-growth-hormone.html

[263] "Court Rules rBGH-Free Milk is Better than the Kind Produced with Artificial Hormones. Now What?", Tom Laskawy, Grist Magazine, Oct 7, 2010, https://grist.org/article/food-2010-10-06-court-rules-on-rbgh-free-milk/

[264] Behind a Corporate Monster: How Monsanto Pushes Agricultural Domination, Food Democracy Now, March 20, 2017, https://www.fooddemocracynow.org/blog/2017/mar/20

[265] Labeling Milk from Cows not Treated with rBST, Libby Moulton, Columbia Law Review, Science and Techology Columbia University, http://stlr.org/2010/10/28/labeling-milk-from-cows-not-treated-with-rbst-legal-in-all-50-states-as-of-september-29th-2010/

[266] *What's In Your Milk?* Dr. Samuel Epstein, M.D., Trafford Publishing, 2006, pages 6,7,13 20,24,25-27,35-37,47,197

[267] Cancer and the Environment, What You Need to Know What You Can Do, US Department of Health and Human Services, Aug 2003, https://www.niehs.nih.gov/health/materials/cancer_and_the_environment_508.pdf

[268] https://www.usda.gov/media/press-releases/2018/12/20/establishing-national-bioengineered-food-disclosure-standard

[269] GMO Free Europe: https://www.gmo-free-regions.org/gmo-free-regions/oceania/newcaledonia.html

[270] Calls to Halt GMO Maize and Cotton Import, News European Parliament, May 17, 2017, http://www.europarl.europa.eu/news/en/press-room/20170509IPR73942/calls-to-halt-gm-maize-and-cotton-import

[271] Health and Environmental Impacts of Glufosinate Ammonium, Topsy Jewell, David Buffin, Pesticide Action Network UK, May 2001, https://friendsoftheearth.uk/sites/default/files/downloads/impacts_glufosinate_ammon.pdf

[272] French Health Regulator Withdraws License for Bayer Weedkiller, Reuters, Oct 26, 2017, https://www.reuters.com/article/us-france-health-glufosinate/french-health-regulator-withdraws-license-for-bayer-weedkiller-idUSKBN1CV2OT

BEES, BIRDS, BATS AND POLLINATORS:

Collony Collapse Disorder: https://www.greenpeace.org/usa/sustainable-agriculture/save-the-bees/

[273] Economic Importance of Bats in Agriculture, Justin G. Boyles, Paul M. Cryan, Gary F. McCracken, Thomas H. Kunz, Science Magazine, March 31, 2011, https://www.biologicaldiversity.org/campaigns/bat_crisis_white-nose_syndrome/pdfs/Boyles2011EconomicsofBats.pdf

[274] Save the Bees, Jon Cooksey, GreenPeace, https://www.greenpeace.org/usa/sustainable-agriculture/save-the-bees/, WhatWould Happen if Bees Went Extinct, BBC,May 2, 2014, video, http://www.bbc.com/future/story/20140502-what-if-bees-went-extinct

[275] Annual Honey Bee Losses Remain Above 40 Percent, Todd Fitchette, May 26, 2018, https://www.westernfarmpress.com/bees/annual-honey-bee-colony-losses-remain-above-40-percent

[276] White Nose Syndrome: Questions and Answers, Center for Biological Diversity, https://www.biologicaldiversity.org/campaigns/bat_crisis_white-nose_syndrome/Q_and_A.html

[277] (see 273) Save the Bees, https://www.greenpeace.org/usa/sustainable-agriculture/save-the-bees/

[278] Neonicotinoid Pesticides are Slowly Killing Bees, Roni Dengler, PBS, June 29, 2017, https://www.pbs.org/newshour/science/neonicotinoid-pesticides-slowly-killing-bees

[279] Forty Percent of the World's Bird Populations Are in Decline, New Study Finds, Yale School of Forestry and Environmental Studies, E360 Digest, April 23, 2018 https://e360.yale.edu/digest/forty-percent-of-the-worlds-bird-populations-are-in-decline-new-study-finds

[280] Importance of Pollinators in Changing Landscapes for World Crops, Alexandra-Maria Klein, Bernard E Vaissiere, James H. Cane, Ingolf Steffan-Dewenter, Saul A Cunningham, Claire Kremen, Teja Tscharntke, Proceedings of the Royal Society B: Biological Sciences, Feb 7, 2007; 274 (1608) 303-313, https://www.ncbi.nlm.nih.gov/pmc/articles/PMC1702377/

[281] USDA Forest Service, Bat Pollination, https://www.fs.fed.us/wildflowers/pollinators/animals/bats.shtml

[282] What Do the Birds and the Bees Have To Do With Global Food Supply, Erica Cirino, March 10, 2016, https://www.audubon.org/news/what-do-birds-and-bees-have-do-global-food-supply

[283] Bird Pollination, USDA Forest Service, https://www.fs.fed.us/wildflowers/pollinators/animals/birds.shtml

[284] Country-Specific effects of Neonicotinoids Pesticides on Honey Bees and Wild Bees, B.A. Woodcok, J.M. Bullock, R.F. Shore, M.S. Heard, M.G. Pereira, J. Redhead, L. Ridding, H. Dean, D. Sleep, June 30, 2017, Science Magazine Vol. 356, Issue 6345, PP 1393-1395, http://science.sciencemag.org/content/356/6345/1393

[285] *Effects of Neonicotinoid Exposure on Human Health, A Systematic Review* Cimino AM, Boyles AL, Thayer KA, Perry MJ, 2017. Environmental Health Perspectives 125: 155-162, https://ehp.niehs.nih.gov/EHP515/

[286] Glyphosate Perturbs the Gut Microbiota of Honeybees, Erick V. S. Motta, Kasie Raymann, and Nancy A. Moran, PNAS October 9, 2018 115 (41) 10305-10310; published ahead of print September 24, 2018 https://doi.org/10.1073/pnas.1803880115 https://www.pnas.org/content/115/41/10305

[287] Mystery Science: More Details on the Strange Organism that Could Destroy Monsanto, Melanie Warner, May 5, 2011, CBS News Moneywatch, https://www.cbsnews.com/news/mystery-science-more-details-on-the-strange-organism-that-could-destroy-monsanto/

[288] New Study Links Pesticide Use to Thyroid Disease in Women, Beyond Pesticides, https://beyondpesticides.org/dailynewsblog/2010/02/new-study-links-pesticide-use-to-thyroid-disease-in-women/

[289] Disruption of Quercetin Metabolism by Fungicide Affects Energy Production in Honey Bees Apis Mellifera), Wenfu Mao, Mary A. Schuler, May R. Berenbaum, March 7, 2017, Proceedings

of the National Academy of Sciences of the United States of America, http://www.pnas.org/content/114/10/2538.abstract

[290] Crop Pollination Exposes Honey Bees to Pesticides Which Alters their Susceptabilty to the Gut Pathogen Nosema Ceranae, Jeffery S. Pettis, Elinor M. Lichtenberg, Michael Andree, Jennie Stitzinger, Robyn Rose, Dennis vanEngelsdorp, July 24, 2013. http://journals.plos.org/plosone/article?id=10.1371/journal.pone.0070182. Research Shows Fungicide Affects Honey Bee Health, Entomology Today, July 25, 2013, https://entomologytoday.org/2013/07/25/research-shows-fungicide-affects-honey-bee-health/

[291] Agricultural Fungicide Attracts Honeybees, Study Finds, Diana Yates, Jan 8, 2018, University of Illinois, Illinois News Bureau, https://news.illinois.edu/view/6367/598033

[292] Alfalfa Pollination, Beatriz Moisset, PhD, Feb 10, 2014, http://pollinators.blogspot.com/2014/02/alfalfa-pollination.html

[293] GMO Alfalfa, What to Know, Oregonians for Farm & Food Rights, https://www.farmandfoodrights.org/current-issues/gmo-alfalfa/

[294] Milkweed Loss in Agricultural Fields Because of Herbicide Use: Effect on the Monarch Butterfly Population, John M. Pleasants, Karen S. Oberhauser, Department of Ecology, Evolution and Organismal Biology, Iowa State University, Department of Fisheries, Wildlife, and Conservation Biology, Univeristy of Minnesota; USDA, National Agricultural Statistics Service, 2011a,b.; Increasing Herbicide Use, 8 Ways Monsanto Fails at Sustainable Agriculture, Roundup Resistance Has Led to Greater Use of Herbicides, with Troubling Implications for Biodiversity, Sustainability, and Human Health,2012, https://www.ucsusa.org/food_and_agriculture/our-failing-food-system/genetic-engineering/increasing-herbicide-use.html#.WnCjm5M-f65

[295] Gardening for Pollinators, USDA Forest Service, https://www.fs.fed.us/wildflowers/pollinators/gardening.shtml
Farm Bill threatens wildlife and pollinators, Poisoned Pollinators Provision, https://thehill.com/opinion/energy-environment/386940-farm-bill-abandons-endangered-wildlife

[296] Disrupting the Balance, Ecological Impacts of Pesticides in California, Susan Kegley, Lars Neumeister, Timothy Martin, Pesticide Action Network, 1997, http://www.panna.org/sites/default/files/DisruptingtheBalance1999.pdf

[297] How to Make a Pest Spray that's Safe and Effective, April 3, 2015, https://www.rodalesorganiclife.com/home/diy-insect-spray-covers-most-pests

[298] Carbofuran Ban Upheld in the USA, http://www.krugerpark.co.za/krugerpark-times-e-9-carbofuran-ban-upheld-in-usa-25358.html

GMO ALFALFA

[299] *The Sand County Almanac,* Aldo Leopold, 1949, Oxford University Press, Oxford

[300] Alfalfa, Wildlife and the Environement, the Importance and Benefits of Alfalfa in the 21st Century, Dan Putnam, Michael Russelle, Steve Orloff, Jim Kuhn, Lee Fitzhugh, Larry Godfrey, Aaron Kiess, Rachael Long, California Alfalfa and Forage Association, 2001, http://agric.ucdavis.edu/files/242006.pdf

[301] (see 293) Aldo Leopold, *Sand County Almanac,* Oxford University Press, 1949

[302] America's Secret Animal Drug Problem, Center for Food Safety, Cristina Stella, Cameron Harsh, Sept 2015, https://www.centerforfoodsafety.org/files/animal_drug_es_10_26_77814.pdf Arsenic in Our Chicken? Nicholas Kristof, New York Times, Aprl 4, 2012, https://www.nytimes.com/2012/04/05/opinion/kristof-arsenic-in-our-chicken.html

FACTORY FARMS (CAFOs)

[303] Farm Animals Need Our Help, American Society for the Prevention of Cruelty to Animals, https://www.aspca.org/animal-cruelty/farm-animal-welfare

[304] (see 302) https://www.aspca.org/animal-cruelty/farm-animal-welfare

[305] GMOs in animal agriculture: time to consider both costs and benefits in regulatory evaluations, Journal of Animal Science Biotechnology, Sept 25, 2013, Alison L Van Eenennaam, https://www.ncbi.nlm.nih.gov/pmc/articles/PMC4015968/

[306] What's Wrong with Factory Farms? Food and Water Watch https://www.factoryfarmmap.org/problems/

[307] "UK Has Nearly 800 Livestock Mega Farms, Investigation Reveals," Andrew Wasley, Fiona Harvey, Madlen Davies, July 17, 2017

[308] The Cost of Cheap Meat, Monica Eng, Sept 24, 2010, Chicago Tribune, https://www.chicagotribune.com/lifestyles/health/ct-met-cheap-protein--20100923-story.html

[309] Antibiotic Resistance Threats, United States 2013, CDC: Antibiotic Resistance, Food and Food Animals, https://www.cdc.gov/drugresistance/pdf/2-2013-508.pdf, https://www.cdc.gov/drugresistance/food.html

[310] National Research Council (US) Committee to Study the Human Health Effects of Subtherapeutic Antibiotic Use in Animal Feeds. The Effects on Human Health of Subtherapeutic Use of Antimicrobials in Animal Feeds. Washington (DC): National Academies Press (US); 1980. Appendix K, Antibiotics In Animal Feeds.Available from: https://www.ncbi.nlm.nih.gov/books/NBK216502/

[311] (see 309) https://www.cdc.gov/drugresistance/pdf/ar-threats-2013-508.pdf

[312] Press Release: US Environmental Protection Agency Sweep's Iowa's Water Crisis Under the Rug, Food and Water Watch, April 10, 2019, https://www.foodandwaterwatch.org/news/us-environmental-protection-agency-sweeps-iowa-water-crisis-under-the-rug

[313] Challenging Factory Farms' Exemption From Pollution Reporting Requirements, Sept 28, 2018, https://aldf.org/case/challenging-factory-farms-exemption-from-pollution-reporting-requirements/ Why Are Cafos Bad, Sierra Club, Michigan Chapter, https://www.sierraclub.org/michigan/why-are-cafos-bad

[314] "Revealed: US-Style Industrial Farms Receive Millions in Subsidies", Andrew Wasley, Alexandra Heal, The Guardian, Dec 28, 2018, https://www.theguardian.com/environment/2018/dec/28/revealed-industrial-scale-farms-receive-millions-in-subsidies

[315] Animal Welfare Act, USDA, https://www.nal.usda.gov/awic/animal-welfare-act

[316] Chickens Used for Eggs, Chickens Used for Meat, Farm Sanctuary Organization, https://www.farmsanctuary.org/learn/factory-farming/chickens/

[317] (See 307) https://www.chicagotribune.com/lifestyles/health/ct-met-cheap-protein--20100923-story.html also see endnote 308, CDC)

[318] How Drugs Pumped Into Supermarket Chickens Pose A Terrifying Threat to Our Health, Tom Rawstorne, Daily Mail, Aug 9, 2013, https://www.dailymail.co.uk/news/article-2388444/How-drugs-pumped-supermarket-chickens-pose-terrifying-threat-health.html

[319] Leanness Enhancing Agents in Pork, Food Safety Focus, Dr. Geraldine LUK, Veterinary Officer, the Government of the Hong Kong Special Administrative Region, Food Safety Focus (14th Issue, September 2007), https://www.cfs.gov.hk/english/multimedia/multimedia_pub/multimedia_pub_fsf_14_01.html

[320] (See 265) Epstein, Samuel S. "Unlabeled Milk from Cows Treated with Biosynthetic Growth Hormones: A Case of Regulatory Abdication." *International Journal of Health Services* 26, no. 1 (January 1996): 173–85. doi:10.2190/EDK8-T5RC-LUMR-B2H7.

[321] "Modern Miracle Men," Rex Beach, U.S. Senate, Washington 1936, https://www.senate.gov/reference/resources/pdf/modernmiraclemen.pdf

[322] Yep, Organic Milk Really is Better For You Than Regular Milk, Melissa Dahl, Dec 10, 2013, NBC News, https://www.nbcnews.com/healthmain/yep-organic-milk-really-better-you-regular-milk-2D11712970

[323] "Organic Factory Farm Investigation," Cornucopia Institute, Dec 2014, https://www.cornucopia.org/organic-factory-farm-investigation/

[324] American Public Health Association: Ban Genetically Engineered Hormonal rBGH Milk Meat Adulterated With Sex Hormones, Dr. Samuel Epstein, Nov 17, 2011, Huffington Post, https://www.huffingtonpost.com/entry/american-publlic-health-a_b_399147.html

[325] Getting Your Omega-3s vs. Avoiding Those PCBs—The Family Health Guide, Harvard Health Publishing, April 2004, http://www.health.harvard.edu/staying-healthy/getting-your-omega-3s-vs-avoiding-those-pcbsthe-family-healthguide

[326] "Salmon Becomes World's First Genetically Modified Animal to Enter Food Supply," David Reid, CNBC, Aug 9, 2017, https://www.cnbc.com/2017/08/09/salmon-becomes-worlds-first-genetically-modified-animal-to-enter-food-supply.html

[327] Here's Why Most of the Meat Americans Eat is Banned in Other Industrialized Countries, Organic Consumers Association, July 9, 2017, https://www.ecowatch.com/antibiotics-meat-2454994122.html

[328] Poultry Inspectors Check More Than 2 Birds Per Second. The Industry Wants Them To Work Faster, Joe Fassler, Sept 14, 2017, The New Food Economy, https://newfoodeconomy.org/npis-birds-per-minute/

[329] Montana Ranchers Are Kicking Up Dust To Bring Back Country of Origin Labels on Meat, Civil Eats, Feb 13, 2019, Public Radio International, PRI, https://www.pri.org/stories/2019-02-13/montana-ranchers-are-kicking-dust-bring-back-country-origin-labels-meat

[330] Steinfeld H, Gerber P, Wassenaar T, Castel V, Rosales M, and de Haan C. 2006. Livestock's long shadow: environmental issues and options, FAO, (Rome: Food and Agriculture Organization of the United Nations, p. 86), http://www.fao.org/3/a-a0701e.pdf

[331] (See 330), Steinfeld H, Gerber P, Wassenaar T, Castel V, Rosales M, and de Haan C. 2006. Livestock's long shadow: environmental issues and options (Rome: Food and Agriculture Organization of the United Nations, (p. 86, p.86, p.88-89, p.99-100, p. 91, p. 92,92) Deforestation taken from p. 91 which also cited:

Mosier A, Wassmann R, Verchot L, King J, and Palm C. 2004. Methane and nitrogen oxide fluxes in tropical agricultural soils: sources, sinks and mechanisms. Environment, Development and Sustainability 6(1-2):11-49.

[332] Iowa Concentrated Animal Feeding Operations Air Quality Study, Feb 2002, https://www.public-health.uiowa.edu/ehsrc/CAFOstudy/CAFO_6-3.pdf, https://www.oregonlegislature.gov/citizen_engagement/Reports/2011_DEQ_Dairy%20Air%20Quality%20Task%20Force%20Appendix%20L%20Iowa%20CAFO%20study.pdf
Back up; Agriculture Sector Emissions, https://www.epa.gov/ghgemissions/sources-greenhouse-gas-emissions#nitrous-oxide

[333] (see 332) Iowa Concentrated Animal Feeding Operations Air Quality Study, Feb 2002, https://www.public-health.uiowa.edu/ehsrc/CAFOstudy/CAFO_6-3.pdf, https://www.oregonlegislature.gov/citizen_engagement/Reports/2011_DEQ_Dairy%20Air%20Quality%20Task%20Force%20Appendix%20L%20Iowa%20CAFO%20study.pdf

[334] Greenhouse Gas Emissions from Animal Agriculture, Humane Society of United States, http://www.humanesociety.org/sites/default/files/archive/assets/pdfs/farm/hsus-fact-sheet-greenhouse-gas-emissions-from-animal-agriculture.pdf,
(see 330) Steinfeld H, Gerber P, Wassenaar T, Castel V, Rosales M, and de Haan C. 2006. Livestock's long shadow: environmental issues and options, FAO, (Rome: Food and Agriculture Organization of the United Nations, p. 114, 103)

[335] (See 330) https://www.humanesociety.org/sites/default/files/archive/assets/pdfs/farm/hsus-fact-sheet-greenhouse-gas-emissions-from-animal-agriculture.pdf

[336] Farm Animals and Methane, Lisa Moore, Tim Male, Environmental Defense Fund, Sept 10, 2007, http://blogs.edf.org/climate411/2007/09/10/livestock_methane/

[337] (See also 251) The Whole Soy Story, The Nutrition Digest, http://americannutritionassociation.org/newsletter/whole-soy-story

[338] (See 334) Greenhouse Gas Emissions From Animal Agriculture, Humane Society, https://www.humanesociety.org/sites/default/files/archive/assets/pdfs/farm/hsus-fact-sheet-greenhouse-gas-emissions-from-animal-agriculture.pdf
(see 330) Steinfeld H, Gerber P, Wassenaar T, Castel V, Rosales M, and de Haan C. 2006. Livestock's long shadow: environmental issues and options (Rome: Food and Agriculture Organization of the United Nations, pp. 97-9).
U.S. Environmental Protection Agency. 2008. Inventory of U.S. greenhouse gas emissions and sinks: 1990-2006, p. 6-8. www.epa.gov/climatechange/emissions/downloads/08_Agriculture.pdf. Accessed July 30, 2008.
U.S. Environmental Protection Agency. 2008. Inventory of U.S. greenhouse gas emissions and sinks: 1990-2006, p. 6-8. www.epa.gov/climatechange/emissions/downloads/08_Agriculture.pdf. Accessed July 30, 2008.

[339] Air Pollution From Factory Farms, Fact Sheet, Environmental Integrity, http://environmentalintegrity.org/wp-content/uploads/FACT-SHEET-on-air-pollution-from-factory-farms.pdf

[340] Other Health Risks of the Meat Industry, PETA, People for the Ethical Treatment of Animals, https://www.peta.org/issues/animals-used-for-food/health-risks-meat-industry/

[341] Methane Capture and Use, EPA, https://www3.epa.gov/climatechange//kids/solutions/technologies/methane.html

[342] Taking Methane from Barn to Biogas, Jim Dickrell, Farm Journal's Milk Magazine, Aug 15, 2018, https://www.milkbusiness.com/article/taking-methane-from-barn-to-biogas

[343] (see 309) Antibiotic Resistance Threats, United States 2013, CDC: Antibiotic Resistance, Food and Food Animals, https://www.cdc.gov/drugresistance/food.html

[344] California Passes Animal Welfare Law, Gregg Henderson, Nov 7, 2018, Ag Web, https://www.agweb.com/article/california-passes-animal-welfare-law/

[345] Animal Feeding Operations (AFOs), EPA, https://www.epa.gov/npdes/animal-feeding-operations-afos#regs

[346] Reducing Environmental Cancer Risk, What We Can Do Now, President's Cancer Panel, 2008-2009 Annual Report, https://deainfo.nci.nih.gov/advisory/pcp/annualreports/pcp08-09rpt/pcp_report_08-09_508.pdf

[347] Dead Zones, Virginia Institute of Marine Science, https://www.vims.edu/research/topics/dead_zones/index.php

FERTILIZER

[348] Factbox: Types of Fertilizer, Their Uses and Hazards, Reuters, April 18, 2013, https://www.reuters.com/article/us-usa-explosion-ammonia/factbox-types-of-fertilizer-their-uses-and-hazards-idUSBRE93H11S20130418

[349] Down to Earth, Jozef Vissner, April 13, 2010, Waginengen University, http://edepot.wur.nl/135448

[350] Anhydrous Ammonia, Green Valley Chemical, http://www.greenvalleychemical.com/Green_Valley_Chemical/Anhydrous_Ammonia.html

[351] Nitric Acid, Jrank, Science Encyclopedia, https://science.jrank.org/pages/4676/Nitric-Acid.html

[352] Mosaic CO: $84 Million Sinkhole Repair Complete in Mulberry, Kevin Bouffard, Mary 30, 2018, The Ledger, https://www.theledger.com/news/20180530/mosaic-co-84-million-sinkhole-repair-complete-in-mulberry

[353] Perchlorate, Technical Fact Sheet, EPA, Jan 2014, https://www.epa.gov/sites/production/files/2014-03/documents/ffrrofactsheet_contaminant_perchlorate_january2014_final.pdf

[354] Fear in the Fields—How Hazardous Wastes Become Fertilizer—Spreading Heavy Metals on Farmland is Perfectly Legal, But Little Research Has Been Done to Find Out Whether It's Safe, Duff Wilson, Seattle Times, 1997, http://community.seattletimes.nwsource.com/archive/?date=19970703&slug=2547772

[355] Wastelands, The Threat of Toxic Fertilizer, Matthew Shaffer, The State PIRGs, Public Interest Research Group, 2001, http://www.pirg.org/toxics/reports/wastelands/WasteLands.pdf

[356] Recycling Plutonium: How the EPA is Disbursing Toxic and Radioactive Waste from the Lowry Landfill to the Sewage System and Onto CO Farmlands and Public Parks, May 4, 2004, Democracy Now, https://www.democracynow.org/2004/5/4/recycling_plutonium_how_the_epa_is

[357] Sludge Happens, Josh Harkinson, Mother Jones Magazine, May/June 2009, http://www.motherjones.com/environment/2009/05/sludge-happens

[358]Agriculture Nutrient Management and Fertilizer, EPA,Fertilizers Made from Waste, https://www.epa.gov/agriculture/agriculture-nutrient-management-and-fertilizer#Wastes
An Amonia Emission Inventory for Fertilizer Application in the United States, Marian Diaz Goebes, Ross Strader, Cliff Davidson, Atmospheric Environment, Jan 30, 2003, https://cfpub.epa.gov/ncer_abstracts/index.cfm/fuseaction/display.files/fileID/13007 2012,

[359] Atrazine Acts as an Endocrine Disruptor by Inhibiting cAMP-Specific Phosphodiesterase-4, Kucka M, Pogrmic-Majkic K, Fa S, Stojikovic SS, Kovacevic R, Toxicology Applied Pharmacology, Nov 15, Atrazine endocrine disruptors: https://www.ncbi.nlm.nih.gov/pubmed/23022511

[360] A Valuable Reputation, Rachel Aviv, The New Yorker, Feb 2, 2014, http://www.newyorker.com/magazine/2014/02/10/a-valuable-reputation

[361] Marie Simonin et al, Engineered nanoparticles interact with nutrients to intensify eutrophication in a wetland ecosystem experiment, *Ecological Applications* (2018). DOI: 10.1002/eap.1742 https://phys.org/news/2018-06-nanomaterials-algae-outbreaks-wetlands-waterways.html#jCp

[362] "Too Much of a Good Thing, Nitrate from Nitrogen Fertilizers and Cancer", President's Cancer Panel, Mary H. Ward, Reviews on Environmental Health, October 21, 2008, https://www.ncbi.nlm.nih.gov/pmc/articles/PMC5987536/?report=classic

[363] Blue Babies and Nitrate Contaminated Water, L Knobeloch, B Salna, A Hogan, J Postle, H Anderson, Environmental Health Perspectives, July 2000, https://www.ncbi.nlm.nih.gov/pmc/articles/PMC1638204/

[364] Too Much of a Good Thing, Nitrate form Nitrogen Fertilizer and Cancer, Presidents Cancer Panel, Mary Ward, Reviews Environmental Health, Oct 21, 2008, https://www.ncbi.nlm.nih.gov/pmc/articles/PMC3068045/

[365] Bioremediation of Groundwater Contaminated by Phosphate Mining and Extraction: A New Approach Using Indigenous Sulfate-Reducing Bacteria, Jill M Whitmer, James A. Saunders, https://doi.org/10.21000/JASMR00010109, https://www.asmr.us/Portals/0/Documents/Conference-Proceedings/2000/0109-Whitmer.pdf

[366] Phosphate Fertilizer Plants, World Bank Group, July 1998, Pollution Prevention and Abatement Handbook, https://www.ifc.org/wps/wcm/connect/eb314980488555a9b78cf76a6515bb18/phosfer_PPAH.pdf?MOD=AJPERES

[367] Red Tide Scientists Speak, But Some People Won't Listen, Nancy Smith, Sunshine State News, Aug 14, 2018, http://www.sunshinestatenews.com/story/red-tide-scientists-take-their-turn-speak

[368] Study Reveals That Nitrogen Fertilizers Deplete Soil Organic Carbon, University of Illinois Urbana, October 29, 2007, https://news.aces.illinois.edu/news/study-reveals-nitrogen-fertilizers-deplete-soil-organic-carbon

[369] Synthetic Nitrogen Fertilizers Alter the Soil Chemistry, Production and Quality of Tea. A Meta-Analysis,"Chunlian Qiao, Burenbayin Xu, Yanting Han, Jing Wang, Xin Wang, Lingli Liu, Weixing Liu, Shiqiang Wan, Hai Tan, Yinzhan Liu, Xinmei Zhao, Environmental Monitoring and Assessment, Feb 1, 2018, https://link.springer.com/article/10.1007/s13593-017-0485-z

[370] Overview of Greenhouse Gases, Nitrous Oxide Emissions, https://www.epa.gov/ghgemissions/overview-greenhouse-gases#nitrous-oxide

[371] Sulfur Dioxide Initiates Global Climate Change in Four Ways, Peter L. Ward, Thin Solid Films Volume 517, Issue 11, April 2, 2009, https://www.sciencedirect.com/science/article/pii/S0040609009000169

[372] Industrial Methane Emissions Are Underreported, Study Finds, Amanda Garris, Cornell University, June 6, 2019, https://news.cornell.edu/stories/2019/06/industrial-methane-emissions-are-underreported-study-finds

[373] Piercing the Haze, Ammonia a Poorly Understood Smog Ingredient Could Be Key to Limiting Deadly Pollution,Sept 13, 2018, Jason Plautz, Science Magazine, https://www.sciencemag.org/news/2018/09/ammonia-poorly-understood-smog-ingredient-could-be-key-limiting-deadly-pollution

[374] Nitrate Intake and the Risk of Thyroid Cancer and Thyroid Disease, Mary H. Ward, Briseis A. Kilfoy, Peter J. Weyer, Kristin E. Anderson, Aaron R. Folsom, James R. Cerhan, Epidemiology, May 2010; 21(3): 389-395, https://www.ncbi.nlm.nih.gov/pmc/articles/PMC2879161/
(see also 364)

[375] Soil Acidification and the Importance of Liming Agricultural Soils with Particular Reference to the United Kingdom, K.W.T. Goulding, Soil Use Management, June 24, 2016, https://www.ncbi.nlm.nih.gov/pmc/articles/PMC5032897/

[376] Radioactive Material From Fertilizer Production, EPA, https://www.epa.gov/radtown/radioactive-material-fertilizer-production

[377] The Clock is Ticking on Florida's Mountains of Hazardous Phosphate Waste,Craig Pittman, Sarasota Magazine, April 26, 2017, https://www.sarasotamagazine.com/articles/2017/4/26/florida-phosphate

[378] Monsanto's Evil Twin, Disturbing Facts About the Fertlizer Industry, Martha Rosenberg, Ronnie Cummins, April 5, 2016, Organic Consumers Association, https://www.organicconsumers.org/essays/monsanto%E2%80%99s-evil-twin-disturbing-facts-about-fertilizer-industry

[379] How the Koch Brothers Are Taking Over the Food Supply, and No One is Noticing, Fritz Kreiss, Occupy.com, March 28, 2013, https://www.occupy.com/article/how-koch-brothers-are-taking-over-food-supply-and-no-one-noticing#sthash.GYE9EwZ4.dpbs

[380] (See 370) Nitrous Oxide, Green House Gas Emissions EPA, https://www.epa.gov/ghgemissions/overview-greenhouse-gases#nitrous-oxide

[381] Carbon Dioxide, Methane, Nitrous Oxide, and the Greenhouse Effect, Conservation in a Changing Climate, http://climatechange.lta.org/get-started/learn/co2-methane-greenhouse-effect/

[382] U.S. Lockheed Martin's Tests on People, Corpwatch, Environmental Working Group, Nov 27, 2000, https://corpwatch.org/article/us-lockheed-martins-tests-humans

[383] Lettuce Samples Found Tainted, Miguel Bustillo, April 28, 2003, Los Angeles Times, http://articles.latimes.com/2003/apr/28/local/me-perc28

[384] **Perchlorate and Diet: Human Exposures, Risks, and Mitigation Strategies.** Maffini MV[1], Trasande L[2,3,4,5], Neltner TG[6]., Current Environmental Health Reports, June 2016, https://www.ncbi.nlm.nih.gov/pubmed/27029550

[385] Stop Tainting Our Produce, Food and Water Watch, https://www.foodandwaterwatch.org/JustBanIt https://www.foodandwaterwatch.org/insight/fact-sheet-toxic-oil-wastewater-our-food

[386] Shonkoff, SBC, Stringfellow, WT, Domen, JK. 2016 (September 2016). Preliminary Hazard Assessment of Chemical Additives Used in Oil and Gas Fields that Reuse Their Produced Water for Agricultural Irrigation in The San Joaquin Valley of California. Technical Report. PSE Healthy Energy, Inc. Oakland, CA, https://www.psehealthyenergy.org/wp-content/uploads/2017/04/Preliminary_Results_13267_Disclosures_FINAL-1.pdf

[387] There Might Be Fracking Wastewater on Your Organic Fruits and Veggies, Josh Harkinson, Mother Jones Magazine, Aug 20, 2015, http://www.motherjones.com/blue-marble/2015/08/organic-crops-can-be-irrigated-fracking-wastewater

[388] Oil and Gas Wastewater As Dust Suppressant Less Thank Ideal, Penn State News, May 30, 2018, https://news.psu.edu/story/523652/2018/05/30/research/oil-and-gas-wastewater-dust-suppressant-less-ideal

[389] EPA Weighs Allowing Oil Companies to Pump Wastewater into Rivers, Streams, James Osborne, Oct 15, 2018, Houston Chronicle, https://www.houstonchronicle.com/business/energy/article/EPA-weighs-allowing-oil-companies-to-pump-13303676.php

[390] Special Report: How the U.S. Government Hid Fracking's Risks to Drinking Water, Neela Banerjee, Inside Climate News, State Impact Pennsylvania, National Public Radio, npr.org, https://stateimpact.npr.org/pennsylvania/2017/11/22/special-report-how-the-u-s-government-hid-frackings-risks-to-drinking-water/

[391] Soil Acidification, Queensland Government, New Zealand, https://www.qld.gov.au/environment/land/management/soil/soil-health/acidification
[392] Study Reveals That Nitrogen Fertilizers Deplete Soil Organic Carbon, University of Illinois Urbana, October 29, 2007, https://news.aces.illinois.edu/news/study-reveals-nitrogen-fertilizers-deplete-soil-organic-carbon

SOIL

[393] Status of the World's Soil Resources, Food and Agriculture Organization of the United Nations, 2015, p. 13, http://www.fao.org/3/a-i5126e.pdf
[394] Why It's Time to Stop Punishing Our Soils with Fertilizers, Richard Schiffman, May 3, 2017, Yale University, https://e360.yale.edu/features/why-its-time-to-stop-punishing-our-soils-with-fertilizers-and-chemicals
[395] Humus, Waksman 1936, Williams and Wilkins Co, p. 7
[396] Bread from Stones, Dr. Julius Hensel, Agricultural Chemist, 1894, (Copy available by Soil and Health Library, July 2009, p. 4)
https://rockdustlocal.com/uploads/3/4/3/4/34349856/bread_from_stones.pdf
Who Was Rudolph Steiner, Biodynamic Association,
https://www.biodynamics.com/steiner.html
[397] (See 321) Modern Miracle Men, Rex Beach US 74th Congress document 264, June 1, 1936
[398] Introduction to Organic Practices, USDA,
http://www.ams.usda.gov/sites/default/files/media/Organic%20Practices%20Factsheet.pdf
[399] Why an Apple Today is Not as Good, the Daily Mail,
https://www.dailymail.co.uk/health/article-207652/Why-apple-today-good.html
[400] (see 369) Synthetic Nitrogen Fertilizers Alter the Soil Chemistry, Production and Quality of Tea. A Meta-Analysis,"Chunlian Qiao, Burenbayin Xu, Yanting Han, Jing Wang, Xin Wang, Lingli Liu, Weixing Liu, Shiqiang Wan, Hai Tan, Yinzhan Liu, Xinmei Zhao, Environmental Monitoring and Assessment, Feb 1, 2018, https://link.springer.com/article/10.1007/s13593-017-0485-z
[401] The Living Soil, Eva Balfour, 1943 Faber and Faber, London.
[402] Organic Foods are Tastier and Healthier Study Finds, Mary Beth Albright, National Geographic, July 14, 2014, https://www.nationalgeographic.com/people-and-culture/food/the-plate/2014/07/14/organic-foods-are-tastier-and-healthier-study-finds/
[403] Hidden Partners, Mycorrhizal Fungi and Plants, New York Botanical Garden, https://sciweb.nybg.org/science2/hcol/mycorrhizae.asp.html
[404] The Formation of Vegetable Mould Through the Action of Worms, Charles Darwin LL.D, F.R.S., London, William Clowes and Sons, Limited, 1881, http://darwin-online.org.uk/content/frameset?itemID=F1357&viewtype=text&pageseq=1
[405] Darwin's Earthworm Experiments Broke New Ground, NPR, February 12, 2009, https://www.npr.org/2009/02/12/100627614/darwins-earthworm-experiments-broke-new-ground.
The Formation of Vegetable Mould Through the Action of Worms, Charles Darwin, 1904, William Clowes and Sons Limited, London, New York Public Library
https://babel.hathitrust.org/cgi/pt?id=nyp.33433044061442;view=1up;seq=9

[406] Taken By Storm, National Wildlife Federation, Melinda Kaslow, April 29, 2013 https://www.nwf.org/Educational-Resources/Reports/2013/04-29-2013-Taken-By-Storm
[407] Managing 2,4-D for No-Till Burndown Treatments
April 29, 2008, Bob Hartzler, Department of Agronomy
https://crops.extension.iastate.edu/cropnews/2008/04/managing-24-d-no-till-burndown-treatments
[408] Glyphosate Fact Sheet, National Pesticide Information Center, http:/npic.orst.edu/factsheets/glyphogen.html
[409] A little Burndown Madness, Glenn Nice, Bill Johnson, Tom Bauman, Purdue University Extension, https://ag.purdue.edu/btny/weedscience/documents/burndownmadness.pdf
[410] The Unintended Consequences of Using Glyphosate (the main ingredient in the herbicide Roundup) By Sharon Rushton, Ann Spake, and Laura Chariton January, 2016, https://content.sierraclub.org/grassrootsnetwork/sites/content.sierraclub.org.activistnetwork/files/teams/documents/The_Unintended_Consequences_of_Using_Glyphosate_Jan-2016.pdf
Carlisle, S.M. and Trevors, J.T. (1988), "Glyphosate in the environment." Water, Air, and Soil Pollution 39:409-420
Levesque, C.A. (1987), "Effects of glyphosate on Fusarium spp.: its influence on root colonization of weeds, propagule density in the soil, and crop emergence." Can. J Microbiol. Vol 33, pp 354-360. 40
Sanogo, S., et al,(2000) "Effects of herbicides on Fusarium solani f. sp glycines and development of sudden death syndrome in glyphosate-tolerant soybean." Phytopathology, v. 90 (N1): 57-66
[411] 41 Levesque, C.A. (1987), "Effects of glyphosate on Fusarium spp.: its influence on root colonization of weeds, propagule density in the soil, and crop emergence." Can. J Microbiol. Vol 33, pp 354-360. https://www.nrcresearchpress.com/doi/10.1139/m87-062#.XOLePpNKgac
Multiplying Microbes, Glyphosate Boosts Fusarium Levels in Missouri Study, Gil Gullickson, Farm Progress, April 24, 2001, https://www.farmprogress.com/multiplying-microbes-glyphosate-boosts-fusarium-levels-missouri-study
[412] "Nitrogen Fertilizers Deplete Soil Organic Carbon," University of Illinois Urbana-Champaign, Live Science, October 30, 2007, https://www.sciencedaily.com/releases/2007/10/071029172809.htm
[413] Carbon Sequestration, Rodale Institute, https://rodaleinstitute.org/why-organic/issues-and-priorities/carbon-sequestration/
[414] Effects of Soil Compaction, Penn State Extension, March 8, 2005, https://extension.psu.edu/effects-of-soil-compaction
[415] Putin Wants Russia to Become World Leader in Organic Food, Philip Case, Dec 4, 2015, Farmers Weekly, https://www.fwi.co.uk/international-agriculture/putin-wants-russia-become-world-leader-organic-food
[416] Biodynamic Principles and Practices, Biodynamic Association, https://www.biodynamics.com/biodynamic-principles-and-practices
[417] Using Plants to Clean Contaminated Soil, Brian Kaller, Resilience, Aug 11, 2014, https://www.resilience.org/stories/2014-08-11/using-plants-to-clean-contaminated-soil/
[418] "How Soil is Destroyed", Hubert W. Kelley, Keeping the Land Alive, Reprinted with FAO Soils Bulletin 50, Soil Erosion and it's Causes, Rome 1990, Permission Food and Agricultural Organization of the United Nations,

http://www.fao.org/3/t0389e/T0389E02.htm#Erosion%20destroyed%20civilizations

FUNGUS RESISTANCE

[419] A Mysterious Infection, Spanning the Globe in a Climate of Secrecy, Matt Richtel and Andrew Jacobs, New York Times, April 6, 2019, https://www.nytimes.com/2019/04/06/health/drug-resistant-candida-auris.html,

[420] Does Agricultural Use of Azole Fungicides Contribute to Resistance in the Human Pathogen Aspergillus Fumigatus?, D.Hollomon, Society of Chemical Industry, Pest Management Science Oct 2017, https://www.ncbi.nlm.nih.gov/pubmed/28485100

[421] Worldwide Emergence of Resistance to Antifungal Drugs Challenges Human Health and Food Security, Matthew C. Fisher, Nichola J. Hawkins, Dominique Sanglard, Sarah J. Gurr, Science, May 18, 2018, https://science.sciencemag.org/content/360/6390/739

[422] Deaths from Fungal Infections Exceeding Malari, say Researchers in New Drug Resistance Warning, Alex Matthews-King, May 17, 2018, The Independent, https://www.independent.co.uk/news/health/fungus-infection-drug-resistance-blood-sepsis-crop-blight-nhs-breast-cancer-malaria-a8356726.html

[423] How Fungi Kills Millions Globallly, CNN, Susie East, Sept 27, 2016, https://www.cnn.com/2016/09/27/health/deadly-fungal-infections/index.html

[424] Field Crop Fungicides for the North Central United States, Daren S. Mueller, Carl A. Bradley, North Central IPM Center, https://www.ncipmc.org/action/Fungicide%20Manual4.pdf

[425] Understudied Fungicides Common in US Streams Draining Agricultural Land, USGS, June 27, 2018, https://toxics.usgs.gov/highlights/fungicides_streams.html

[426] Bayer Golf Products and Resources, Golf Course Management, https://www.backedbybayer.com/turf-and-ornamentals-management/golf-course-management?filter=fungicide

[427] White Nose Syndrome Response Team, https://www.whitenosesyndrome.org/

[428] Fungicides Market Research Report, Forecast till 2023, ID: MRFR/F-B & N/3405-HCRR | May, 2019 | Region: Global | 110 pages, https://www.marketresearchfuture.com/reports/fungicides-market-4832

[429] The Still Underestimated Problem of Fungal Diseases Worldwide, Fausto Almeida, Marcio L. Rodrigues, Carolina Coelho, Frontiers in Microbiology, Feb 12, 2019, https://www.ncbi.nlm.nih.gov/pmc/articles/PMC6379264/

CLIMATE CRISIS

[430] Tackling Climate Change Through Livestock, Key Facts and Findings, Food and Agriculture Organization of the United Nations, http://www.fao.org/news/story/en/item/197623/icode/

[431] Global Warming—Agriculture's Impact on Greenhouse Gas Emissions, Iowa State University Extension and Outreach, Eugene Takle, Don Hofstrand, https://www.extension.iastate.edu/agdm/articles/others/takapr08.html

[432] Changes in Agriculture Could Cut Sector Non-Carbon Dioxide Greenhouse Gas Emissions By Up to 50 Percent, International Institute of Applied Systems Analysis, phys.org, Dec 17, 2018, https://phys.org/news/2018-12-agriculture-sector-non-carbon-dioxide-greenhouse.html

[433] Latest Agriculture Emissions Data Show Rise of Factory Farms, Institute for Agriculture and Trade Policy IATP, Ben Lilliston, March 26, 2019, https://www.iatp.org/blog/201904/latest-agriculture-emissions-data-show-rise-factory-farms

[434] Inventory of U.S. Greenhouse Gas Emissions and Sinks 1990-2017, EPA, https://www.epa.gov/sites/production/files/2019-04/documents/us-ghg-inventory-2019-main-text.pdf, p. 364

[435] Can We Feed 10 Billion People on Organic Farming Alone, John Reganold, Aug 14, 2016, The Guardian, https://www.theguardian.com/sustainable-business/2016/aug/14/organic-farming-agriculture-world-hunger

[436] Animal Feeding Operations, USDA, CAFOs and AFOs, https://www.nrcs.usda.gov/wps/portal/nrcs/main/national/plantsanimals/livestock/afo/

[437] Gassy Cows Are Warming the Planet, and They're Here to Stay, Maanvi Singh, National Public Radio, WBEZ Chicago, The Salt April 12, 2014, https://www.npr.org/sections/thesalt/2014/04/11/301794415/gassy-cows-are-warming-the-planet-and-theyre-here-to-stay

[438] Possible health impacts of Bt toxins and residues from spraying with complementary herbicides in genetically engineered soybeans and risk assessment as performed by the European Food Safety Authority EFSA, Christoph Then and Andreas Bauer-Panskus, Environmental Sciences Europe, Jan 11, 2017, https://www.ncbi.nlm.nih.gov/pmc/articles/PMC5236067/

[439] Palm Oil is the Elephant in the Greenhouse, Stephanie Searle, International Council on Clean Transportation, ICCT, June 6, 2018, https://www.theicct.org/blog/staff/palm-oil-elephant-greenhouse

[440] Third of Earth's Soil is Acutely Degraded Due to Agriculture, Jonathan Watts, The Guardian, Sept 12, 2017, https://www.theguardian.com/environment/2017/sep/12/third-of-earths-soil-acutely-degraded-due-to-agriculture-study

[441] Organic Farming is on the Rise in the U.S., Kristen Bialik, Kristi Walker, Pew Research Center, http://www.pewresearch.org/fact-tank/2019/01/10/organic-farming-is-on-the-rise-in-the-u-s/

[442] Livestock Grazing on Public Lands, Bureau of Land Management, https://www.blm.gov/programs/natural-resources/rangelands-and-grazing/livestock-grazing

[443] Animal Feeding Operations (AFO) and Concentrated Animal Feeding Operations (CAFO), USDA Natural Resources Conservation Service, https://www.nrcs.usda.gov/wps/portal/nrcs/main/national/plantsanimals/livestock/afo/

[444] (see 443) https://www.nrcs.usda.gov/wps/portal/nrcs/main/national/plantsanimals/livestock/afo/

[445] Possible health impacts of Bt toxins and residues from spraying with complementary herbicides in genetically engineered soybeans and risk assessment as performed by the European Food Safety Authority EFSA, Christoph Then and Andreas Bauer-Panskus, Environmental Sciences Europe, Jan 11, 2017, https://www.ncbi.nlm.nih.gov/pmc/articles/PMC5236067/

[446]Increasing Herbicide Use, 8 Ways Monsanto Fails at Sustainability, Union of Concerned Scientists, https://www.ucsusa.org/food_and_agriculture/our-failing-food-system/genetic-engineering/increasing-herbicide-use.html#.WnCjm5M-f65

[447] The Hidden Dangers of Chemical Fertilizers, Laura Buckler, April 1, 2018, OH&S Occupational Health & Safety, https://ohsonline.com/Articles/2017/12/07/The-Hidden-Dangers-of-Chemical-Fertilizers.aspx

[448] Rise of Mega Farms: How the US Model of Intensive Farming is Invading the World, Fiona Harvey, Andrew Wasley, Madlen Davies, David Child, The Guardian, July 18, 2017, https://www.theguardian.com/environment/2017/jul/18/rise-of-mega-farms-how-the-us-model-of-intensive-farming-is-invading-the-world

[449] GMOs in Animal Agriculture: Time to consider Both Costs and Benefits in Regulatory Evaluations, Alison L Van Eenennaam, Journal of Animal Science and Biotechnology, Sept 25, 2013, https://www.ncbi.nlm.nih.gov/pmc/articles/PMC4015968/

[450] Status of the World's Soil Resources, FAO of the United Nations, 2015, http://www.fao.org/3/a-i5126e.pdf

[451] We Don't Have Enough Organic Farms, Why Not? Rachel Cernansky, National Geographic, Nov 20, 2018, https://www.nationalgeographic.com/environment/future-of-food/organic-farming-crops-consumers/

[452] Reduce Your Exposure to Pesticides, Soil Association, https://www.soilassociation.org/organic-living/whyorganic/reduce-your-exposure-to-pesticides/

[453] Organic Standards, USDA, https://www.ams.usda.gov/grades-standards/organic-standards

[454] 2018 Farm Bill & Legislative Principles, https://www.usda.gov/sites/default/files/documents/2018-farm-bill-and-legislative-principles.pdf

[455] Farm Subsidies with Pros, Cons, and Impact, Kimberly Amadeo, March 21, 2019, https://www.thebalance.com/farm-subsidies-4173885

[456] Open The Books, Harvesting U.S. Farm Subsidies, Adam Andrzejewski, Thomas W Smith, Sept 29, 2018, https://www.openthebooks.com/openthebooks_oversight_report_%E2%80%93_harvesting_us_farm_subsidies/, full report: https://issuu.com/openthebooks/docs/usfarmsubsidies_08072018?e=31597235/63670406

[457] The Rich and Famous at the Farm Bill Trough, Diane Katz, The Daily Signal, May 29, 2013, https://www.dailysignal.com/2013/05/29/the-rich-and-famous-at-the-farm-bill-trough/

[458] Tragedy and Transformation: Deforestation in the Amazon, Steve Schwartsman, Environmental Defense Fund, March 20, 2013, https://www.edf.org/blog/2013/03/20/tragedy-and-transformation-deforestation-amazon

[459] 11 of the World's Most Threatened Forests, World Wildlife Fund, Jill Schwartz, April 27, 2015, https://www.worldwildlife.org/stories/11-of-the-world-s-most-threatened-forests

[460] US Plush Toilet Paper Use Wiping Out Canada's Forests, Flushing Away The Future: Report, Adrian Humphreys, National Post, Feb 25, 2019, https://nationalpost.com/news/canada/u-s-plush-toilet-paper-use-wiping-out-canadas-forests-flushing-away-the-future-report

[461] 10 Years Ago the Amazon Was Being Bulldozed for Soy—Then Everything Changed, Greenpeace, https://www.greenpeace.org/usa/victories/amazon-rainforest-deforestation-soy-moratorium-success/

[462] Palm Oil, Rainforest Rescue, https://www.rainforest-rescue.org/topics/palm-oil#start

[463] Palm Oil, World Wildlife Fund, www.worldwildlife.org/pages/which-everyday-products-contain-palm-oil

[464] Bethany Lindsay, "It blows my mind': How B.C. destroys a key natural wildfire defense every year," CBC News · Nov 17, 2018, https://www.cbc.ca/news/canada/british-columbia/it-blows-my-mind-how-b-c-destroys-a-key-natural-wildfire-defence-every-year-1.4907358

[465] Viktoria Wagner, Pedro M. Antunes, Michael Irvine, Cara R. Nelson, Herbicide usage for invasive non-native plant management in wildland areas of North America, Journal of Applied Ecology, 29 June 2016, https://missoulian.com/news/local/um-researchers-find-lack-of-government-accountability-on-widespread-herbicide/article_a13ac9e9-f535-51ef-a8ce-b398b6c29e62.html
[466] (see 464) Bethany Lindsay, It Blows my mind: How B.C. Destroys a Key Natural Wildfire Defense Every Year," CBC News, https://www.cbc.ca/news/canada/british-columbia/it-blows-my-mind-how-b-c-destroys-a-key-natural-wildfire-defence-every-year-1.4907358
[467] Sharon Rushton, Ann Spake, Laura Chariton, "The Unintended Consequences of Using Glyphosate", Sierra Club, January 2016, https://content.sierraclub.org/grassrootsnetwork/sites/content.sierraclub.org.activistnetwork/files/teams/documents/The_Unintended_Consequences_of_Using_Glyphosate_Jan-2016.pdf
[468] Chemical Composition of Wildland Fire Emissions, Shawn P. Urbanski, Wei Min Hao, Stephen Baker, Developments in Environmental Science, Volume 8, 2009, Elsevier B.V., US Forest Service, https://www.fs.fed.us/rm/pubs_other/rmrs_2009_urbanski_s001.pdf
[469] Dianna Farsetta, Pesticides and Forest Service Fires, The Center for Media and Democracy's PR Watch, Oct 7, 2005, https://prwatch.org/spin/2005/10/4054/pesticides-and-forest-service-fires
[470] Rachel Carson, Silent Spring, 1962, Houghton Mifflin Harcourt Publishing, USA, p 253
[471] Peatlands and Climate Change, IUCN, https://www.iucn.org/resources/issues-briefs/peatlands-and-climate-change
[472] The Issue with Tissue, NRDC Natural Resources Defense Council, Feb 2019, https://www.nrdc.org/sites/default/files/issue-tissue-how-americans-are-flushing-forests-down-toilet-report.pdf
[473] Save Food: Global Initiative on Food Loss and Waste Reduction, Key Facts on Food Loss and Waste You Should Know!Food and Agriculture Organization of the United Nations, http://www.fao.org/save-food/resources/keyfindings/en/
[474] Pesticides and Climate Change, Californians for Pesticide Reform, http://www.pesticidereform.org/climate-change/
[475] (see 437) Grassy Cows are Warming the Planet, npr.org, https://www.npr.org/sections/thesalt/2014/04/11/301794415/gassy-cows-are-warming-the-planet-and-theyre-here-to-stay
[476] https://www.latimes.com/science/sciencenow/la-sci-sn-ethanol-ozone-levels-brazil-20140501-story.html

ADDITIVES IN FOOD

[477] GRAS: The Hidden Substances in Your Food, Jeneen Interlandi, Aug 17, 2016, https://www.consumerreports.org/food-safety/gras-hidden-ingredients-in-your-food/
[478]Ed Markey,Senator Markey: FDA's Final Rule On Food Safety Process Is A Missed Opportunity https://www.markey.senate.gov/news/press-releases/senator-markey-fdas-final-rule-on-food-safety-process-is-a-missed-opportunity
[479] Jawdroppingly Toxic Food Ingredients & Artificial Additives to Avoid, Masters in Public Health Programs List, Advocates for Public Health Education, https://mphprogramslist.com/50-jawdroppingly-toxic-food-additives-to-avoid/

[480] Diet and Nutrition, the Artificial Food Dye Blues, Carol Potera, https://www.ncbi.nlm.nih.gov/pmc/articles/PMC2957945/

[481] Eating with Your Eyes, the Chemistry of Food Colorings, American Chemical Society, Brian Rohrig, October 2015, https://www.acs.org/content/acs/en/education/resources/highschool/chemmatters/past-issues/2015-2016/october-2015/food-colorings.html

[482] The Problem with Sugar Free Kids, Alice Park, Time Magazine, http://time.com/the-trouble-with-sugar-free-kids/

[483] Possible Neurologic Effects of Aspartame, a Widely Used Food Additive, TJ Maher, RJ Wurtman, Environmental Health Perspectives, Nov 1987, https://www.ncbi.nlm.nih.gov/pmc/articles/PMC1474447/

[484] Aspartame: Decades of Science Point to Serious Health Risks, Stacy Malkin, US Right to Know, Sug 14, 2017, https://usrtk.org/sweeteners/aspartame_health_risks/

[485] Is Fructose Bad For You?, Rachel Nall, Medical News Today, Nov 28, 2018, https://www.medicalnewstoday.com/articles/323818.php

[486] Abundance of Fructose Not Good for the Liver, Heart, Harvard Health Publishing, Heart Letter,Sept 2011, https://www.health.harvard.edu/heart-health/abundance-of-fructose-not-good-for-the-liver-heart

[487] Why You Should Never Eat High Fructose Corn Syrup, Dr. Mark Hyman MD, Huffington post, Nov 12, 2013, https://www.huffingtonpost.com/dr-mark-hyman/high-fructose-corn-syrup_b_4256220.html

[488] High-Fructose Corn Syrup Promotes Colon Tumor Growth in Mice, Weill Cornell Medicine Sandra and Edward Meyer Cancer Center, March 21, 2019, https://meyercancer.weill.cornell.edu/news/2019-03-21/high-fructose-corn-syrup-promotes-colon-tumor-growth-mice

[489] Mercury in Corn Syrup? Food Made with Ingredient May Have Traces of Toxic Metal, Michael Hawthorne, Chicago Tribune, Jan 27, 2009, https://www.chicagotribune.com/lifestyles/chi-mercury-corn-syrupjan27-story.html

[490] Study Reveals Possible Connection Between High Fructose Corn Syrup and Opioid Addiction, David DiSalvo, Forbes Magazine, Nov 16, 2017, https://www.forbes.com/sites/daviddisalvo/2017/11/16/how-high-fructose-corn-syrup-could-be-fueling-opioid-addiction/#49ab087039f6

[491] Ensure and Boost May Be Harmful to Cancer Patients, American Cancer Society, Aug 10, 2015, https://csn.cancer.org/node/296019

[492] Our Toxic Air, Michael Hawthorne, Darnell Little, Chicago Tribune, Sept 29, 2008, https://www.chicagotribune.com/news/ct-xpm-2008-09-29-0809290162-story.html

[493] Neotame: Is This More-Dangerous-Than-Aspartame-Sweetener Hiding In Your Food? Dr. Mercola, March 28, 2012, https://articles.mercola.com/sites/articles/archive/2012/03/28/neotame-more-toxic-than-aspartame.aspx

[494] Additional Information About High-Intensity Sweeteners Permitted For Use In Food In the United States,FDA, http://www.fda.gov/Food/IngredientsPackagingLabeling/FoodAdditivesIngredients/ucm397725.htm

[495] Splenda: The Artificial Sweetener That Explodes Internally, https://thepeopleschemist.com/splenda-the-artificial-sweetener-that-explodes-internally/

[496] Gut Microbiome Response to Sucralose and its Potential Role in Inducing Liver Inflammation in Mice, Xiaoming Bian, Liang Chi, Bei Gao, Pengcheng Tu, Hongyu Ru, Kun Lu, Frontiers in Physiology, July 24, 2017, https://www.ncbi.nlm.nih.gov/pmc/articles/PMC5522834/

[497] The Dangers of Sucralose: Why is It Considered Diabetic Friendly?, Christopher Noftall, Diabetes Daily, Aug 18, 2016, https://www.diabetesdaily.com/blog/the-dangers-of-sucralose-why-is-it-considered-diabetic-friendly-300777/

[498] Splenda: Is it Safe?, Natalie Butler RD, LD, Medical News Today, Feb 7, 2017, https://www.medicalnewstoday.com/articles/262475.php

Sucralose Administered in Feed, Beginning Prenatally Through Lifespan, Induces Hematopoietic Neoplasias in Male Swiss Mice, Soffritti M., Padovani M, Tibaldi E, Falconi L, Manservisi F, Lauriola M, Internation Journal of Occupational and Environmental Health, Vol 22, 2016, Issue 1, Jan 29, 2016, https://www.tandfonline.com/doi/abs/10.1080/10773525.2015.1106075?journalCode=yjoh20&

[499] Carcinogenicity of Saccharin, MD Reuber, Environmental Health Perspectives, Aug 25, 1978, https://www.ncbi.nlm.nih.gov/pmc/articles/PMC1637197/

[500] S. 1750—95th Congress: Saccharin Study, Labeling and Advertising Act." www.Govtrack.us, 1977, https://www.govtrack.us/congress/bills/95/s1750

[501] Truvia vs. Stevia, Janine Grant, Livestrong, https://www.livestrong.com/article/366165-truvia-vs-stevia/

[502] Food Safety : FDA Should Strengthen Its Oversight of Food Ingredients Determined To Be Generally Recognized As Safe, Nanoparticles: https://www.gao.gov/products/GAO-10-246

FATS

[503] Recent Advances In Canola Meal Utilization In Swine Nutrition, G Mejicanos, N. Sanjayan, I.H. Kim, C.M. Nyachoti, Journal of Animal Science and Technology, Feb 16, 2016, https://www.ncbi.nlm.nih.gov/pmc/articles/PMC4754856/

[504] Which Everyday Products Contain Palm Oil? www.worldwildlife.org/pages/which-everyday-products-contain-palm-oil

[505] The Palm Oil Industry and Noncommunicable Diseases, Sowmya Kadandale, Robert Marten, Richard Smith, July 15, 2018, World Health Organization, https://www.who.int/bulletin/volumes/97/2/18-220434/en/

Bulletin of the World Health Organization 2019; 97:118-128

[506] Mayo Clinic Staff, "Trans Fat is Double Trouble for Your Heart Health," March 1, 2017, https://www.mayoclinic.org/diseases-conditions/high-blood-cholesterol/in-depth/trans-fat/art-20046114

[507] Trans Fat, American Heart Organization, https://www.heart.org/en/healthy-living/healthy-eating/eat-smart/fats/trans-fat

PROCESSED FOODS

[508] Ashley Parrish, "What is a Processed Food?", Michigan State University Extension, Nov 26, 2014, https://www.canr.msu.edu/news/what_is_a_processed_food

[509] Agricultural Subsidies and the American Obesity Epidemic, Caroline Franck MSc, Sonia M. Grandi MSc, Mark J. Eisenberg, MD, September 2013, American Journal of Preventative Medicine, https://www.ajpmonline.org/article/s0749-3797(13)00320-6/fulltext

[510] Taylor Wolfram, "Processed Foods: What's Ok and What to Avoid," Academy of Nutrition and Dietetics, Feb 11, 2019, https://www.eatright.org/food/nutrition/nutrition-facts-and-food-labels/processed-foods-whats-ok-and-what-to-avoid

[511] Dr. Samuel Epstein, *The Politics of Cancer*, Sierra Club Books, San Francisco, 1978, pages. 288-289.
[512] Dietary Nitrates, Nitrites, and Nitrosamines Intake and the Risk of Gastric Cancer: A Meta-Analysis
Peng Song, Lei Wu, Wenxian Guan
Nutrients. 2015 Dec; 7(12): 9872–9895. Published online 2015 Dec 1. doi: 10.3390/nu7125505
PMCID: PMC4690057, https://www.ncbi.nlm.nih.gov/pmc/articles/PMC4690057/ .
Tricker A.R., Preussmann R. Carcinogenic *N*-nitrosamines in the diet: Occurrence, formation, mechanisms and carcinogenic potential. Mutat. Res. 1991; 259:277–289. doi: 10.1016/0165-1218(91)90123-4.
Anderson L.M., Souliotis V.L., Chhabra S.K., Moskal T.J., Harbaugh S.D., Kyrtopoulos S.A. *N*-nitrosodimethylamine-derived O (6)-methylguanine in DNA of monkey gastrointestinal and urogenital organs and enhancement by ethanol. Int. J. Cancer. 1996; 66:130–134. doi: 10.1002/(SICI)1097-0215(19960328)66:1<130:AID-IJC22>3.0.CO;2-G
[513] "Personal Health, Nitrites and Nitrates Are So Widespread It's Hard to Find Food Brands That Don't Contain Them", Jane Brody, New York Times, August 15, 1979, https://www.nytimes.com/1979/08/15/archives/personal-health.html
[514] Bee Wilson, "Yes Bacon Really is Killing Us. Decades' worth of research proves that chemicals used to make bacon do cause cancer. So how did the meat industry convince us it was safe?, The Guardian, March 1, 2018, https://www.theguardian.com/news/2018/mar/01/bacon-cancer-processed-meats-nitrates-nitrites-sausages

REFINED WHITE FLOUR

[515] Against the Grain, Michael Specter, The New Yorker, Oct 27, 2014, https://www.newyorker.com/magazine/2014/11/03/grain
[516] Glyphosate, Pathways to Modern Diseases II: Celiac Sprue and Gluten Intolerance, Anthony Samsel, Stephanie Seneff, Interdisciplinary Toxicology, Dec 6, 2013, DOI: 10/2478/intox-2013-0026, https://www.ncbi.nlm.nih.gov/pmc/articles/PMC3945755/
[517] What is Celiac Disease? Celiac Disease Foundation, https://celiac.org/about-celiac-disease/what-is-celiac-disease/
[518] Vitamin and Mineral Deficiences Are Highly Prevalent in Newly Diagnosed Celiac Disease Patients, Nicolette J Wierdsma, Marian AE van Bokhorst-de van der Schueren, Marijike Berkenpas, Chris J.J. Mulder, Ad A.van Bodegraven, Nutrients, Oct 5, 2013, https://www.ncbi.nlm.nih.gov/pmc/articles/PMC3820055/
[519] William Davis MD, *Wheat Belly*, Rodale Books, New York, 2011, p.21-22, 53, 63,139
[520] Migraine Associated with Gastrointestinal Disorders: Review of the Literature and Clinical Implications, Saskia van Hemert, Anne C. Breedveld, Jorgen M.P. Rovers, Jan P.W. Vermeiden, Ben J.M. Witteman, Marcel G. Smits, Nicole M. de Roos, Frontiers in Neurology, Nov 21, 2014, https://www.ncbi.nlm.nih.gov/pmc/articles/PMC4240046/
Microscopic Colitis, Crohn's and Colitis Foundation, https://www.crohnscolitisfoundation.org/resources/microscopic-colitis.html
[521] Sugar Blues, William Dufty, p. 120-121, Chilton Book Company, PA
[522] The Truth About Potassium Bromate, Luke Yoquinto, Live Science, March 16, 2012, https://www.livescience.com/36206-truth-potassium-bromate-food-additive.html
[523] Acute Exposure Guideline Levels for Select Airborne Chemicals, National Research Council of the National Academies, 2007, https://www.epa.gov/sites/production/files/2014-11/documents/chlorinedioxide_final_volume5_2007.pdf

[524] The Little Known Secrets about Bleached Flour, Dr. Mercola, March 26, 2009, https://articles.mercola.com/sites/articles/archive/2009/03/26/The-Little-Known-Secrets-about-Bleached-Flour.aspx

[525] Rise in Diabetes 'to Cause Surge in Heart Disease and Strokes,' Alex Therrian, BBC News, Aug 23, 2018, https://www.bbc.com/news/health-45270141

Diabetes, Heart Disease, and Stroke, National Institute of Diabetes and Digestive and Kidney Diseases, U.S. Health and Human Services National Institutes of Health, https://www.niddk.nih.gov/health-information/diabetes/overview/preventing-problems/heart-disease-stroke

[526] Dead Doctors Don't Lie, Dr. Joel Wallach, Dr. Ma Lan, 1999, Wellness Publications LLC p. 310

REFINED WHITE SUGAR

[527] Endocrine System: Facts, Functions, and Diseases, Kim Ann Zimmerman, Feb 15, 2018, https://www.livescience.com/26496-endocrine-system.html

[528] Is Sugar Sabotaging Your Hormones, Dr. Sarika Arora MD, Women's Health Network, https://www.womenshealthnetwork.com/hormonalimbalance/hormonal-imbalance-caused-by-sugar.aspx

[529] *Sugar Blues*, William Dufty, p. 137, 148, 1975, Chilton Book Company, PA

[530] *Sugar Blue, William Dufty,* p. 70, 71, 79, Chilton Book Company, PA

[531] Sugar Sweetened Cigarettes: Added Sugars in American Cigarette Brands, AB Seidenberg, LE van Nierop, EN Lindblom, KM Ribisl, March 2018, Cancer Epidemiology, Biomarkers & Prevention, http://cebp.aacrjournals.org/content/27/3/357.1

FOOD SAFETY

[532] Factory Farms, Farm Animals Need Our Help, https://www.aspca.org/animal-cruelty/farm-animal-welfare

[533] They Eat What? What Are They Feeding Animals at Factory Farms? Organic Consumers Association, https://www.organicconsumers.org/news/they-eat-what-what-are-they-feeding-animals-factory-farms,

Doug Gurian Sherman, Union of Concerned Scientist, Cafos Uncovered, April 2008, https://www.ucsusa.org/sites/default/files/legacy/assets/documents/food_and_agriculture/cafos-uncovered.pdf

[534] Andrea Beck, All the Recent Food Recalls You Need to Know About, Good Housekeeping, April 5, 2019, https://www.bhg.com/news/food-recalls/

[535] Flood of Food Imported to U.S., but Only 2 Percent Inspected, Brad Racino, 10/3/2011, NBC News, http://www.nbcnews.com/id/44701433/ns/health-food_safety/t/flood-food-imported-us-only-percent-inspected/#.XHvDvM9Kg3o

[536] Trump Administration Gives More Power Over Meat Inspections to Pork Industry, April 3, 2019, the Daily Beast, https://www.thedailybeast.com/trump-administration-to-give-more-power-over-meat-inspections-to-pork-industry

[537] New Investigation Highlights Dangers of High-Speed Slaughter, ASPCA,Nov 29, 2018, https://www.aspca.org/news/new-investigation-highlights-dangers-high-speed-slaughter

[538] Viveth Karthikeyan, Adam Garber, "How Safe Is Our Food," US PIRG Education Fund, https://uspirgedfund.org/feature/usf/how-safe-our-food
[539] What is HAACP, Modern Meat, Public Broadcasting Corporation, Frontline, 2014, https://www.pbs.org/wgbh/pages/frontline/shows/meat/evaluating/haccp.html
[540] Matthew Wald, "Meat Packer Admits Slaughter of Sick Cows," New York Times, March 13, 2008
[541] Martha Rosenberg, Death of Meat Inspector Highlights Conditions at Nation's Slaughterhouses, Intrepid Report, June 26, 2013, http://www.intrepidreport.com/archives/10015
[542] Frances Russell, The Costs of Factory Farming, Winnepeg Free Press, Nov 26, 2004, https://newspaperarchive.com/winnipeg-free-press-nov-26-2004-p-14/
[543] Jennifer Frazer, The Case for Transmissible Alzeheimer's Grows, Scientific American, Feb 7, 2019, https://blogs.scientificamerican.com/artful-amoeba/the-case-for-transmissible-alzheimers-grows/
[544] Institute of Medicine (US) Food and Nutrition Board. Cattle Inspection: Committee on Evaluation of USDA Streamlined Inspection System for Cattle (SIS-C). Washington (DC): National Academies Press (US); 1990. 2, INTRODUCTION AND HISTORICAL REVIEW OF MEAT INSPECTION. Available from: https://www.ncbi.nlm.nih.gov/books/NBK235649/
[545] Harvey W. Wiley, FDA Consumer Magazine, Centennial Edition 2006, https://www.fda.gov/AboutFDA/History/FOrgsHistory/Leaders/ucm2016811.htm
[546] Parasites in Food, CDC, https://www.cdc.gov/parasites/food.html
[547] "Uh-Oh Your Salmon Might Be Filled with Tapeworms," Christa Sgobba, Men's Health, Jan 12, 2017, https://www.menshealth.com/health/a19536655/salmon-and-tapeworms/
[548] Fish and Fishery Products Hazards and Controls Guidance, FDA, Ch. 5 Parasites, https://www.fda.gov/media/80777/download
[549] Food Safety for Pregnant Women, FDA, https://www.fda.gov/media/83740/download
[550] Freezing Fish, Killing Parasites, C. Claiborne Ray, New York Times, https://www.nytimes.com/2015/05/19/science/freezing-fish-killing-parasites.html

MOLDS IN FOOD

[551] *The Cure for All Diseases*, Hulda Clark, New Century Press, 1995 pages 348,382-390, 422-423

LABELING FOOD

[552] BE Disclosure, USDA, https://www.ams.usda.gov/rules-regulations/be
[553] USDA Outlines First-Ever Rule for GMO Labeling, Sees Implementation in 2020, Reuters, Dec 20, 2018, https://www.reuters.com/article/us-usa-gmo-labeling/usda-outlines-first-ever-rule-for-gmo-labeling-sees-implementation-in-2020-idUSKCN1OJ2TF
[554] USDA Announces GMO Labeling Standard, Food Business News, Dec 20, 2018, https://www.foodbusinessnews.net/articles/13064-usda-announces-gmo-labeling-standard
[555] Here's a First Look at the Label That Must Appear on All GMO Foods by 2020, Sam Bloch, The New Food Economy, Dec 20, 2018, https://newfoodeconomy.org/gmo-label-rule-usda-bioengineered/
[556] American Farm Bureau Supports National GMO Pre-Emption Bill, June 27, 2016, American Farm Bureau, https://www.fb.org/newsroom/american-farm-bureau-supports-national-gmo-pre-emption-bill
[557] New GMO Food Labels Are Already Creating Havoc, Phil Lempert, Winsight Grocery Business, March 26, 2019, https://www.winsightgrocerybusiness.com/fresh-food/new-gmo-food-labels-are-already-creating-havoc
[558] WTO Shoots Down US Meat Labeling Rule, Lydia Wheeler, The Hill, May 18, 2015, https://thehill.com/regulation/242385-wto-rules-against-us-appeal-to-keep-country-of-origin-labeling-rule
[559]Removal of Mandatory Country of Origin Labeling Requirements for Beef and Pork Muscle Cuts, Ground Beef, and Ground Pork, A Rule by the Agricultural Marketing Service USDA, March 2, 2016, Office

of the Federal Register, https://www.federalregister.gov/documents/2016/03/02/2016-04609/removal-of-mandatory-country-of-origin-labeling-requirements-for-beef-and-pork-muscle-cuts-ground

560 CRISPR Plants Now Subject to Tough GM Laws in European Union, Ewen Callaway, Nature International Journal of Science, July 25, 2018, https://www.nature.com/articles/d41586-018-05814-6

561 Genes and Chromosomes, David N. Finegold, MD University of Pittsburgh, Merck Manual, https://www.merckmanuals.com/home/fundamentals/genetics/genes-and-chromosomes

562 Gene-Edited Food Quietly Arrives in Restaurant Cooking Oil, Candace Choi, AP News, March 12, 2019, https://www.apnews.com/17f0f799580a483fbd1b2d69bcf2ba18

IRRADIATION

563 Irradiation and Food Safety Answers to Frequently Asked Questions, USDA, https://www.fsis.usda.gov/wps/portal/fsis/topics/food-safety-education/get-answers/food-safety-fact-sheets/production-and-inspection/irradiation-and-food-safety/irradiation-food-safety-faq

564 Food Irradiation, What You Need to Know, FDA, https://www.fda.gov/food/buy-store-serve-safe-ood/food-irradiation-what-you-need-know

565 Francis Raul, Francine Gossé, Henry Delincé, Andrea Hartwig, Eric Marchioni, Michel Miesch, Dalal Werner & Dominique Burnouf (2002) Food-Borne Radiolytic Compounds (2-Alkylcyclobutanones)May Promote Experimental Colon Carcinogenesis, Nutrition and Cancer, 44:2, 189-191, DOI: 10.1207/S15327914NC4402_11

566 What's Wrong with Food Irradiation? Organic Consumers Association, https://www.organicconsumers.org/sites/default/files/what%27s%20wrong%20with%20food%20irradiation.pdf

567 Food Irradiation, the Problems and Concerns, July 2002, http://www.foodcomm.org.uk/campaigns/irradiation_concerns/

568 All About Organics, Whole Foods, https://www.wholefoodsmarket.com/organic

PESTICIDE RESIDUES

569 New Data on Pesticides in Food Raises Safety Questions, US Right to Know, Carey Gillam, Nov 23, 2016, https://usrtk.org/gmo/before-the-holiday-feast-new-data-on-pesticides-in-food-raises-safety-questions/

570 Weedkiller Found in Granola and Crackers, Internal FDA Emails Show, Carey Gillam The Guardian, April 30, 2018, https://www.theguardian.com/us-news/2018/apr/30/fda-weedkiller-glyphosate-in-food-internal-emails

571 California Scientists: Safe Level of Roundup is 100x Lower Than EPA Allowance, Environmental Working Group, June 21, 2017, Eco Watch, https://www.ecowatch.com/california-monsanto-glyphosate-2445606387.html

572 About Pesticide Tolerances, EPA, https://www.epa.gov/pesticide-tolerances/about-pesticide-tolerances

573 (see 538) https://usrtk.org/gmo/before-the-holiday-feast-new-data-on-pesticides-in-food-raises-safety-questions/

ENDOCRINE DISRUPTORS

574 Endocrine Disruption, The Endocrine Disruptor Exchange, https://endocrinedisruption.org/interactive-tools/endocrine-basics

[575] Rachel Carson, *Silent Spring* page 242, Houghton Mifflin Harcourt Publishing, 1962

[576] Who gets Cancer, American Cancer Society, https://www.cancer.org/treatment/understanding-your-diagnosis/after-diagnosis/who-gets-cancer.html

FOOD PACKAGING

[577] BPA is Fine, If You Ignore Most Studies About It, Douglas Main, Newsweek, March 4, 2015, https://www.newsweek.com/2015/03/13/bpa-fine-if-you-ignore-most-studies-about-it-311203.html

[578] Prolonged Exposure to Bisphenol A from Single Dermal Contact Events, Jiaying Liu, Jonathan W. Martin, University of Alberta, Stockholm University, July 31, 2017, Environmental Science and Technology, 51 (17), pp 9940-9949 DOI: 10.1021/acs.est.7b03093, https://pubs.acs.org/doi/pdfplus/10.1021/acs.est.7b03093

[579] BPA in Thermal Paper, Minnesota Pollution Control Agency, https://www.pca.state.mn.us/green-chemistry/bpa-thermal-paper

PFAS/PFCs

[580] PFC Wrappers Chart, Environmental Working Group, https://www.ewg.org/research/many-fast-food-wrappers-still-coated-pfcs-kin-carcinogenic-teflon-chemical

[581] Many Fast Food Wrappers Still Coated In PFCs, Kin To Carcinogenic Teflon Chemical, Dave Andrews, Bill Walker, Environmental Working Group, Feb 1, 2017, https://www.ewg.org/research/many-fast-food-wrappers-still-coated-pfcs-kin-carcinogenic-teflon-chemical

[582] The Nasty Ingredient in Fast-Food Wrappers, Maddie Oatman, Mother Jones, Feb 1, 2017, https://www.motherjones.com/environment/2017/02/fast-food-wrappers-chemicals/

[583] For Those Exposed to GenX, An Agonizing Wait for Answers, The Fayetteville Observer, Greg Barnes, Mar 27, 2018, https://www.fayobserver.com/news/20180327/for-those-exposed-to-genx-agonizing-wait-for-answers

[584] (see 548) https://www.ewg.org/research/many-fast-food-wrappers-still-coated-pfcs-kin-carcinogenic-teflon-chemical

FLAME RETARDANTS (PFOE)

[585] Detecting WEEE Contamination in Recycled FCM Plastics, Ksenia Groh, June 2, 2017, Food Packaging Forum, https://www.foodpackagingforum.org/news/detecting-weee-contamination-in-recycled-fcm-plastics

PHTHALATES

[586] Dirty Dozen Endocrine Disruptors, Hormone Altering Chemicals and How to Avoid Them, Environmental Working Group, Oct 28, 2013, https://www.ewg.org/research/dirty-dozen-list-endocrine-disruptors

PERCHLORATE

[587] FDA is dragging its feet while children continue to be exposed to perchlorate in food Tom Neltner, January 11, 2019, Environmental Defense Fund, http://blogs.edf.org/health/2019/01/11/fda-perchlorate-in-food/

[588] Blount BC, Valentin-Blasini L, Osterloh JD, Mauldin JP, Pirkle JL. 2006a. Perchlorate exposure of the US population, 2001-2002. Journal of Exposure Science and Environmental Epidemiology 17(4): 400-07. https://www.ncbi.nlm.nih.gov/pubmed/17051137

Blount BC, Pirkle JL, Osterloh JD, Valentin-Blasini L, Caldwell LK. 2006b. Urinary perchlorate and thyroid hormone levels in adolescent and adult men and women living in the United States. Environmental Health Perspectives 114(12): 1865-71. https://www.ncbi.nlm.nih.gov/pubmed/17185277

STYRENE

[589] National Human Adipose Tissue Survey, EPA, August 1990, https://nepis.epa.gov/Exe/ZyNET.exe/9100CFRU.txt?ZyActionD=ZyDocument&Client=EPA&Index=1986%20Thru%201990&Docs=&Query=&Time=&EndTime=&SearchMethod=1&TocRestrict=n&Toc=&TocEntry=&QField=&QFieldYear=&QFieldMonth=&QFieldDay=&UseQField=&IntQFieldOp=0&ExtQFieldOp=0&XmlQuery=&File=D%3A%5CZYFILES%5CINDEX%20DATA%5C86THRU90%5CTXT%5C00000020%5C9100CFRU.txt&User=ANONYMOUS&Password=anonymous&SortMethod=h%7C-&MaximumDocuments=1&FuzzyDegree=0&ImageQuality=r75g8/r75g8/x150y150g16/i425&Display=hpfr&DefSeekPage=x&SearchBack=ZyActionL&Back=ZyActionS&BackDesc=Results%20page&MaximumPages=1&ZyEntry=9

[590] The Long Battle Over "White Pollution," China File, May 1, 2013, http://www.chinafile.com/reporting-opinion/media/long-battle-over-white-pollution

PLASTIC

[591] MicroPlastics Are Turning Up Everywhere, Even in Human Excrement, Jill Neimark, NPR, WBEZ, https://www.npr.org/sections/thesalt/2018/10/22/659568662/microplastics-are-turning-up-everywhere-even-in-human-excrement

[592] In A First, Microplastics Found in Human Poop, Laura Parker, National Geographic, Oct 22, 2018, https://www.nationalgeographic.com/environment/2018/10/news-plastics-microplastics-human-feces/

[593] Styrene, ToxNet, National Institutes of Health, https://toxnet.nlm.nih.gov/cgi-bin/sis/search/a?dbs+hsdb:@term+@DOCNO+171

[594] What Are Microplastics? National Oceanic and Atmospheric Administration, National Ocean Service, https://oceanservice.noaa.gov/facts/microplastics.html

[595] Understanding Endocrine Disruption, TEDX, The Endocrine Disruption Exchange, https://endocrinedisruption.org/assets/media/documents/EDC%20Fact%20Sheet%2020180130.pdf

[596] Cooking Safely in Microwave Oven, USDA, https://www.fsis.usda.gov/wps/portal/fsis/topics/food-safety-education/get-answers/food-safety-fact-sheets/appliances-and-thermometers/cooking-safely-in-the-microwave/cooking-safely-in-the-microwave-oven

FISH AND WATERWAYS

[597] Overfishing and Pollution Have Trashed the Mediterranean, Agata Mrowiec, Aug 16, 2018, Oceana, https://oceana.org/blog/overfishing-and-pollution-have-trashed-mediterranean

[598] (see 586) Microplastics https://www.npr.org/sections/thesalt/2018/10/22/659568662/microplastics-are-turning-up-everywhere-even-in-human-excrement

[599] These US Communities are Most at Risk from Ocean Acidification, Robert F. Service, Science, Feb 23, 2015, https://www.sciencemag.org/news/2015/02/these-us-communities-are-most-risk-ocean-acidification

[600] Stockholm Convention, Protecting Human Health and the Environment from Persistent Organic Pollutants, United Nations Environment Program, http://chm.pops.int/TheConvention/Overview/tabid/3351/Default.aspx

[601] 2 EPA Studies Confirm Threat to Fish of Dioxin from Paper Plants, March 14, 1989, New York Times, https://www.nytimes.com/1989/03/14/science/2-epa-studies-confirm-threat-to-fish-of-dioxin-from-paper-plants.html

[602] Red tides on the Rise Worldwide, Laurie Ann Peach, Christian Science Monitor, July 21, 1992, https://www.csmonitor.com/1992/0721/21121.html

[603] Potential Disaster at Huge St. James Waste Pile Has Crews Racing to Prevent Massive Wall Collapse, David J. Mitchell, The Advocate, Jan 30, 2019, https://www.theadvocate.com/baton_rouge/news/article_3cf05134-233a-11e9-aa0f-17aeb020318d.html

[604] The Clock is Ticking on Florida's Mountains of Hazardous Phosphate Waste, Craig Pittman, Sarasota Magazine, April 26, 2017, https://www.sarasotamagazine.com/articles/2017/4/26/florida-phosphate

[605] About Radioactive Material from Fertilizer Production, EPA, https://www.epa.gov/radtown/radioactive-material-fertilizer-production

[606] Very Large Deadzone Forecast for Gulf of Mexico, University of Michigan News, June 10, 2019, https://news.umich.edu/very-large-dead-zone-forecast-for-gulf-of-mexico/

The Gulf Could See One of the Largest Dead Zones in History This Year, Jen Christensen, CNN, June 10, 2019, https://www.cnn.com/2019/06/10/health/gulf-dead-zone-study-climate-scn/index.html

[607] What Does Big Sugar Have to Do With Florida's Red Tide, Biana Graulau, WTSP News, Sept 6, 2018, https://www.wtsp.com/article/news/local/what-does-big-sugar-have-to-do-with-floridas-red-tide/67-587820301

EPA Takes Over Mississippi Phosphates' Huge Mounds of Acidic Byproduct, Karen Nelson, Sun Herald, March 7, 2017, https://www.sunherald.com/news/local/counties/jackson-county/article137021948.html

[608] Mosaic Plant Sinkhole Dumpa 215 Million Gallons of Reprocessed Water into Floridan Aquifer, Christopher O'Donnell, Tampa Bay Times, Sept 17, 2016, https://www.tampabay.com/news/environment/water/mosaic-plant-sinkhole-dumps-215-million-gallons-of-reprocessed-water-into/2293845

[609] State Can Dump Water in Gulf, Dale White, Herald Tribune, April 4, 2003, https://www.heraldtribune.com/article/LK/20030404/News/605247753/SH/

[610] Red Tide is Devastating Florida's Sea Life, Are Humans to Blame? Maya Wei-Haas, National Geographic, Aug 8, 2018, What's more, recent exceptional red tide years seem to follow massive storms,

[611] Florida Red Tide FAQs, Mote Marine Laboratory and Aquarium, https://mote.org/news/florida-red-tide

[612] What is the Loop Current? National Ocean Service, National Oceanic and Atmospheric Administration, https://oceanservice.noaa.gov/facts/loopcurrent.html

[613] U.S. Researchers Find Roundup Chemical in Water, Air, Carey Gillam, Reuters, Aug 31, 2011, https://www.reuters.com/article/us-glyphosate-pollution/u-s-researchers-find-roundup-chemical-in-water-air-idUSTRE77U61720110831

[614] Atrazine Found in Water of Dozens of Midwest Communities, May 3, 2012, http://www.panna.org/press-release/atrazine-found-water-dozens-midwest-communities

[615] Dieldrin Dilemma, How Dated Science and Fish-Eating Advisories May Be Putting Brains At Risk, Sam Totoni, Oct 22, 2018, Environmental Health News, https://www.ehn.org/dieldrin-lingers-and-harms-brains-2613317049.html?rebelltitem=1#rebelltitem1

[616] Facts and Figures About the Great Lakes, EPA, https://www.epa.gov/greatlakes/great-lakes-facts-and-figures

[617] Pesticides as Water Pollutants, FAO Food and Agriculture Organization of the United Nations, http://www.fao.org/docrep/w2598e/w2598e07.htm

DRINKING WATER

[618] Cancer Trends Progress Report, Nitrate, National Cancer Institute, Summary of Trends in US Cancer Control Measures, Feb 2019, https://progressreport.cancer.gov/prevention/nitrate

[619] Near Record Farm Pollution Found in Missippi River, June 15, 2016, Emily Cassidy, Environmental Working Group Ag Mag, https://www.ewg.org/agmag/2016/06/near-record-farm-pollution-found-mississippi-river

[620] Dr. Hirzy Testifies Before Congress, United States Senate, June 29, 2000, https://www.nofluoride.com/hirzy_senate.cfm

[621] Hydrofluorosilicic Acid, Mosaic Co, http://www.mosaicco.com/products/industrial_products_hfs.htm

[622] The Phosphate Fertilizer Industry: An Environmental Review, https://fluoridealert.org/articles/phosphate01/

[623] Water Fluoridation: A Critical Review of the Physiological Effects of Ingested Fluoride as a Public Health Intervention, Stephen Peckham, Niyi Awofeso, Scientific World Journal, Feb 26, 2014, https://www.ncbi.nlm.nih.gov/pmc/articles/PMC3956646/

[624] (See 623) https://www.ncbi.nlm.nih.gov/pmc/articles/PMC3956646/

[625] EPA Union, Why EPA's Headquarters Professionals' Union Opposes Fluoridation, Dr. J. William Hirzy, Senior Vice President, EPA Headquarters Union 2000, http://fluoridealert.org/articles/epa-union/
Fluoride and IQ, 53 Studies, http://fluoridealert.org/studies/brain01/

[626] Fluoridation, Dialysis & Osteomalacia, Fluoride Alert, http://fluoridealert.org/studies/kidney04/

[627] Water Fluoridation Status in OECD Nations, Fluoride Alert, http://fluoridealert.org/content/oecd_nations/

[628] Erin Brokavich Chemical in Tap Water of more Than 200 Million Americans, David Andrews, Bill Walker, Environmental Working Group, Sept 20, 2016, https://www.ewg.org/research/chromium-six-found-in-us-tap-water

[629] Chromium 6 in Gas Drilling Wastes? Nils Bruzelius, Environmental Working Group, March 17, 2011, https://www.ewg.org/enviroblog/2011/03/chromium-6-gas-drilling-wastes
Drilling Down, Natural Gas's Toxic Waste, New York Times, https://archive.nytimes.com/www.nytimes.com/interactive/2011/02/27/us/natural-gas-documents-1.html#document/p375/a9929

[630] Erin Brokovich Weighs in on California's Removal of Limits on Chemical Made Famous in Movie, Dale Kasler, Ryan Sabalow, The Sacramento Bee, Aug 1, 2017, https://www.sacbee.com/news/state/california/water-and-drought/article164863427.html

[631] Go Easy on The Salt, Brian Palmer, NRDC, Feb 11, 2016, https://www.nrdc.org/onearth/go-easy-salt

[632] MX in Drinking Water, World Health Organization, 2004, http://www.who.int/water_sanitation_health/dwq/chemicals/mx.pdf
MX is the common name for 3-chloro-4-dichloromethyl-5-hydroxy-2(5H)-furanone)

[633] Byproduct of Water-Disinfection Process Found To Be Highly Toxic, Jim Barlow, University of Illinois, Sept 14, 2004, https://news.illinois.edu/view/6367/207503

[634] National Primary Drinking Water Regulations, EPA, https://www.epa.gov/ground-water-and-drinking-water/national-primary-drinking-water-regulations
The Precautionary Principle, World Commission on the Ethics of Scientific Knowledge and Technology, SHS.2005/WS/21, https://unesdoc.unesco.org/ark:/48223/pf0000139578

[635] President's Cancer Panel Report, 2008-2009, https://deainfo.nci.nih.gov/advisory/pcp/annualreports/pcp08-09rpt/pcp_report_08-09_508.pdf

[636] Wingspread Statement, https://www.healthandenvironment.org/environmental-health/social-context/history/precautionary-principle-the-wingspread-statement
Precautionary Principle, A Working Definition, https://unesdoc.unesco.org/ark:/48223/pf0000139578

DISEASE TRENDS

[637] "Omnivore's Dilemma," Michael Pollan, 2006, The Penguin Press p.

[638] GMOS and Cancer, Jeffrey Smith, Institute for Responsible Technology, https://responsibletechnology.org/gmos-and-cancer/

[639] Nitrogen Management on U.S. Corn Acres, 2001-10, USDA, Marc Ribaudo, Michael Livingston, James Williamson, Economic Brief Number 20, November 2012, https://www.ers.usda.gov/webdocs/publications/42865/33561_eb20.pdf?v=41228

[640] J.S. Knapp, K.C.A. Bromley-Challoner, in Handbook of Water and Wastewater Microbiology, 2003, 2.1.2. Xenobiotic
Tim J. Evans DVM, MS, PhD, DACT, DABVT, in Small Animal Toxicology (Third Edition), 2013, Xenobiotic Storage Depots,
Learn More About Xenobiotics: www.sciencedirect.com/topics/immunology-and-microbiology/xenobiotic,
[641] Cancer Prevention, World Health Organization, The World Cancer Report 2014 http://www.who.int/cancer/prevention/en/ ,
[642] Cancer, Key Facts, Sept 12, 2018, http://www.who.int/mediacentre/factsheets/fs297/en/
[643]Environmental and Heritable Factors in the Causation of Cancer—Analyses of Cohorts of Twins from Sweden, Denmark, and Finland, Paul Lichenstein, Niels V. Holm, Pia K. Verkasola, Anastasi Ilisadou, Jaakko Kaprio, Markku Koskenvuo, Eero Pukkala, Axel Skytthe, Kari Hemminki, New England Journal Of Medicine, July 13, 2000, DOI: 10.1056/NEJM200007133430201, http://www.nejm.org/doi/full/10.1056/NEJM200007133430201
[644] Cancer and the Environment, What You Need to Know, National Institutes of Health, August 2003, https://www.niehs.nih.gov/health/materials/cancer_and_the_environment_508.pdf
[645] Reduce Your Exposure to Pesticides, The Soil Association, https://www.soilassociation.org/organic-living/whyorganic/reduce-your-exposure-to-pesticides/
[646] (see 592) https://www.niehs.nih.gov/health/materials/cancer_and_the_environment_508.pdf
[647] Reducing Environmental Cancer Risk, President's Cancer Panel Annual Report 2008-2009, https://deainfo.nci.nih.gov/advisory/pcp/annualreports/pcp08-09rpt/pcp_report_08-09_508.pdf
[648] Glyphosate; Tolerances for Residues, Electronic Code of Federal Regulations, Glyphosate, May 23, 2019, https://www.ecfr.gov/cgi-bin/retrieveECFR?gp=1&SID=2d508200c2a0994fc9e3c41911ee4cc1&ty=HTML&h=L&mc=true&r=SECTION&n=se40.26.180_1364
[649] Genetically Engineered Crops, Glyphosate and the Deterioration of Health in the United States, Nancy L. Swanson, Andre Leu, Jon Abrahamson, Bradley Wallet, Journal of Organic Systems 9(2), 2014, http://www.organic-systems.org/journal/92/JOS_Volume-9_Number-2_Nov_2014-Swanson-et-al.pdf
Kruger, M., Schledorn, P., Schrödl, W., Hoppe, H.W., Lutz, W. and Shehata, A.A., 2014. Detection of glyphosate residues in animals and humans. Journal of Environmental and Analytical Toxicology, 4(2): 210-15. http://www.stopsprayingnb.ca/resources/23.pdf
[650] (see 596) Glyphosate; tolerances for residues 180.364, Electronic Code of Federal Regulations, https://www.ecfr.gov/cgi-bin/retrieveECFR?gp=1&SID=2d508200c2a0994fc9e3c41911ee4cc1&ty=HTML&h=L&mc=true&r=SECTION&n=se40.26.180_1364
[651] (see 597) http://www.organic-systems.org/journal/92/index.html
[652] National Water Quality Assessment Projecct, Pesticide National Synthesis Project, US Geological Survery, USGS, https://water.usgs.gov/nawqa/pnsp/usage/maps/show_map.php?year=2016&map=GLYPHOSATE&hilo=L
[653] Because Some Foods Carry Organophosphate Residues, Janet Raloff, Science News, April 21, 2011, https://www.sciencenews.org/blog/science-public/because-some-foods-carry-organophosphate-residues

REMEDIES: NOURISH

[654] Robert McCarrison, Nutrition and Health, the Cantor Lectures, p. 24, the McCarrison Society, 1953, Faber and Faber, London.
[655] 5 Blue Zones: Where the World's Healthiest People Live, April 6, 2017, National Geographic, https://www.nationalgeographic.com/books/features/5-blue-zones-where-the-worlds-healthiest-people-live/

[656] Theodore Zava, David Zava "Assessment of Japanese Iodine Intake Based on Seaweed Consumption in Japan, A literature based Analysis", Thyroid Research, Oct 5, 2011, https://www.ncbi.nlm.nih.gov/pmc/articles/PMC3204293/

PREPARE TO RISE

[657] Remarks Intended for Delivery tot he Texas Democratic State Committee in the Municipal Auditorium in Austin, November 22, 1963 (Undeliverable), https://www.jfklibrary.org/archives/other-resources/john-f-kennedy-speeches/austin-tx-undelivered-19631122

[658] Media Release: Nature's Dangerous Decline 'Unprecedented, Species Extinctin Rates 'Accelerating,' IPBES, May 2019, https://www.ipbes.net/news/Media-Release-Global-Assessment

[659] What is Happening to Agrobiodiversity, FAO, http://www.fao.org/docrep/007/y5609e/y5609e02.htm

[660] Big Ag's Dirty Little Secret, Pesticide Action Network North America, http://www.panna.org/gmos-pesticides-profit/big-ags-dirty-little-secret

[661] How Billions in Tax Dollars Subsidize the Junk Food Industry, Eric Planin, The Fiscal Times, July 25, 2012, https://www.businessinsider.com/billions-in-tax-dollars-subsidize-the-junk-food-industry-2012-7

[662] Sam Roberts, "Dr. Epstein, 91, Cassandra of Cancer Prevention Dies", The New York Times, April 25, 2018, https://www.nytimes.com/2018/04/25/obituaries/dr-samuel-epstein-91-cassandra-of-cancer-prevention-dies.html

[663] Farewell to the Delaney Amendment, Donella Meadows, Sept 26, 1996, http://donellameadows.org/archives/farewell-to-the-delaney-amendment/

[664] Organic Farms Become a Winner in Putin's Feud with the West, Neil MacFarquhar, Nov 8, 2014, New York Times, https://www.nytimes.com/2014/11/19/world/europe/russia-food-sanctions-european-union-farmers.html

[665] What's in the 2018 Farm Bill? The Good, The Bad, and The Offal, Farm Aid, Dec 2018, https://www.farmaid.org/issues/farm-policy/whats-in-the-2018-farm-bill-the-good-the-bad-and-the-offal/

[666] The Snack Food and Corn Syrup Lobbyist Shaping Trump's Dietary Guidelines for Americans, Laura Peterson, Pogo, Aug 23, 2018, https://www.pogo.org/investigation/2018/08/the-snack-food-and-corn-syrup-lobbyist-shaping-trumps-dietary-guidelines-for-americans/

[667] Epigenetic Mechanisms of Integrative Medicine, by Riya R.Kanherkar, Susan E. Stair, Naina Bhatia-Dey, Paul J. Mills, Deepak Chopra, Antonei B. Csoka, Evidence-Based Complementary and Alternative Medicine, Volume 2017 (2017), Article ID 4365429, 19 pages, https://doi.org/10.1155/2017/4365429

[668] Cancer Chemoprevention by Dietary Polyphenols: Promising Role for Epigenetics, Alexander Link, Francesc Balaguer, Ajay Goel, Biochemical Pharmacology, Dec 15, 2010, 80(12): 1771-1792, https://www.ncbi.nlm.nih.gov/pmc/articles/PMC2974019/#R5

[668] Foodborne Illness: What Consumers Need to Know, USDA Food Safety and Inspection Service, https://www.fsis.usda.gov/wps/portal/fsis/topics/food-safety-education/get-answers/food-safety-fact-sheets/foodborne-illness-and-disease/foodborne-illness-what-consumers-need-to-know/ct_index

[669] (See 592) Cancer and The Environment, What Your Need to Know, https://www.niehs.nih.gov/health/materials/cancer_and_the_environment_508.pdf

[670] Rare Earths, Forbidden Cures, Dr. Joel Wallach, Dr. Ma Lan, Dr. William H. Moore, Double Happiness Publishing, Bonita, CA, 1994, p. 8

[671] (See 670) Rare Earths, Forbidden Cures, Dr. Joel Wallach, Dr. Ma Lan, 1994, p, 19

[672] Epigenetics, Dr. Joel Wallach, Dr. Ma Lan, Dr. Gerhard N. Schrauzer, SelectBooks Inc, New York, 2014, p.371

[673] A Low Salt Diet Could Be the True Cause of Heartburn, Salt Sense, Sept 5, 2012, https://www.saltsense.co.uk/a-low-salt-diet-could-be-the-true-cause-of-heartburn/

[674] Microplastics Found in 90 Percent of Table Salt, Laura Parker, National Geographic, Oct 17, 2018, https://www.nationalgeographic.com/environment/2018/10/microplastics-found-90-percent-table-salt-sea-salt/

The Inaugural Address, JFK, https://www.jfklibrary.org/learn/about-jfk/historic-speeches/inaugral-address
[675] The Basics of the Regulatory Process, EPA, http://www.epa.gov/laws-regulations/basics-regulatory-process
[676] Summary of the Federal Food, Drug and Cosmetic Act, FDA, http://www.epa.gov/laws-regulations/summary-federal-food-drug-and-cosmetic-act
[677] Adulterated Food, https://www.gpo.gov/fdsys/pkg/USCODE-2010-title21/html/USCODE-2010-title21-chap9-subchapIV-sec342.htm
[678] 21 U.S. Code S348. Food Additives, Cornell Law School, Legal Information Institute, https://www.law.cornell.edu/uscode/text/21/348
[679] Farewell to the Delaney Amendment, Donella Meadows, Sept 26, 1996, Academy for Systems Change, The Donella Meadows Project, http://www.donellameadows.org/archives/farewell-to-the-delaney-amendment/
[680] Dietary Supplement Health and Education Act of 1994, www.health.gov/dietsupp/ch1.htm
[681] Food Modernization Act, FSMA, FDA, https://www.fda.gov/Food/GuidanceRegulation/FSMA/
[682] (see 623) Summary of the FD&C Act, https://www.epa.gov/laws-regulations/summary-federal-food-drug-and-cosmetic-act
[683] Generally Recognized as Secret, Chemicals Added to Food in the United States, Tom Neltner, Maricel Maffini, Natural Resources Defense Council, April 2014, http://www.nrdc.org/food/files/safety-loophole-for-chemicals-in-food-report.pdf
[684] Organic Production/Organic Food: Informatin: USDA, Mary V. Gold, June 2007, https://www.nal.usda.gov/afsic/organic-productionorganic-food-information-access-tools
[685] The National List, USDA, https://www.ams.usda.gov/rules-regulations/organic/national-list/
[686] Consumer Info About Food from Genetically Engineered Plants, FDA, https://www.fda.gov/food/ingredientspackaginglabeling/geplants/ucm461805.htm
[687] Pesticide Laws and Regulations, National Pesticide Information Center, http://npic.orst.edu/reg/laws.html
[688] PRN 97-6: Use of Term "Inert" in the Label Ingredients Statement, EP, https://www.epa.gov/pesticide-registration/prn-97-6-use-term-inert-label-ingredients-statement
[689] Safer Chemicals, Environmental Defense Fund, https://www.edf.org/health/policy/chemicals-policy-ref
[690] CERCLA, Summary of the Comprehensive Response, Compensation, and Liability Act (Superfund), 42 U.S.C. S9601 et seq, http://www.epa.gov/laws-regulations/summary-comprehensive-environmental-response-compensation-and-liability-act
[691] RCRA, Summary of the Resource Conservation and Recovery Act, http://www.epa.gov/laws-regulations/summary-resource-conservation-and-recovery-act
[692] Proposition 65, State of California OEHHA, https://oehha.ca.gov/proposition-65/about-proposition-65
[693] History of the Clean Water Act, EPA, http://www.epa.gov/laws-regulations/history-clean-water-act
[694] Summary of the Safe Drinking Water Act, EPA, http://www.epa.gov/laws-regulations/summary-safe-drinking-water-act
[695] Ron paul, HENRY LAMB EXPOSES THE DANGERS OF CODEX HON. RON PAUL OF TEXAS IN THE HOUSE OF REPRESENTATIVES Monday, July 11, 2005 https://www.govinfo.gov/content/pkg/CRECB-2005-pt11/pdf/CRECB-2005-pt11-Pg15560.pdf

INDEX

Thank you for reading the Green Handbook.
Together anything is possible.
To learn more please visit:
www.preparetorise.com.

Made in the USA
Coppell, TX
16 March 2026

73966456R00143